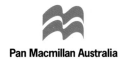 THE CSIRO
LOW-CARB DIET

BY ASSOCIATE PROFESSOR GRANT BRINKWORTH
AND PENNIE TAYLOR

Foreword by Prof. Manny Noakes and Dr. Rob Grenfell

Photography by
Jeremy Simons

Pan Macmillan Australia

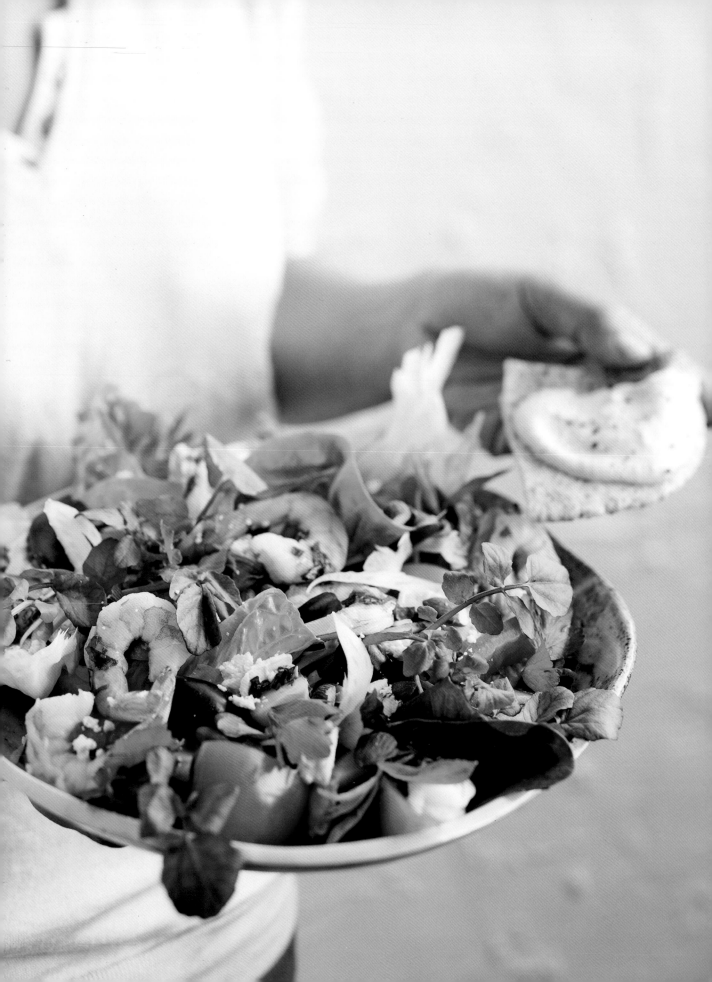

FOREWORD

Over many years, the CSIRO's nutrition and health laboratories have gained an international reputation as leaders in nutrition and lifestyle research. One of our strategic goals has been to develop and deliver scientifically validated lifestyle solutions to help Australians improve their health through diet and exercise. Rigorous scientific research has always been the bedrock of our approach, underpinning many practical applications that can positively impact people's lives.

In 2005, CSIRO produced the first of a series of books advocating a scientifically proven eating and exercise plan known as the Total Wellbeing Diet. Ten years on, we released the diet online and the Impromy pharmacy-based programs. These products, containing advice, exercises and recipes, have helped hundreds of thousands of Australians lose weight and improve their health, and continue to be relevant after more than a decade.

Nutritional science is constantly evolving, and CSIRO scientists are at the forefront of research that explores how different food combinations and dietary patterns affect our health, both in terms of weight loss and the management of weight-related disease such as type 2 diabetes and heart disease.

For many years, the CSIRO has been investigating the health effects of a much lower carbohydrate diet. Between 2012 and 2014, CSIRO researchers undertook one of the largest nutritional intervention studies conducted in Australia, funded by the National Health and Medical Research Council of Australia, the premier government health body in Australia. From these results they developed the CSIRO Low-carb Diet, a new lifestyle program for type 2 diabetes which is lower in carbohydrate and higher in healthy fats than the Total Wellbeing Diet. Both diets are high in protein, which has advantages for body composition and appetite control.

Where this new low-carbohydrate diet stood out was the degree to which it helped participants manage their weight and normalise their blood glucose levels. The diet does not exclude carbohydrates entirely, but in the early stages limits them to 50 grams a day. Compared to a traditional high-carbohydrate approach, this low-carbohydrate diet dramatically blunts blood-sugar levels after meals, improves blood-cholesterol profiles and helps to reduce requirements for diabetes medications.

The results of this exciting research show that the CSIRO Low-carb Diet can achieve important improvements in health markers, and it is anticipated that this diet may have a wider application than just type 2 diabetes management. Presented here in this comprehensive lifestyle guide complete with menu plans, recipes and exercises, the diet is nutritionally balanced and contains a unique combination of foods that are high in lean protein as well as healthy fats.

No single diet suits every individual; differences in individual taste, genetic makeup, culture, age, gender and beliefs need to be considered. Nutritional science has to adapt to new discoveries, and also deal with the complexities of the vastly different needs of the population. Although low-carbohydrate diets have been popular for a very long time, concerns have been raised about their safety and nutritional quality. Our research shows that the scientifically formulated CSIRO Low-carb Diet is nutritionally rich and can be very effective in improving weight and metabolic health.

Prof. Manny Noakes
Research Program Director,
Nutrition and Health,
CSIRO Health and Biosecurity

Dr. Rob Grenfell,
Health Director,
CSIRO Health and Biosecurity

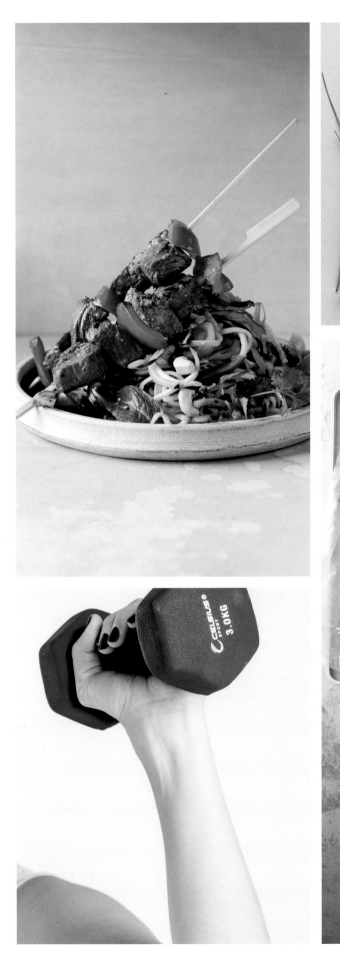
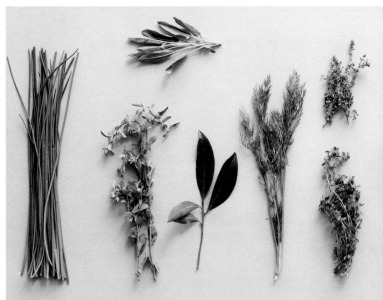
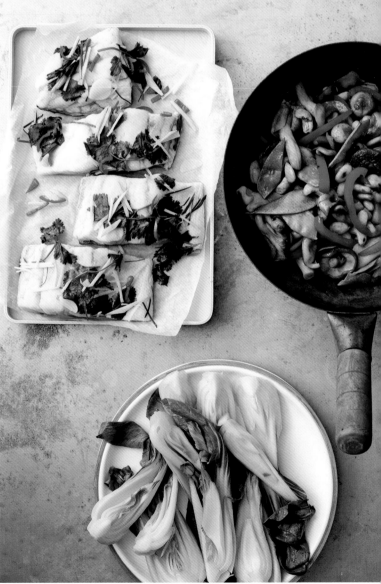

CONTENTS

AUTHOR AND CONTRIBUTOR PROFILES

Authors

Associate Professor Grant Brinkworth

Grant is a principal research scientist in Clinical Nutrition and Exercise at CSIRO Health and Biosecurity. He has a PhD and expertise in diet, nutrition and exercise science. He has more than 15 years' experience leading large-scale, multidisciplinary clinical research teams and studies evaluating the effects of dietary patterns, foods, nutritional components and physical exercise on weight loss, metabolic disease risk management, health and performance.

Grant has particular interests in developing effective lifestyle solutions for achieving optimal weight, metabolic health and diabetes management, and understanding the role of lower-carbohydrate dietary patterns for health management. He has published more than 70 peer-reviewed research papers on the topic of diet and lifestyle management of obesity and related diseases. He also holds an MBA degree, and has interests in innovation and the commercialisation of science outcomes and lifestyle programs for large-scale uptake and community adoption.

Pennie Taylor

Pennie is the senior research dietitian at CSIRO Health and Biosecurity. She is a contributor to the CSIRO and Baker IDI Diabetes Diet and Lifestyle plan and the CSIRO Total Wellbeing Diet range of programs, which aim to maximise health and wellbeing through better nutrition, physical activity and weight management.

Pennie's expertise is in dietary patterns and design, nutrition and obesity. She has managed and supported many clinical trials exploring the influence of dietary patterns and dietary composition on health outcomes, including weight loss, appetite and metabolic variables among morbidly obese people with pre-existing co-morbidities such as diabetes and heart disease. Pennie is also a private practitioner for EvolvME and an active committee member for the Dietitians Association Australia and the Obesity Surgery Society of Australia and New Zealand. For her PhD she is investigating novel strategies to optimise glucose control, appetite responses and feeding behaviour in people with type 2 diabetes.

Contributors

Dr Natalie Luscombe-Marsh Natalie is a research scientist at CSIRO Health and Biosecurity, and an Adjunct Senior Lecturer at the University of Adelaide. She has a PhD in nutrition and disease, and more than 12 years' experience in designing clinical trials determining the acute and longer-term effects of different dietary patterns, particularly those higher in protein and unsaturated fat, on cardiometabolic risk in obesity and type 2 diabetes. A major focus of her research has been understanding the role gut mechanisms play in the regulation of energy intake and glycaemia in response to protein, in young and older adults. Natalie has authored 50 peer-reviewed papers, two book chapters, and numerous industry reports, and has received several awards recognising the novelty and impact of her work.

Dr Tom Wycherley Tom is a research scientist at the University of South Australia, and an honorary research scientist at the Menzies School of Health Research in Darwin. He is an accredited exercise scientist and holds a PhD in nutrition and exercise science, and a master's degree in epidemiology. He has more than 10 years' experience researching the role of dietary intake and physical activity in regulating body weight and cardiometabolic disease risk. He has published more than 20 peer-reviewed research articles, and is passionate about translating research findings into improved public health.

Professor Campbell Thompson Campbell is a senior consultant in medicine at the Flinders Medical Centre and the Royal Adelaide Hospital. He has spent more than ten years on metabolic research using magnetic resonance and other biochemical techniques to monitor high-energy and fat metabolism at rest and during exercise in adults, elite athletes and children. He has a particular interest in metabolic syndrome, insulin resistance and diabetes. Since 2009, Campbell has worked in the Comprehensive Metabolic Care Centre at the Royal Adelaide Hospital, where weight-management strategies such as bariatric (weight-loss) surgery are offered to overweight people. He has written more than 150 peer-reviewed research articles.

Professor Manny Noakes Manny is the Research Director for the Nutrition and Health Program at the CSIRO. She was instrumental in the development and release of five editions of *The CSIRO Total Wellbeing Diet* (TWD), launched in 2004, which has been translated into 17 languages and has sold over 1 million copies in Australia.

Manny is a former executive member of the Federal Government Food and Health Dialogue, which influences nutrition reformulation targets for manufactured foods in order to improve the nutritional quality of the Australian food supply. She is also a member of the Heart Foundation Food and Nutrition Advisory Committee, and the Woolworths Healthier Australia Taskforce, amongst other industry bodies.

Manny is the recipient of three CSIRO Medals, is a Distinguished Alumni of Flinders University, holds a research excellence award from the University of Adelaide and is a recipient of the Zonta Club Woman of International Achievement award.

Megan Rebuli Megan is a Research Dietitian at CSIRO Health and Biosecurity and an accredited practising dietitian with the Dietitians Association of Australia. She has a background in public health nutrition and epidemiology, as well as experience in dietary assessment and analysis in practice. Megan has worked on clinical trials delivering diet interventions targeting health outcomes including weight loss, cardiovascular disease, and diabetes, as well as enhancing overall health.

Dr Gilly Hendrie Gilly is a research scientist at CSIRO Health and Biosecurity. She has a PhD and expertise in diet, nutrition and obesity prevention. She has worked extensively on the development of new tools to measure dietary intake, and methods to quantify dietary patterns, including the development of indexes to assess diet quality. Gilly has a deep understanding of dietary patterns and how these impact on global concerns such as obesity, food security and climate change. She has published more than 50 peer-reviewed research papers in the areas of nutrition, dietary patterns and lifestyle programs.

Danielle Baird Danielle is a Research Dietitian at CSIRO Health and Biosecurity. Her expertise lies in analysing dietary data across a number of diverse and complex research areas. Danielle has analysed dietary data from National Nutrition Surveys collected over the past 30 years to gain a comprehensive understanding of Australia's food choices and dietary behaviour, and how these impact on important issues such as obesity, food security, climate change and the need for policy reform.

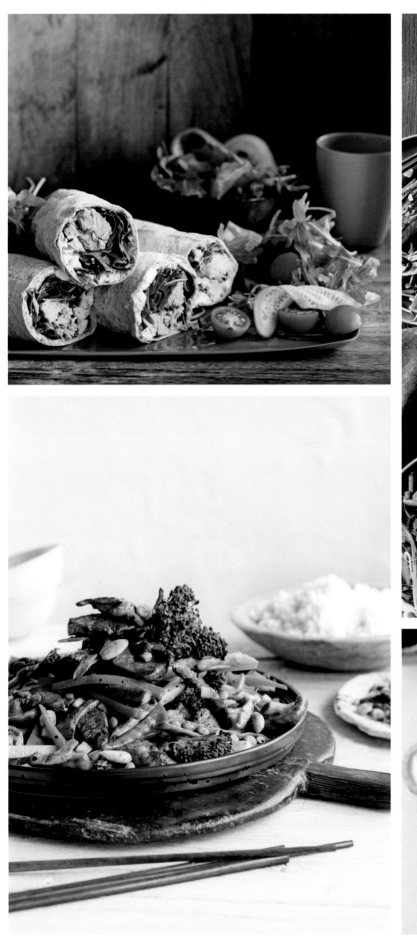
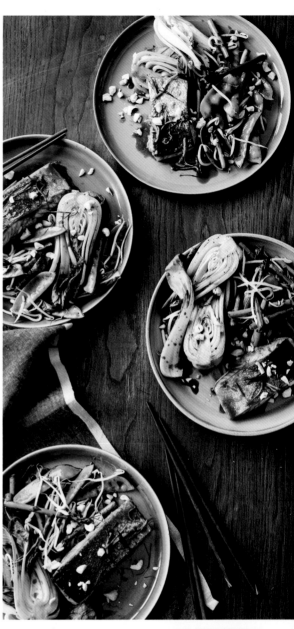
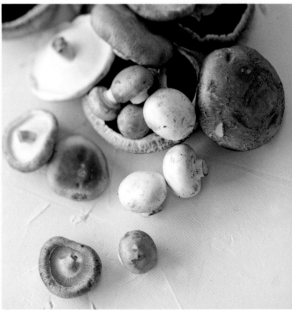

INTRODUCTION

All over the world there are concerns about human health and chronic (long-term) disease, and the effects these will have in terms of both physical and financial suffering. We've all grown used to hearing about the 'obesity epidemic', but many of us have little idea what that actually means, even if we're tipping the scales in that direction ourselves.

Numerous diets promise weight loss and improvements in health. If you've picked up this book, the chances are you've tried a variety of diets over the years. So how, and why, is this one different? For a start, it's much more than just a diet – it's a complete lifestyle program that can revitalise your health and wellbeing.

The CSIRO Low-carb Diet limits carbohydrates while raising levels of healthy fats and protein. Many traditional diets suggest a carbohydrate intake of 200–300 grams per day; with the low-carb approach outlined in this book, however, the amount of carbohydrates per day is reduced to 50 grams, with small increases in later weeks for flexibility. This diet isn't about saying no to carbohydrates, it's about choosing the right types and the right amounts. It also suits the way we eat today.

There are many versions and/or variations of low-carb diets, but the principles and daily practice of this diet are based on targeted, original CSIRO research backed by scientific evidence and proven dietary principles from around the world, such as the proven healthiness of the Mediterranean diet. This emerging research has led to a paradigm shift in how we think obesity and related diseases, particularly diabetes, should be treated.

Why cut down on carbohydrates?

We live in a carbohydrate-rich environment. A visit to any shopping centre, airport or staff canteen will tell you how difficult it is to find low-carb options. Many of the ingredients we buy to cook with at home are high in carbohydrates, and the dishes we've grown up with often feature them as a key component.

One reason for this is that carbohydrates – rice, breads, pasta, potatoes, pastries and biscuits – have emerged as a cheap, accessible and energy-dense modern food source. To add to the complexity, carbohydrates have been heavily promoted by industry and health bodies as an essential part of a healthy diet.

But there's no such thing as a one-size-fits-all diet. A physically active teenager will have different energy and nutritional requirements from a 50-year-old office worker. As a society, we're probably consuming too many carbohydrates overall. This becomes a problem for many people because the carbohydrate rich foods we favour are high in kilojoules with low nutritional quality and stop us eating more nutritionally replete foods. For younger, fitter and healthier people, it's probably just a matter of getting a better dietary balance by replacing nutritionally poor high-carb – and often sugary – foods with nutritionally dense carbohydrate foods, such as whole grains.

For people who are overweight, however, the benefits of adopting a structured low-carb diet are significant, not just in terms of weight loss, but for improved metabolic health and general wellbeing. This is because high-carb foods can cause rapid elevation of blood sugar levels, which can ultimately lead to type 2 diabetes, heart disease and their associated health consequences.

The research and results

In our 2012–14 clinical trial, participants were randomly assigned to one of two groups. One group consumed an energy-reduced, low-carbohydrate, higher protein and high-healthy-fat diet – the diet upon which the CSIRO Low-carb Diet is now based. The other group consumed a traditional energy-reduced, higher carbohydrate, low-fat diet. Both groups also participated in a structured program of 60 minutes of combined aerobic exercise and resistance (strength) training three times a week. The participants followed the diet and exercise regime for at least 12 months. Both groups experienced significant weight loss of 10 kilograms in the first 12 months, which proves a tried-and-tested weight-loss formula: reducing calories and increasing exercise will result in weight loss that can be sustained over the long term (in this case two years).

But the low-carb approach resulted in greater health improvements and helped to normalise blood cholesterol levels and blood glucose levels. Indeed, participants in the low-carb group reduced their diabetes medication by an average of 40 per cent. This research shows just how effective the low-carb approach can be, not only for weight loss but as a potent strategy for improving the key health targets your GP measures.

Being overweight is fairly normal now in Australia. It's estimated that 60–70 per cent of us are heavier than we should be. Many of us don't view this as a serious problem; we're just carrying a few extra kilos – three or four – around the middle. It's worth knowing, though, that a few extra kilos can significantly increase our chance of developing a metabolic disease such as type 2 diabetes down the track. Research shows that for every kilo of weight gained over 10 years, our risk of developing diabetes increases by 49 per cent in the subsequent 10 years. Weight gain and metabolic disease are inextricably linked; a dietary approach that's the most effective not only for weight loss but also reducing the risk factors for weight-related diseases, makes the best sense.

The diet in practice

The Low-carb Diet is a tasty, nutritionally complete, tailored plan offering 6000–9000 kilojoules (depending on individual needs), with a focus on whole foods. The majority of the kilojoules come from healthy unsaturated fats (nuts, seeds, oils, avocado, olives and fish) and lean protein foods (red meats, poultry, fish, eggs and tofu), with some dairy allowances. It encourages eating an abundance of low-carb vegetables and reducing starchy vegetables (potatoes, sweet potatoes, pumpkin and carrots). Bread, cereals and fruits are restricted but allowed.

Dramatically reducing your carbohydrate intake while living in a carbohydrate-rich environment isn't necessarily straightforward. But to help you make the transition, we've provided:

- clear descriptions of high-carb foods and low-carb alternatives
- a comparison of various dietary approaches
- an outline of daily allowances of carbohydrates, healthy fats and protein
- weekly prescriptive meal plans to reduce your carbohydrate intake initially, then increase it slightly for dietary flexibility as you reach your target weight
- 80 delicious recipes with all the daily allowances calculated and explained
- shopping and pantry-staple lists for better organisation
- extensive photography that provides a visual snapshot of how the diet works.

The exercise plan

The companion exercise plan is an essential component of this approach and aims to provide a complete lifestyle solution. An appropriate level of physical activity is an important factor in weight loss and weight maintenance, as well as improved health. The structured plan incorporates aerobic exercise, resistance (strength) training and flexibility exercises to deliver comprehensive health and wellbeing. All the resistance and flexibility exercises are photographed and fully described, and all can be done at home with minimal equipment.

Medical advice

Throughout this book, readers will be encouraged to seek medical advice. Although our dietary program has been scientifically tested by medical researchers, we each have different medical and dietary requirements that call for an individual approach. Doctors across Australia understand that lifestyle changes (i.e. diet and exercise) are the most important first step in improving anyone's overall health, and will generally encourage a patient who wishes to follow a responsible and proven dietary approach. People on blood pressure, cholesterol and diabetes medication may find that their need for medication falls significantly as a result of this diet and lifestyle program. Regular monitoring is therefore essential to avoid over-medication (see Appendix A for details).

Sustaining the diet

Weight loss and weight maintenance need a long-term approach. Many people lose weight successfully but find it hard to keep the weight off. By necessity, the Low-carb Diet reduces reliance on energy-dense processed food and encourages eating plentiful amounts of food that's nutritionally rich and satisfying. You may find, at first, that it's a dramatically different way of eating, but most people who try it can adjust to the principles as time goes on, or experiment with adaptations. The recipes have been written to maximise flavour and interest, and help you stay the course. We at the CSIRO hope that once you get to know and appreciate the flavours and health benefits of this diet, you'll willingly adopt it in the long term. The benefits will be better health and improved quality of life. It really is worth giving it a try.

HOW TO USE THIS BOOK

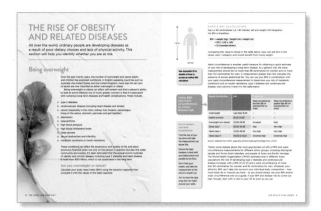

First, to learn how excess carbs in our diet are doing damage to our health, turn to pages 8–9.

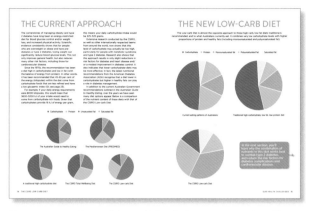

For an overview of how this diet compares to other diets, see pages 14–15.

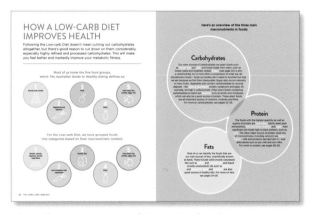

Then, for a summary of the main food groups and how they relate to macronutrients such as carbohydrates, see pages 20–21.

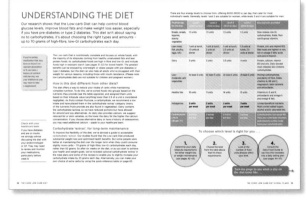

Pages 38–39 are your starting point for working out which level of the diet is best for you.

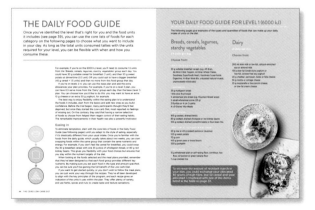

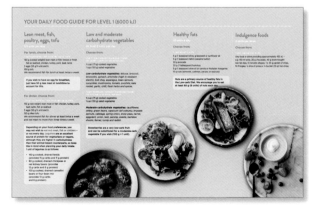

Pages 44–47 list the core foods in each category, to help you choose what you can eat for each meal.

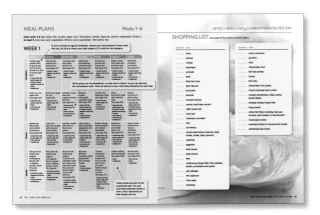

Page 48 onwards puts this all together in 12 weeks of tailored meal plans, including shopping lists!

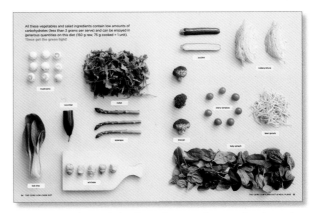

For a snapshot of the best low-carb veggies to eat, see pages 54–55.

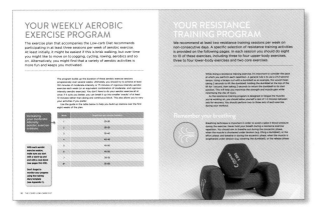

You're almost off and running! Refer to pages 92–93 for details of the exercise plans.

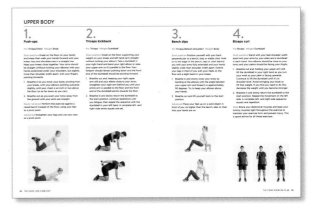

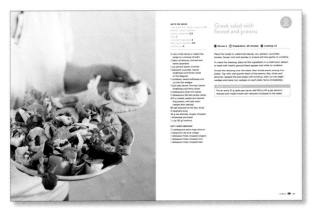

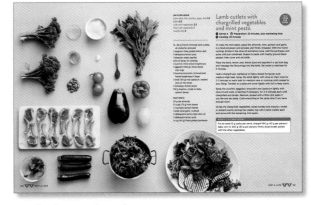

Then turn to page 110 for a collection of delicious, easy-to-make low-carb recipes.

PART 1

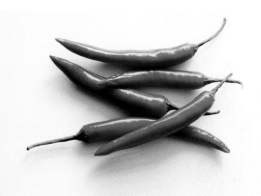

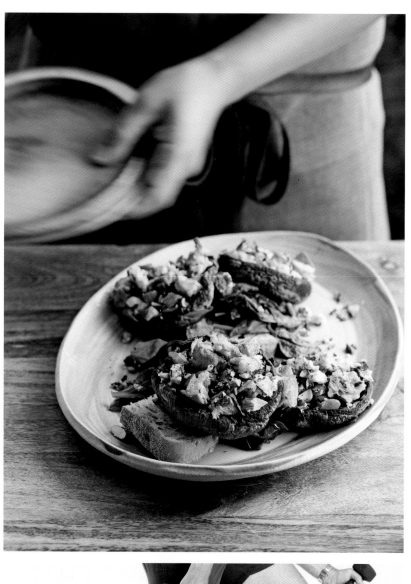

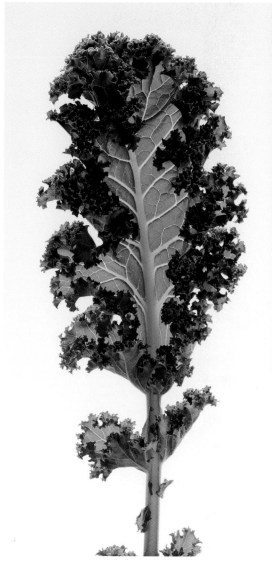

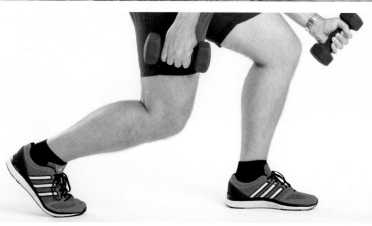

Our Health Challenges

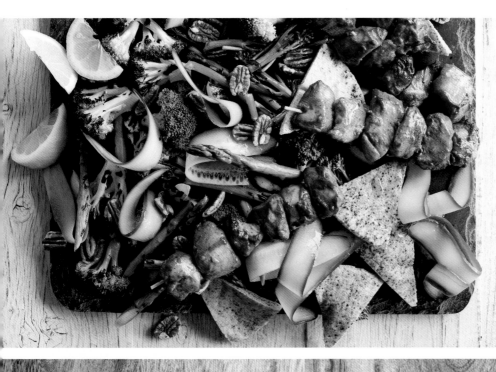

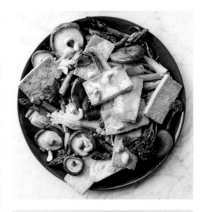

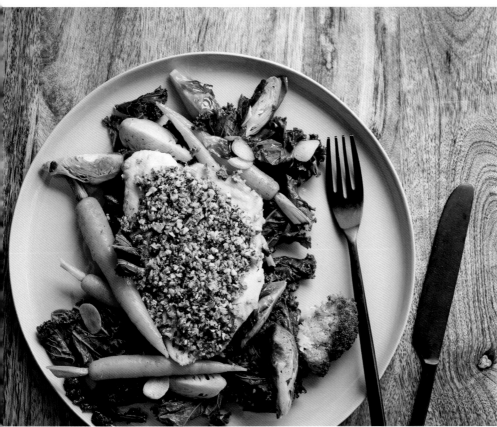

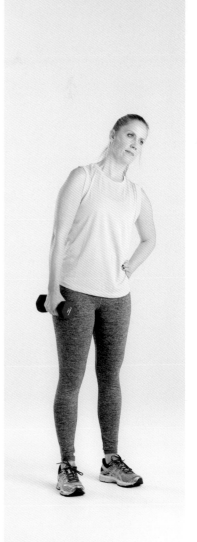

THE RISE OF OBESITY AND RELATED DISEASES

All over the world, ordinary people are developing diseases as a result of poor dietary choices and lack of physical activity. This section will help you identify whether you are at risk.

Being overweight

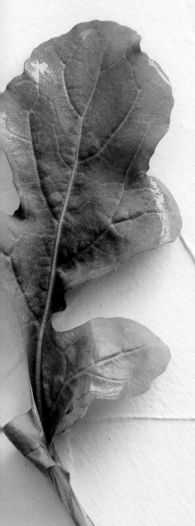

Over the past twenty years, the number of overweight and obese adults and children has exploded worldwide. In English-speaking countries such as Australia, the United States and the United Kingdom, more than 65 per cent of adults are now classified as either overweight or obese.

Being overweight or obese can affect self-esteem and limit a person's ability to lead an active lifestyle, but of much greater concern is that it's associated with numerous long-term diseases and health complications. These include:

- type 2 diabetes
- cardiovascular disease (including heart disease and stroke)
- cancer (especially in the colon, kidney, liver, breasts, oesophagus, lining of the uterus, stomach, pancreas and gall bladder)
- depression
- osteoarthritis
- high blood pressure
- high blood cholesterol levels
- sleep apnoea
- sexual dysfunction and infertility
- metabolic syndrome or insulin resistance.

These conditions can affect life expectancy and quality of life, and place enormous financial strain not only on the person in question but also the wider community and society. It's been estimated that the annual cost to Australia of obesity and chronic disease, including type 2 diabetes and heart disease, is more than $130 billion, which is not sustainable in the long term.

Are you overweight or obese?

Calculate your body mass index (BMI) using the equation opposite then compare it with the values in the table opposite.

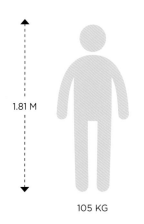

1.81 M

105 KG

See Appendix B for details of how to access an online BMI calculator.

Using BMI and waist circumference to assess disease risk

How to measure your waist circumference:

Find the top of your hip bone and take the measurement just above this.

Ensure the tape measure is level with your belly button and parallel to the floor.

Don't hold your breath, and take the measurement at the end of a breath out.

Aim to have the tape snug (but not tight) around your waist.

SAMPLE BMI CALCULATION

Gary is 181 centimetres (i.e. 1.81 metres) tall and weighs 105 kilograms. His BMI is therefore:

BMI = weight (kg) / height (m) x height (m)
= 105 / (1.81 x 1.81)
= 32 (rounded down)

Comparing this value to those in the table below, Gary can see he's in the obese class 1 category and would benefit from losing weight.

Waist circumference is another useful measure for obtaining a quick estimate of your risk of developing a long-term disease. As a general rule, the waist measurement should be no more than 88 centimetres for women and no more than 102 centimetres for men. A measurement greater than this indicates the presence of excess abdominal fat. You can use your BMI in combination with your waist circumference measurement to determine your risk of metabolic conditions such as insulin resistance, type 2 diabetes and cardiovascular disease. Use columns 3 and 4 in the table below.

Weight classification	BMI	Disease risk	
		Waist circumference less than 88 cm (women)/102 cm (men)	Waist circumference greater than 88 cm (women)/102 cm (men)
Underweight	Less than 18.49	—	—
Healthy (normal)	18.50–24.99	—	—
Overweight (pre-obese)	25.00–29.99	Increased	High
Obese class I	30.00–34.99	High	Very high
Obese class II	35.00–39.99	Very high	Very high
Obese class III	40.00 or more	Extremely high	Extremely high

Source: Adapted from WHO, apps.who.int/bmi/index.jsp?introPage=intro_3.html

There's some debate about the most appropriate cut-offs of BMI and waist circumference measurements for different ethnic groups, including Aboriginal people and Torres Strait Islanders, and people of Asian and Pacific heritage. The World Health Organization (WHO) estimates that in different Asian populations the risk of developing type 2 diabetes and cardiovascular disease increases with a BMI of 22–25 and a waist circumference of more than 80 centimetres for women and 90 centimetres for men. Whatever your ethnicity, BMI can't take into account your individual body composition – how much body fat or muscle you have – so you should always use your BMI and/or waist circumference only as a guide. If your BMI and disease risk do come out high, though, start with a visit to your GP as soon as you can.

Metabolic syndrome

This is the name given to a cluster of conditions – excess abdominal fat, high levels of unhealthy blood fats (triglycerides and low-density lipoprotein or LDL cholesterol) and low levels of good blood fats (high-density lipoprotein or HDL cholesterol), high blood pressure, high blood glucose and insulin resistance (see Appendix A for more information). Doctors have grouped these conditions together because in combination they increase the risk of developing type 2 diabetes and cardiovascular disease. In fact, people with metabolic syndrome have a five times higher risk of developing type 2 diabetes than people who are overweight but otherwise healthy, and an increased risk of developing cardiovascular disease by a factor of two to four. If you have just one of these conditions and a large waist circumference, your GP should check regularly whether you also have cardiovascular disease or type 2 diabetes.

Cardiovascular disease

There are often no early warning signs to indicate increasing risk of cardiovascular disease. To help, the Australian National Vascular Disease Prevention Alliance has developed an online risk calculator (see Appendix B) to help you estimate your risk.

Cardiovascular disease is an umbrella term for diseases that affect the circulatory system – i.e. the heart and blood vessels. It includes heart disease (and heart attack) and stroke, and is used by doctors as a shorthand for all these conditions because their risk factors are the same and they can all result from a condition called atherosclerosis (better known as hardening or narrowing of the arteries).

Cardiovascular disease affects one in six Australians – in other words, 3.72 million of us! In 2010 it accounted for 25.8 per cent of the burden of disease in Australia measured in years of life lost. While treatment of cardiovascular disease and some of its risk factors has advanced significantly, it's still our most expensive disease; in 2004–05 it cost the Australian Government about $5.9 billion.

Chronic kidney disease

Age

High blood pressure

Sex (male)

Family history* of heart attack, stroke or high cholesterol

Irregular heartbeat

Smoking   High cholesterol

Diabetes

Being overweight (large waist circumference)

Each individual's risk of developing cardiovascular disease and type 2 diabetes depends on a combination of modifiable factors (such as smoking, poor eating and exercise habits), and non-modifiable factors (such as age, gender, and a family history of diabetes or cardiovascular disease). Take a look at the main risk factors above and consider how they apply to you.

*mother, father or sibling under the age of 55 years

Type 2 diabetes

About 80 per cent of people with type 2 diabetes are also overweight or obese. Given the rising global obesity rates, the world is now bracing itself for a tsunami of preventable type 2 diabetes. In 2013, 382 million people worldwide had diabetes; this is expected to rise to 592 million by 2035. In Australia, approximately 1 million people currently know they have diabetes, and about the same number again remain undiagnosed. This is the important point about type 2 diabetes: you could have it and not know, while all the time it's slowly doing damage to your body.

How does obesity lead to type 2 diabetes?

❝ This is the important point about type 2 diabetes: you could have it and not know, while all the time it's slowly doing damage to your body. ❞

Obesity disrupts the way our body uses and stores glucose, the carbohydrate we use as fuel. In simple terms, when we eat, the digestive process turns the carbohydrate in our food into glucose, which then circulates in the blood to fuel every cell in the body. (For more on carbohydrate-containing foods, see pages 21–23.) When we eat carbohydrates, this conversion process is very rapid and leads to a sudden rise in the levels of glucose in the blood (also called blood glucose). In response to this blood glucose spike, the pancreas (an organ next to the stomach) produces insulin, a hormone that tells cells throughout the body to take up the glucose to use as fuel or to store for later (in fat, muscle or the liver). Over time, particularly in people who are overweight or obese, insulin can no longer efficiently move glucose into cells – this is *insulin resistance* (see the graph below). This makes it increasingly difficult for the body to control blood glucose levels.

In response, the pancreas produces even more insulin to compensate, which can lead not only to high blood glucose levels (hyperglycaemia) but also high blood insulin levels (hyperinsulinemia). In some cases, this puts so much stress on the pancreas that its ability to produce and release insulin declines. Ultimately, this means the body is left in a permanent state of hyperglycaemia unless insulin medication is used.

> The progression of type 2 diabetes

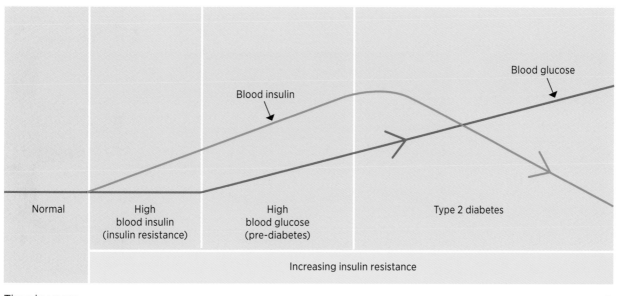

Normal | High blood insulin (insulin resistance) | High blood glucose (pre-diabetes) | Type 2 diabetes

Increasing insulin resistance

Time in years

Pre-diabetes

Type 2 diabetes is diagnosed when blood glucose levels are consistently high (see the table below). It's usually preceded by a condition called pre-diabetes, where glucose levels tend to rise to just above the normal range, which means that diabetes can be expected to develop unless something is done to reduce blood glucose levels. Pre-diabetes can be present over a period of several years, a lead-in time that allows preventative strategies, such as weight loss and increased physical activity, to be put in place.

Initially, someone with type 2 diabetes might feel tired, sleepy after meals, unwell and thirsty, and may need to urinate frequently. In extreme cases, where blood glucose levels are very high, they may even become unconscious. In many cases, though, they may be blissfully unaware they have the condition.

In the long term, if type 2 diabetes remains undiagnosed or isn't well managed, consistently high levels of blood glucose can cause blood vessel damage which leads to serious complications including nerve damage (diabetic neuropathy), kidney damage (diabetic nephropathy) and loss of sight (diabetic retinopathy). Diabetes also substantially increases the risk of cardiovascular disease, such as heart attack or stroke. In other words, every time your blood glucose is abnormally high, it's doing you damage.

Getting a diagnosis

Doctors can diagnose pre-diabetes and diabetes relatively easily by measuring blood glucose levels and comparing them to the values given in the table below. Separate blood samples can be taken after fasting (first thing in the morning, before breakfast) and after drinking a liquid containing a standardised amount of glucose. Diabetes will be diagnosed if fasting blood glucose levels are high or if blood glucose rises higher than a certain level after the glucose drink (this is called post-prandial glucose).

Another blood test used to diagnose diabetes measures glycosylated haemoglobin (HbA1c), which is a very fancy way of describing the amount of glucose that has become bound to haemoglobin (the oxygen-carrying molecule in red blood cells) over the past three months (which is the lifespan of a red blood cell). This test indicates whether your blood glucose levels have been unusually high during those past three months.

How diabetes is diagnosed →

Condition	Fasting blood glucose (mmol/L)	Blood glucose 2 hours after ingestion of 75 g glucose (mmol/L)*	HbA1c levels	
			(per cent)	(mmol/mol)
Normal	3.9–5.5	less than 7.8	less than 5.7	less than 39
Pre-diabetes	5.6–6.9	7.8–11	5.7–6.4	39–47
Diabetes	7.0 or more	more than 11	6.5 or more	48 or more

Note: HbA1c levels will be given either as a percentage (old unit) or as mmol/mol (new unit). Only one of these is required for a diagnosis of diabetes. *Oral glucose tolerance test.

If you've calculated your BMI and it indicates that you're overweight or obese, see your GP for blood glucose tests. If your GP has already indicated you don't have type 2 diabetes, but you'd like to determine your risk of developing it in the next five years, you can complete the risk assessment tool in Appendix B.

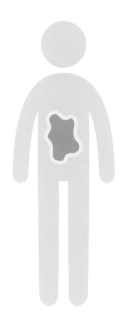

THIN ON THE OUTSIDE

While there's a close relationship between obesity and type 2 diabetes, it's possible to develop diabetes even if you're not overweight or obese. Other factors, including our individual genetics and the foods we eat, can influence our risk of developing type 2 diabetes and our ability to control it. In Asia, where the rates of obesity have not increased dramatically, the greatest explosion of diabetes is predicted, because people with Asian heritage tend to store body fat around their vital organs and abdominal region, where it's not as visible but still does enough damage to cause diabetes. This is why having a large waist circumference can be a useful indicator of diabetes risk.

So even if your weight is normal and your risk factors seem relatively low, take a moment to consider your diet and activity levels, and whether these could be improved. If so, the Low-carb Diet and exercise plan could not only improve your overall wellbeing but also help you manage your long-term risk of developing metabolic syndrome and type 2 diabetes.

The good news

If you've been diagnosed with pre-diabetes or type 2 diabetes, or you need to lose some weight and have any of the modifiable risk factors for metabolic syndrome and cardiovascular disease, the good news is there is help at hand.

There are a number of key health targets that you can work towards, and addressing these will not only dramatically reduce your risk of developing health complications, but will improve your overall wellbeing, making you feel great and allowing you to live the active, healthy life you deserve.

These targets are:
- reducing your weight and waist circumference
- lowering your blood pressure
- improving your blood fat profile (by decreasing your triglycerides and LDL cholesterol levels, and increasing your HDL cholesterol levels)
- better controlling your blood glucose levels. For example, reducing HbA1c and fasting glucose levels, post-meal glucose spikes and glycaemic fluctuations throughout the day (the degree to which glucose levels go up and down; also known as glycaemic variability.)

In fact, these are among the key factors that your GP will consider in improving your health and wellbeing, and by making the changes outlined in this book you can improve all of them, in addition to gaining many other benefits, providing you with a complete wellness solution.

Importantly, if you have diabetes, or suspect you may have it, you will gain particular benefit from using this plan in collaboration with your GP's diabetes management plan. More detailed information on how doctors treat diabetes is included in Appendix A; this section will show you how the CSIRO Low-carb Diet perfectly complements the medical management of diabetes to assist you in putting together the best treatment plan.

THE CURRENT APPROACH

The cornerstones of managing obesity and type 2 diabetes have long been an energy-restricted diet for blood glucose control and/or weight loss, and increased physical activity. Scientific evidence consistently shows that for people who are overweight or obese and have pre-diabetes or type 2 diabetes, losing weight can significantly reduce blood glucose levels. This not only improves general health, but also reduces many other risk factors, including those for cardiovascular disease.

Since the 1970s, the recommendation has been a diet high in carbohydrates and low in fat (with the balance of energy from protein). In other words, it has been recommended that 45–65 per cent of the energy (kilojoules) within the diet come from carbohydrate foods that are less refined and have a low glycaemic index (GI; see page 23).

For example, if your daily energy requirements were 8000 kilojoules, this would mean that 3600–5200 kJ of your intake would need to come from carbohydrate-rich foods. Given that carbohydrates provide 16 kJ of energy per gram,

this means your daily carbohydrate intake would be 225–325 grams.

Extensive research conducted by the CSIRO, as well as other internationally respected teams from around the world, now shows that this level of carbohydrate may actually be too high, particularly for people with metabolic syndrome and type 2 diabetes. Research also shows that this approach results in only slight reductions in risk factors for diabetes and heart disease and/or a modest improvement in diabetes control. It also indicates that lower-carbohydrate diets may be more effective. In fact, the latest nutritional recommendations from the American Diabetes Association (ADA) recognise that a diet lower in carbohydrates but higher in healthy fats can play a role in diabetes management.

In addition to the current Australian Government recommendations outlined in the *Australian Guide to Healthy Eating*, over the years we have seen many diet options appear. Below is a comparison of the nutrient content of these diets with that of the CSIRO Low-carb Diet.

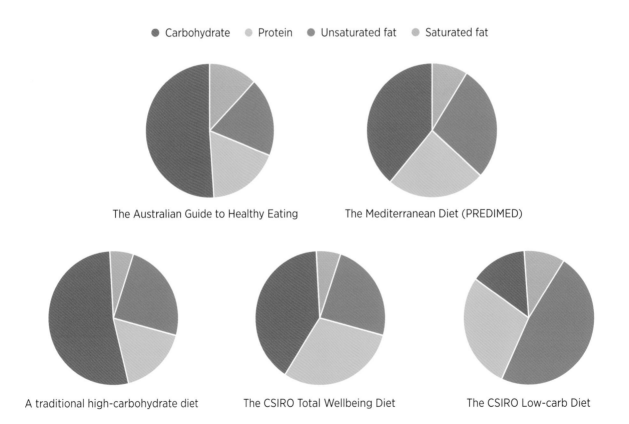

● Carbohydrate   ● Protein   ● Unsaturated fat   ● Saturated fat

The Australian Guide to Healthy Eating

The Mediterranean Diet (PREDIMED)

A traditional high-carbohydrate diet

The CSIRO Total Wellbeing Diet

The CSIRO Low-carb Diet

THE NEW LOW-CARB DIET

The Low-carb Diet is almost the opposite approach to those high-carb, low-fat diets traditionally recommended, and to what Australians currently eat. It combines very low carbohydrate levels with higher proportions of protein and healthy fats (including monounsaturated and polyunsaturated fat).

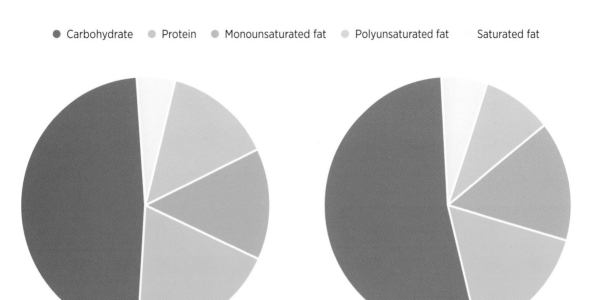

● Carbohydrate   ● Protein   ● Monounsaturated fat   ● Polyunsaturated fat   Saturated fat

Current eating patterns of Australians

Traditional high-carbohydrate, low-fat, low-protein diet

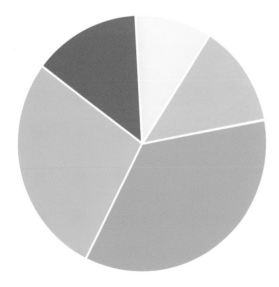

The CSIRO Low-carb Diet

In the next section, you'll learn why the combination of nutrients in this diet works best to combat type 2 diabetes, and reduce the risk factors for diabetes complications and cardiovascular disease.

PART 2

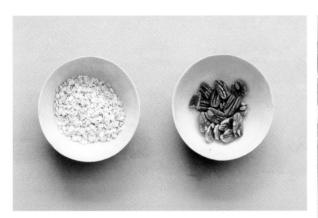

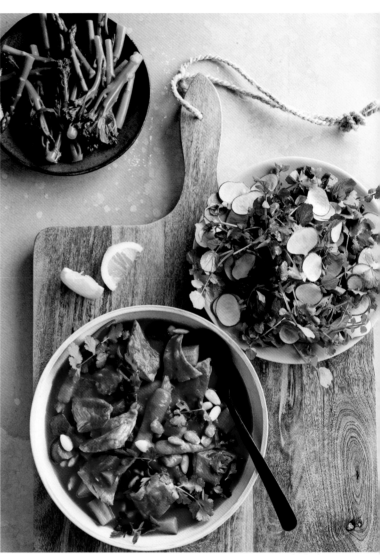

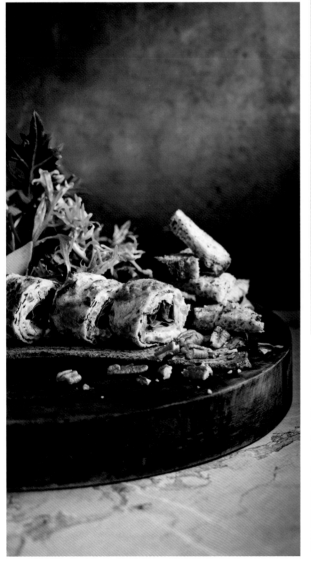

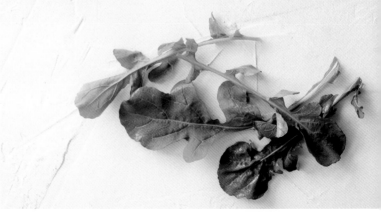

Why the CSIRO Low-carb Diet Works

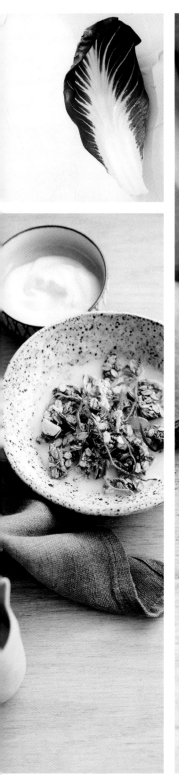

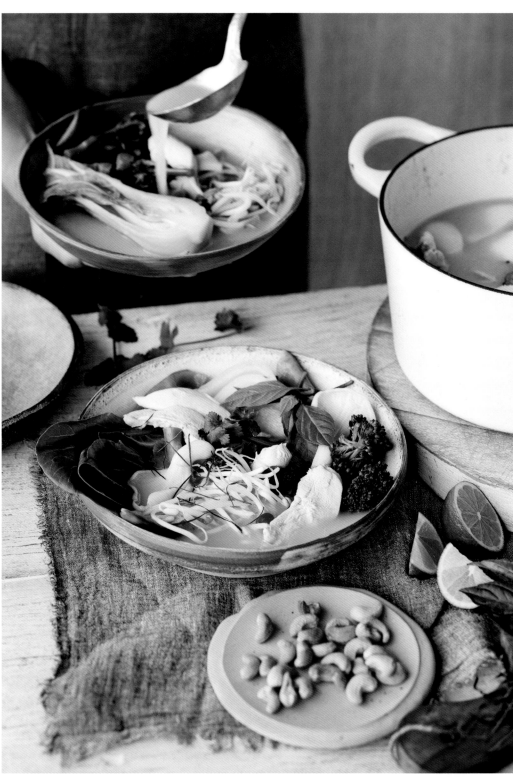

THE SCIENCE BEHIND THE LOW-CARB DIET

This diet is the culmination of more than 20 years of research by the CSIRO and other leading institutions into the health benefits of low-carbohydrate, high-protein and high-unsaturated-fat dietary patterns.

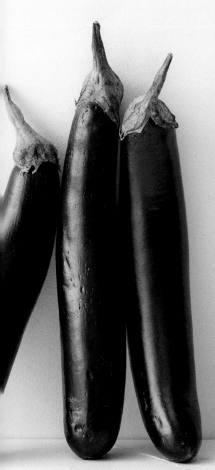

The Low-carb Diet combines the latest evidence to create a nutritionally complete, very low-carbohydrate, high-protein and high-unsaturated-fat eating plan. The results of our rigorous clinical research trial of the diet show that the benefits it provides are huge.

In this clinical study, 115 overweight or obese adults with type 2 diabetes were divided into two groups. Those in the first group were to consume an energy-restricted, very low-carbohydrate, high-protein, high-unsaturated-fat and low-saturated-fat diet (14 per cent high-quality carbohydrate, 28 per cent protein and 58 per cent fat with less than 10 per cent saturated fat) – in other words, the Low-carb Diet. Those in the second group ate an equally energy-restricted, high-carbohydrate, low-fat diet (53 per cent high-quality carbohydrate, 17 per cent protein and 30 per cent fat with less than 10 per cent saturated fat). Both groups participated in a structured physical activity program of 60 minutes of combined aerobic and resistance exercise three times a week. The trial ran for 52 weeks. During the trial, each participant's weight, body composition (to monitor reductions in fat mass), blood glucose control, cardiovascular disease risk, markers of kidney function and psychological wellbeing were assessed regularly.

The number of people who completed the full 52 weeks of the trial was similar for the two groups: 41 people (71 per cent) from the Low-carb Diet group completed the trial compared with 37 people (65 per cent) from the high-carbohydrate group.

As the table opposite shows, the Low-carb Diet group experienced a reduction in diabetes medication requirements **twice** that for the high-carbohydrate group. This means fewer side effects, a lower risk of hypoglycaemia and reduced costs. Similarly, the reduction in glycaemic variability in the Low-carb Diet group was **three times** that in the high-carbohydrate group. Blood triglycerides also decreased more on the Low-carb Diet, while HDL (good) cholesterol increased more.

Health measure	Average change in the Low-carb Diet group	Average change in high-carbohydrate group
Medication requirements*	–40%	–20%
Glycaemic variability	–30%	–10%
Blood triglycerides	–0.4 mmol/L	–0.01 mmol/L
HDL cholesterol	+0.1 mmol/L	+0.06 mmol/L

*Medications for controlling blood glucose levels

Both groups enjoyed substantial reductions in body weight, fat mass, blood pressure, Hb1Ac and fasting glucose, as well as improved mood and quality of life.

Benefits enjoyed by both groups

Health measure	Average change in Low-carb Diet group	Average change in high-carbohydrate group
Body weight	–9.1% (10 kg)	–9.1 per cent (10 kg)
Fat mass	–8.3 kg	–8.3 kg
Blood pressure	–6/6 mmHg	–6/6 mmHg
HbA1c	–1% (-12.6 mmol/mol)	–1% (-12.6 mmol/mol)
Fasting glucose	–1.4 mmol/L	–1.4 mmol/L
LDL cholesterol	–0.1 mmol/L	–0.2 mmol/L
Mood and quality of life	about 30%	about 30%

The significance of our results

Each change in one of the measures seen above has an important effect on our health. Average figures from large population studies show that a drop in blood pressure of 5/5 mmHg (say from 140/95 to 135/90) reduces the risk of stroke by more than 30 per cent and reduces the risk of dementia or heart failure, or dying from cardiovascular disease, by 20 per cent. This means that the participants in our study who averaged a reduction of 6/6 mmHg improved their risk factors considerably.

In the same way, a drop in HbA1c of 1 per cent or -12.6 mmol/mol (say from 7.5 to 6.5 per cent or 59 to 48 mmol/mol) reduces the risk of heart attack by 14 per cent, of developing microvascular disease by one-third, of limb amputation by almost half and of diabetes-related death by 21 per cent.

And finally, for every 1 per cent increase in HDL cholesterol, the risk of cardiovascular disease falls by 3 per cent. The increase enjoyed by our trial participants following the Low-carb Diet and exercise plan was 8 per cent, which means a 24 per cent decrease in cardiovascular disease risk.

The other major benefit of the Low-carb Diet and exercise plan was the large reduction in dependence on medications. In other words, by following the Low-carb Diet and exercise plan, you can be confident that you're becoming healthier, regardless of how much weight you lose.

HOW A LOW-CARB DIET IMPROVES HEALTH

Following the Low-carb Diet doesn't mean cutting out carbohydrates altogether, but there's good reason to cut down on them considerably, especially highly refined and processed carbohydrates. This will make you feel better and markedly improve your metabolic fitness.

Most of us know the five food groups, which *The Australian Guide to Healthy Eating* defines as:

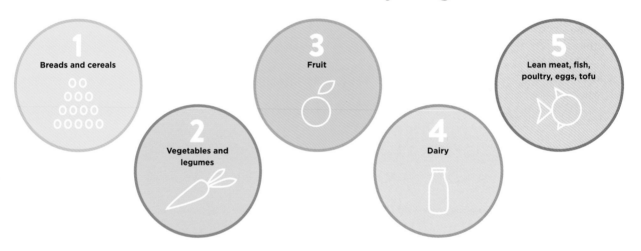

1. Breads and cereals
2. Vegetables and legumes
3. Fruit
4. Dairy
5. Lean meat, fish, poultry, eggs, tofu

For the Low-carb Diet, we have grouped foods into categories based on their macronutrient content:

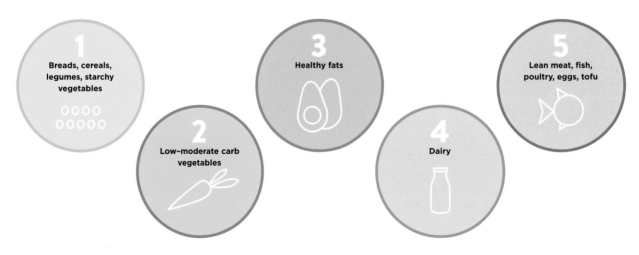

1. Breads, cereals, legumes, starchy vegetables
2. Low-moderate carb vegetables
3. Healthy fats
4. Dairy
5. Lean meat, fish, poultry, eggs, tofu

Here's an overview of the three main macronutrients in foods:

Carbohydrates

Our main sources of carbohydrates are grain foods such as **wheat**, **rice** and **oats**, and foods made from them, such as bread, pasta and breakfast cereals. **Sugar** (see page 32) is also a carbohydrate, but is most often a component of what we call discretionary foods – foods our bodies don't need to function but that we eat because we find them pleasurable. Sugar also occurs naturally in many fruits. Vegetables also contain carbohydrates to varying degrees – the **starchy vegetables** potato, sweetcorn and peas, for example, are high in carbohydrate. Other plant foods containing carbohydrate as starch are **legumes** such as lentils and chickpeas, which can also be a good source of protein. These plant foods are all important sources of vitamins, minerals and fibre. For more on carbohydrates, see pages 22–23.

Protein

The foods with the highest quantity as well as quality of protein are **lean meats** (lamb, beef, pork and poultry), **fish and other seafood** and **eggs**. Also significant are foods high in plant proteins, such as **tofu**. The other major source of protein (and lots of micronutrients, including calcium) are **dairy foods** – milk and products derived from it – and alternatives such as soy milk and nut milks. For more on protein, see pages 28–29.

Fats

Most of us can identify the foods that are our main sources of fats, scientifically known as lipids. These include solid (mostly saturated) fats such as **butter** and **coconut oil**, and liquid (mostly unsaturated) oils such as **olive oil** and **peanut oil**. **Nuts** and **avocado** are also good sources of healthy fats. For more on fats, see pages 24–26.

WHAT ARE CARBOHYDRATES?

The simplest carbohydrates are sugars, which are sweet, soluble in water and made of short carbon chains or rings. The simplest of these are monosaccharides (single or simple sugars), of which the three main types in food are glucose, fructose (fruit sugar) and galactose.

Disaccharides (double sugars) are made up of two monosaccharides bonded together: each molecule of sucrose (table sugar) is made of one glucose bound to one fructose molecule; lactose (milk sugar) is one glucose bound to one galactose; and maltose is two glucose molecules bound together. Polyols are sugar alcohols, some of which occur naturally, but they are most often encountered as additives in processed foods.

Oligosaccharides (made up of six to ten simple sugars) are the most complex of the sugars, and some occur naturally in fruits and vegetables. Maltodextrin is an artificial oligosaccharide used in processed foods.

Polysaccharides are the complex carbohydrates, made up of many simple sugars bonded together. These include starch, cellulose and pectin, which are found in abundance in rice, wheat, maize and potatoes.

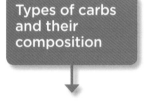

Types of carbs and their composition

Class	Subgroup	Types	Composition
Sugars	Monosaccharides	Glucose, galactose, fructose	n/a
	Disaccharides	Sucrose	Glucose + fructose
		Lactose	Glucose + galactose
		Maltose	Glucose + glucose
	Polyols	Erythritol, glycerol, maltitol, mannitol, sorbitol, xylitol	n/a
Oligosaccharides	Malto-oligosaccharides	Maltodextrins	Made from starch
	Other oligosaccharides	Raffinose	Galactose + glucose + fructose
		Fructo-oligosaccharides	1 glucose + numerous fructose
Polysaccharides	Starch	Natural starch	Amylose + amylopectin (both made up of several glucose molecules)
		Modified starches (food additives)	Made from starch
	Non-starch polysaccharides	Cellulose, hemicellulose, pectin, hydrocolloids	Numerous

What happens when we eat carbohydrates?

The carbohydrates we eat can have a profound effect on our blood glucose levels and glycaemic variability (see page 11). This is because all carbohydrates, including fructose (fruit sugar), are broken down into simple sugar and released into the bloodstream as glucose. The higher the total carbohydrate content of a food and the more refined and highly processed the carbohydrate it contains, the more it will increase blood glucose.

Two measures provide a quick means of determining whether carbohydrate foods will produce a significant increase in blood glucose levels: glycaemic index and glycaemic load.

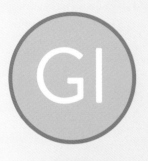

Glycaemic index

The glycaemic index (GI) was developed as a means of comparing food types based on their likelihood of raising blood glucose. Foods are given a GI of 1 to 100 based on the total rise in blood glucose after they're eaten, compared to pure glucose, which is set at 100. Low GI is up to 55, medium is 56–69 and high 70+. Although the GI tells us how likely it is that different food types will cause a significant rise in blood glucose, we need to determine the glycaemic load of a meal in order to know how great that rise is likely to be, and how long it will last.

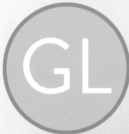

Glycaemic load

The increase in blood glucose (the size of the spike) caused by eating a carbohydrate food is determined by the total carbohydrate contained in the portion of that food eaten at a sitting. This is known as the glycaemic load (GL). A ranking system of GL from low to high has not been established, but the higher the GL, the higher the blood glucose will rise. This means that keeping the GL of your meals low will help control your blood glucose response and improve your health.

GL is determined by multiplying the GI of a food by the amount of carbohydrate (in grams) in the portion of the food to be eaten:

> **GL = GI/100 x total amount of carbohydrate eaten (grams)**

While selecting lower-GI foods will reduce the GL of your meal, it's possible for a food to be high in GI but have a low GL because you might only eat a small amount of it in any one sitting. Keeping an eye on both the type and amount of carbohydrate you eat, and how often, can have a marked influence on the rise in your blood glucose after eating, but *altering the total amount will have the greater effect*.

Reduce your carbohydrate portions throughout the day, every day!

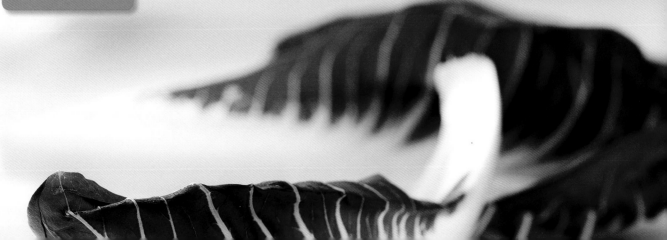

HOW 'GOOD' FATS IMPROVE OUR HEALTH

We all grew up with the notion that a diet high in fat will lead to weight gain and increase our risk of heart disease. For decades now, health authorities around the world have advocated a high-carbohydrate, low-fat diet to reduce the risk of heart disease, and for weight and diabetes management. However, more recent research suggests that this recommendation may not offer the greatest health benefits.

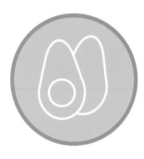

Over the past 20 years, several high-quality, large-scale clinical trials have demonstrated that a structured, energy-controlled diet that derives more of its energy from unsaturated fat results in a similar weight loss to a structured, energy-controlled diet that derives a high proportion of its energy from carbohydrate. In other words, it has become clear that a blanket low-fat message may not be the answer.

In fact, the best way to improve our health and reduce our risk of cardiovascular disease and type 2 diabetes is to focus on fat *quality* rather than fat quantity. The best approach now seems to be increasing our intake of monounsaturated and polyunsaturated (good) fats while limiting our intake of saturated (bad) fats. This is because these good fats help to:

- slow down the rate at which digested food leaves our stomach, which lowers our blood glucose response and reduces glycaemic variability
- improve our blood fat levels
- make us feel full and stop us overeating
- provide the creamy or fatty mouthfeel that heightens the pleasure of a meal.

Fats are an essential part of our dietary intake for many reasons. They're the main structural component of the membranes that enclose our cells; they carry fat-soluble vitamins such as vitamin A, D, E and K; they assist with appetite control; and, when used in appropriate amounts, they blunt the blood glucose response after eating.

There are three main types of fats in the diet: saturated, monounsaturated and polyunsaturated fats. It's important to note that the foods we eat as fat sources contain a mixture of these fat types. In red meat, for example, which is generally considered a source of saturated fat, half the fat is, in fact, monounsaturated.

❝ It has become clear that a blanket low-fat message may not be the answer. ❞

Saturated fats

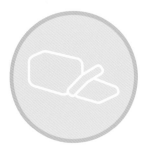

Unlike the other types of fats, saturated fats have no double bonds in their chemical structure, which makes them *saturated* with hydrogen atoms. This structure is more rigid, which means these fats are generally solid at room temperature. They predominate, for example, in butter, lard (pig fat), tallow (beef fat) and coconut oil. Saturated fat is found in very high quantities in processed and discretionary foods.

For many years now, *The Australian Guide to Healthy Eating* has recommended reducing our intake of saturated fat. This is because saturated fat has been shown to increase bad blood fat levels and thus increase the risk of cardiovascular disease. A number of studies have also shown that replacing saturated fat with monounsaturated and polyunsaturated fat can reduce the risk of cardiovascular disease. There's now growing debate about whether saturated fat in itself is bad for us, and some recent studies have even disputed any association between saturated-fat intake and risk of cardiovascular disease or type 2 diabetes.

Having said all that, most health professionals currently agree that high intakes of saturated fat (more than 10 per cent of total energy intake) could increase the risk of cardiovascular disease and type 2 diabetes by:

- promoting insulin resistance
- elevating LDL (bad) cholesterol, which leads to atherosclerosis (hardening of the arteries)
- impairing blood-vessel function, particularly in the heart.

❝ It's still a good idea to limit your intake of saturated fat. ❞

This means it's still a good idea to limit your intake of saturated fat (with the exception of saturated fat from most dairy foods, which does not appear to increase heart disease risk), or replace foods high in saturated fat with small amounts of foods containing unsaturated fats. For this reason, we've limited the saturated-fat content of the Low-carb Diet to no more than 10 per cent of total daily energy intake.

Unsaturated fats

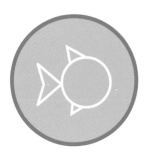

Unsaturated fats have at least one double bond, which means fewer hydrogen atoms are attached. Monounsaturated fats have one double bond, while polyunsaturated fats have two or more. Unsaturated fats are more likely to be liquids at room temperature. Olive oil is high in monounsaturated fatty acids, while many vegetable oils such as sunflower and peanut oil are high in polyunsaturated fatty acids.

The scientific evidence for monounsaturated and polyunsaturated fats demonstrates that they have the opposite effect of saturated fat on metabolic risk factors for cardiovascular disease, by:

- improving insulin sensitivity and producing a lower blood glucose response
- reducing LDL cholesterol, total cholesterol and triglyceride levels
- increasing HDL (good) cholesterol levels
- improving the functioning of the blood vessels in the heart.

These effects occur with higher intakes of dietary unsaturated fats, provided the level of saturated fat remains low. This means higher intakes of unsaturated fats would be particularly beneficial for people with insulin resistance, metabolic syndrome or type 2 diabetes. The Low-carb Diet takes advantage of these effects by deriving a high proportion of its energy from monounsaturated and polyunsaturated fats, while keeping saturated fat intake low. This enables optimal blood glucose control while also improving cardiovascular health.

The two main types of essential polyunsaturated fats are *omega-3* and *omega-6* fats. (The designations omega-3 and omega-6 indicate the position of the first double bond in the fatty acid molecule.) Omega-6 fats are readily available in Western diets, while the main sources of omega-3 fats are fatty fish such as salmon, and some plant-based foods such as flaxseeds. Because it's important to maintain a one-to-one balance between these two types of polyunsaturated fats, omega-3 fats are an essential part of a healthy diet. Populations that consume a diet high in omega-3 fats, such as the Mediterranean-style diet, have been shown to have less chronic disease, including diabetes.

Fats in food

Saturated fat

Dairy foods: butter, milk, cream, cheese

Meat: chicken skin, processed meats, mince, fatty meat cuts including marbled red meats

Baked goods: cakes, biscuits, sweet and savoury pastries, pies

Takeaway foods: pizza, burgers

Fats: ghee, coconut oil, palm oil

Polyunsaturated fat

Omega-3

Fish: salmon, sardines

Nuts and seeds: flaxseed

Omega-6

Nuts and seeds: walnuts, pine nuts, pecans, brazil nuts, sunflower seeds

Oils: sunflower oil, sesame oil

Soy beans

Monounsaturated fat

Avocados

Nuts and seeds: almonds, cashews, macadamias, hazelnuts, pecans, peanuts

Oils: olive oil, canola oil

Meats: lean fish and chicken

Olives

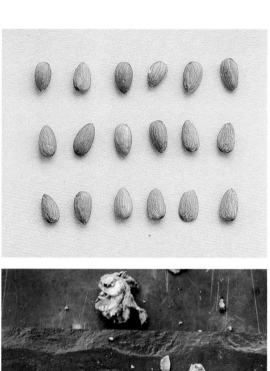

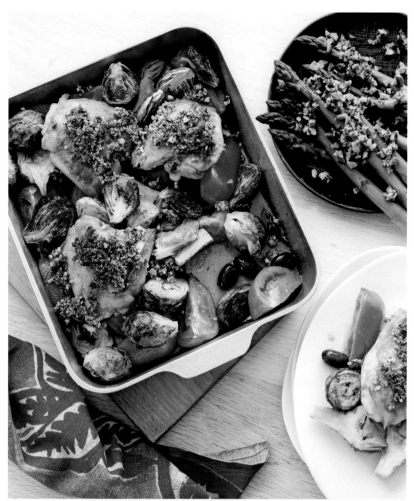

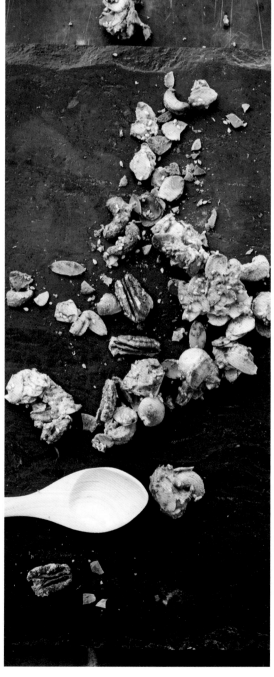

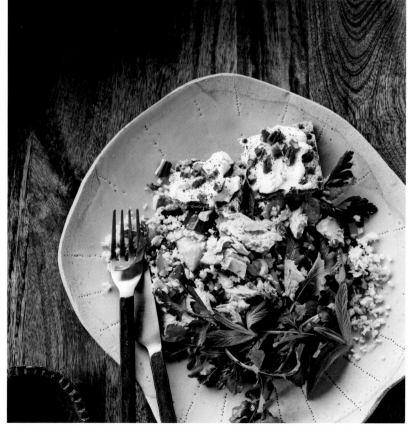

HOW A HIGHER PROTEIN INTAKE HELPS

As we all know from experience, one of the biggest challenges in achieving weight loss and maintaining a healthy body weight over the long term is controlling our appetite and hunger.

❛ **Protein will help you feel fuller for longer.** ❜

What if a diet could make you less hungry? That would be perfect, because if you don't feel hungry all the time, you're less likely to overeat. You're in luck, because research conducted at CSIRO and around the world has repeatedly shown that compared to carbohydrates and fat, protein will help you feel fuller for longer. This means that the Low-carb Diet, with its higher proportion of protein, will help you stay full after each meal and reduce feelings of hunger and the desire to snack throughout the day.

Burning energy as we digest our food

It may come as a surprise that about 10 per cent of our total daily energy expenditure is the energy required to digest, absorb, transport and store food. In other words, we need to eat food in order to digest it. This is known as the *thermic effect of food* or thermogenesis. The thermic effect of food is influenced by several factors, including how much protein, fat and carbohydrates a meal contains.

Research shows that it takes more energy to digest and absorb protein than either carbohydrates or fat. This means that by eating meals with a higher proportion of energy from protein, you'll expend more energy on digestion. This may help you control your weight.

Maintaining muscle during weight loss

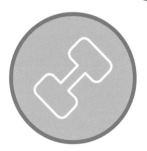

We lose weight when we reduce our energy intake below our daily energy needs. When this happens, the majority of the weight loss occurs as a reduction in body fat, but we also lose some other weight – what we call *fat-free mass* – which is predominantly muscle tissue.

If you wish to maintain a healthier lower body weight in the long term, however, it's important to retain as much fat-free mass and muscle as possible. This is because the majority of our daily energy expenditure comes from maintaining the body during rest, which is known as the *resting metabolic rate*. Our resting metabolic rate is largely determined by our level of fat-free mass, so retaining fat-free mass and muscle tissue during weight loss means we can achieve and maintain a higher daily resting energy expenditure and therefore a lower body weight.

Research has shown that losing weight using a diet higher in protein can increase the proportion of weight loss from fat tissue rather than fat-free mass and muscle tissue. This effect can be further magnified by combining a higher-protein diet with increased physical exercise, particularly resistance or strength training exercise, which is also part of the exercise plan in this book (see pages 92–109). With higher-protein diets, protein production in the muscle tissue (which is largely protein) has also been shown to increase, which improves the retention of fat-free mass during weight loss. While this helps maintain muscle mass and strength, it has the added benefit of maintaining the resting metabolic rate, which enhances overall energy expenditure. This means that a higher-protein diet can make it easier to maintain body weight in the longer term.

Maintaining fat-free mass and muscle tissue is also important for achieving good insulin sensitivity (i.e. fighting insulin resistance) and blood glucose control, which as we have seen are particularly important for people with type 2 diabetes. Muscle mass is one of the body's major storage sites for glucose, so maintaining a larger muscle mass will make it easier for your body to transport and store glucose from the blood, leading to better blood glucose control.

Aiding in glucose control

Increasing the proportion of protein in your diet while reducing the total amount of carbohydrates and the glycaemic load, can make the rise in blood glucose after a meal smaller. This will assist with blood glucose control and reduce glycaemic variability.

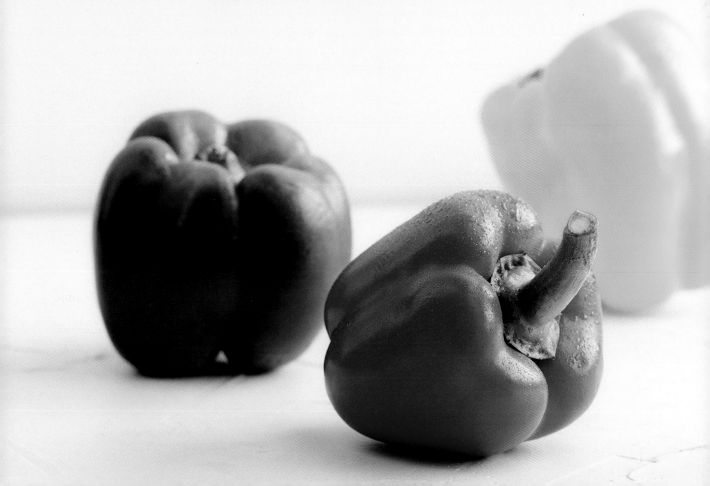

MORE REASONS TO ENJOY THE CSIRO LOW-CARB DIET

When you start the Low-carb Diet and exercise plan, people around you might have questions about this approach. Using this information as a guide, you'll be able to answer their questions based on scientific evidence, and illustrate the many benefits you can enjoy.

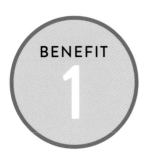

It improves your mood and quality of life

Feelings of low mood and depression have been associated with numerous poor health outcomes, including type 2 diabetes, weight gain and an inability to stick to diet and lifestyle changes.

At CSIRO we have examined the long-term effects on mood and quality of life of our Low-carb Diet compared to more traditional high-carbohydrate diets. The results from validated questionnaires indicate that both styles of diet markedly improve psychological mood and perceived quality of life. This cheerful news has important implications for reducing the risk of diabetes-related complications, because it means people will be more likely to stick with the Low-carb Diet and exercise plan.

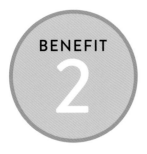

It maintains your brain function

Transitioning from high-carb to low-carb eating may not be smooth sailing for everyone. Eating reduced amounts of carbs means the body needs to switch to burning fat for energy more frequently and, while we feel the benefits on the scales, some people may also experience tiredness or have difficulty concentrating initially. However, these symptoms are short-lived and disappear relatively quickly. Research shows that other small changes in cognitive performance may occur during the first few weeks of a low-carb diet, but that these, too, are short-lived.

Our own investigations, which included testing task-processing speed, memory, reasoning ability and verbal fluency, have shown that both a high-carbohydrate, low-fat weight-loss diet and the Low-carb Diet improved or maintained cognitive function over the course of a year. This is because, in adults, almost all of the brain's glucose needs are supplied by the liver, and not from eating continuously. It is only during periods when blood glucose is very low (hypoglycaemia) that cognitive performance may be impaired.

Science also shows that the restricted carbohydrate intake of a very low-carbohydrate diet does not cause hypoglycaemia. This is because the body adapts by using other stored fuel sources, most importantly fat, which means the body can maintain its glucose stores for brain function.

If you have type 2 diabetes with pre-existing complications, it's important for your healthcare team to monitor your mental ability and performance closely, as unfortunately you're at greater risk of cognitive decline. If you're taking any glucose-lowering medication and you make changes to your lifestyle, you should also consult your healthcare team, to ensure your dosages are appropriate to prevent medication-induced hypoglycaemia.

BENEFIT

3

It provides adequate fibre

Traditionally, low-carbohydrate diets tended to offer less fibre because they called for the restriction of fibre-containing carbohydrate-rich foods, such as wholegrains, starches and legumes. The great diversity of our modern food supply, however, has allowed us to create the Low-carb Diet in such a way as to still deliver the recommended daily fibre intake of 25–30 grams.

This dietary fibre comes from both the liberal amounts of low-carbohydrate vegetables, such as cabbage, brussels sprouts and broccoli, and the small amount of high-fibre grains, including legumes, allowed within the Low-carb Diet. Low-carb need not mean no-carb. In fact, the people following the Low-carb Diet in our trials had an average fibre intake of 26 grams a day.

Although Australians generally consume adequate amounts of dietary fibre, this doesn't mean we're consuming sufficient amounts of active fibre, better known as fermentable fibre or resistant starch. On average we consume as little as 4–6 grams per day, when we actually need 15–20 grams per day to maintain gut health. Resistant starch is the fraction of starch we consume that escapes digestion in the small intestine, and is made up of components that act as a nutritional source for the gut microbiome, preferentially feeding the friendly sub-population of microbes. This helps ensure we retain a healthy balanced microbiome that, in turn, promotes a healthy gut. Resistant starch is processed by our gut bacteria to produce short-chain fatty acids including acetate, propionate and, most importantly, butyrate, which is the preferred energy source for the cells that line the gut. Butyrate also promotes blood flow through the blood vessels of the gut and repair of the gut lining, and assists in the prevention of colorectal cancer as well as giving us a feeling of satiety.

If you have a history of bowel complaints, you should consult your GP, and it's particularly important to eat more foods that are high in resistant starch, such as chickpeas, bananas or high-fibre, bran-based cereals.

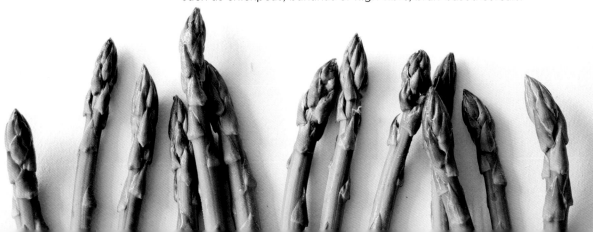

Food	Resistant starch content (grams)
30 g unprocessed raw oats	3.5
100 g baked potato (baked, then chilled and reheated to increase resistant starch content)	19
100 g green banana	12
100 g ripe banana	5
100 g cooked cannellini beans	4
40 g slice of rye or pumpernickel bread	1.4–1.8
100 g broad beans	12.7
120 g fresh garden peas	17.4

Note: These are average values and will vary with different food brands and varieties.

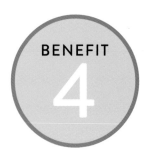

BENEFIT 4

It is rich in important nutrients

We specifically designed the Low-carb Diet to ensure that it's nutritionally complete, and provides adequate intakes of all essential vitamins, minerals and trace elements. What's more, our research has shown that when overweight and obese people with type 2 diabetes follow a low-carb diet such as ours, they maintain good blood levels of the key micronutrients – including copper, zinc, selenium, sodium, potassium, calcium, magnesium and iron. These levels were similar to those of people following a traditional high-carbohydrate, low-fat diet.

If you're a vegetarian, however, or have specific food preferences or a history of deficiencies (such as an iron deficiency), or even if you're at risk of deficiency because of your age, you'll need to discuss specific food choices with your dietitian to ensure your diet provides all the nutrients you need. In some cases, you might also require a supplement.

As we age, our capacity to absorb and effectively utilise nutrients decreases. This is notable for vitamins A and B12, and calcium. Interactions can also occur between medications and nutrients that make the nutrients less available for uptake within the body. Many people with obesity take acid reducers for reflux, for example, which can decrease the body's levels of vitamin B12, calcium and magnesium. People with type 2 diabetes who take the diabetes drug metformin over the long term are at risk of vitamin B12 deficiency, which can mimic nerve damage in the hands and feet. Ask your endocrinologist or GP for a blood test if you think you're at risk of any deficiencies at all.

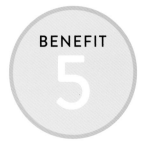

BENEFIT 5

It restricts your intake of refined sugar

Limiting your intake of carbohydrate-rich foods will in turn lower your consumption of refined sugar. Refined (or processed) sugar is almost completely devoid of nutrients and makes blood glucose rise very sharply. Eating too much sugar without doing enough exercise can contribute to excess weight gain and obesity, and lead to a range of other health problems, from tooth decay to diabetes. Restricting your intake of refined sugar only magnifies the health benefits that can be achieved with this diet.

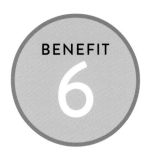

BENEFIT
6

It sustains physical performance

Our bodies store a limited amount of glucose in the liver and muscles in the form of glycogen, which is used primarily to maintain blood glucose levels between meals and fuel physical activity. When blood glucose levels start to become low, the body breaks the stored glycogen down into glucose, releasing it into the blood to maintain stable blood glucose levels. When we eat carbohydrates, our glycogen stores are replenished first and then surplus carbohydrates are converted into fat.

During rest and low-intensity physical activity, our bodies use mostly stored fat for energy. As the intensity of exercise increases, a greater proportion of our energy needs are supplied by glucose. When consuming a low-carbohydrate diet, within days our bodies are able to adapt to increase the proportion of fat used for fuel during both rest and exercise. This means that most people will not experience any sustained negative effects of a low-carbohydrate diet on physical performance.

Our research suggests that people following the Low-carb Diet and exercise plan are very unlikely to feel greater fatigue or loss of physical ability. Over a one-year period, our trial participants experienced no adverse effects on physical performance, including aerobic capacity and muscle strength, and could still undertake regular exercise. A high carbohydrate intake isn't essential for maintaining physical performance. There's no reason why the Low-carb Diet should affect your ability to lead an active lifestyle or maintain your daily living activities. It's generally only in extreme exercise conditions, when high-intensity exercise is performed for several continuous hours, that the body depletes its glycogen stores and an increased carbohydrate intake could possibly help prolong the exercise session.

ONE EXCEPTION

People who are using insulin or taking medication that triggers the pancreas to release insulin, such as sulfonylureas (e.g. gliclazide or glimepiride) or GLP analogues (e.g. exenatide), may need more carbohydrate during exercise. If this applies to you, speak to your healthcare team before you start a new exercise program, and monitor your blood glucose levels before, during and after exercise. You may need a change in your medication timing and/or dosage to take the effect of exercise into account. You might also need to ensure you eat the carb-rich foods in the Low-carb Diet before exercise.

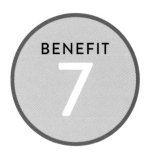

BENEFIT
7

It maintains kidney function

A traditional high-carbohydrate, low-fat diet derives only 18–20 per cent of its energy from protein. In contrast, a very low-carbohydrate diet derives 25–35 per cent of its energy from protein. A diet high in protein is believed to place excessive strain on the kidneys and lead to poor kidney function. This is only the case, however, for extremely high protein intakes. Although the *proportion* of energy from protein in the Low-carb Diet is high, its total amount of dietary protein is similar to that of the typical Australian diet – about 100 grams per day – and has no damaging effect on the kidneys.

Our research has also shown that for people who are overweight or obese and have type 2 diabetes and an increased risk of kidney disease, weight loss has a similar effect on kidney function, whether it results from a traditional high-carbohydrate, low-protein, low-fat diet or the Low-carb Diet. Other studies have produced similar results, and have shown that diets with similar levels of protein to the Low-carb Diet have no detrimental effect on kidney function in people with type 2 diabetes and pre-existing early stage kidney disease.

We can confidently say, therefore, that the Low-carb Diet will maintain kidney function in people wihout established kidney disease. It's important, however, to start the Low-carb Diet and exercise plan in close consultation with your healthcare team, so that they can monitor your kidney health. This is particularly important if you already have type 2 diabetes and/or known kidney impairment or poor kidney function.

DOES KETOSIS PLAY A ROLE?

Ketosis occurs when the body burns its own fat for energy rather than the carbohydrates (or glucose) from a meal. When we're in ketosis, we derive our energy from ketones, small molecules created when fat stores are broken down. When the body is in ketosis we tend to feel less hungry and thus may eat less than we would otherwise.

Some people say that a very low-carbohydrate diet is beneficial because it triggers an increase in the production of ketones from fat deposits. It's not clear from the current evidence, however, whether this is actually the case. When we first start a very low-carbohydrate diet, the levels of ketones in our blood do increase. But over the long term, these higher ketone levels dissipate, possibly because they're being increasingly used as a fuel source.

It's also unclear from research how great the carbohydrate restriction must be before ketosis kicks in. There's no evidence, however, that the benefits of a very low-carbohydrate diet depend on elevated ketone levels.

Although we know that ketosis can suppress appetite, we don't yet know the minimum level of ketosis required to achieve this.

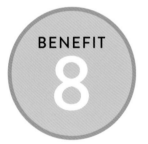

BENEFIT 8

It maintains bone health

Some people say that very low-carbohydrate diets can lead to compromised bone health and increase the risk of osteoporosis. They claim that these diets increase ketone levels in the blood and that this, combined with the higher proportional protein intake, increases sulfuric acid levels in the blood. The concern has been that the body will remove calcium from the bones to buffer the blood against this increased acidity, thus reducing bone mass and increasing the risk of bone fracture.

We're pleased to say that our trial, along with other recent long-term scientific studies, shows this needn't be the case. After one to two years on either a diet like ours or a traditional high-carbohydrate, low-protein, low-fat diet, there were no differences in several markers of bone health, including mineral density, mineral content and bone turnover. Whether this is the case for all low-carbohydrate diets is not yet known. If you have any pre-existing bone conditions that require medical treatment, you should, of course, consult your healthcare team so that they can closely monitor your bone health.

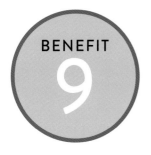

It is environmentally sustainable

As consumers, we're all increasingly interested in sustainable eating. The CSIRO's research suggests that the two most effective strategies for securing a healthy food supply for future generations is to focus on diet *quantity* and diet *quality*. This means eating to our energy needs, and consuming foods that promote health and wellbeing rather than discretionary or junk foods.

Most research into sustainable diets has focused on greenhouse gas emissions. Most emissions from the typical Australian diet can be attributed to foods from the five core food groups – fruit, vegetables, meat, dairy and grains. But almost 30 per cent of our dietary emissions come from energy-dense discretionary foods that provide minimal nutritional value. These include fried foods, sugar-sweetened beverages and confectionery. And of course, the more kilojoules we consume, the greater the greenhouse gas emissions from our diet.

If more of us ate only what we needed, following a nutritionally complete dietary pattern and decreasing our intake of discretionary foods, we'd enjoy a net nutritional benefit at no additional environmental expense. In fact, this could reduce emissions due to diet by 15–30 per cent while providing significant health benefits.

The composition of our diet also directly affects the total greenhouse gas emissions. Our analysis shows that for men, the Low-carb Diet produces lower greenhouse gas emissions than the average Australian diet and similar emissions to the traditional dietary recommendations. For women, it produces lower greenhouse gas emissions than both the average Australian diet and the traditional recommendations.

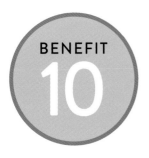

It is affordable

Many people think that because very low-carbohydrate diets have a higher proportion of protein, they're expensive and only an option for the rich, but this isn't the case. Our analysis shows that although a low-carb diet is more expensive than the traditional high-carbohydrate, low-fat diet, the difference is only around $3 a day – about the price of a cup of coffee. Not only that, but improved health, reduced healthcare costs and less reliance on medication could leave you in front financially.

PART 3

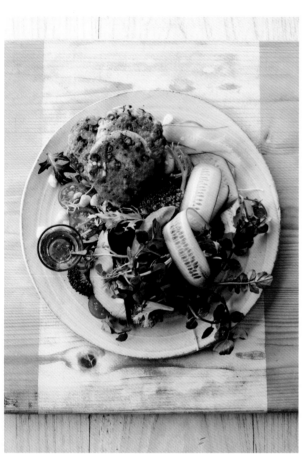

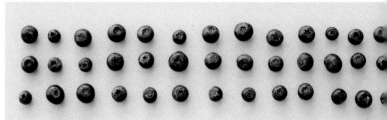

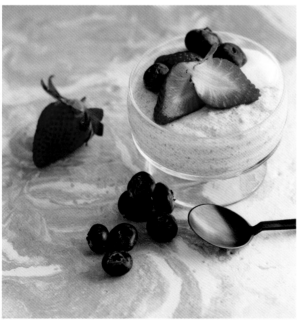

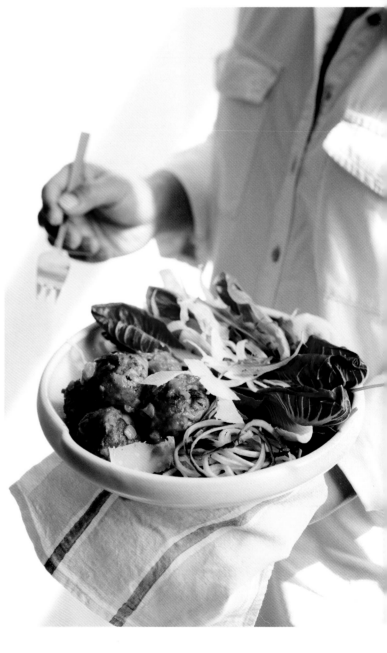

The CSIRO Low-carb Diet & Meal Plans

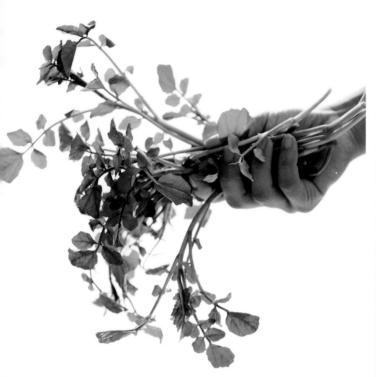

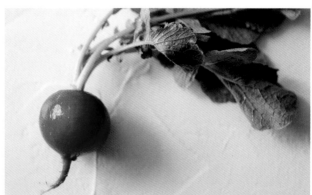

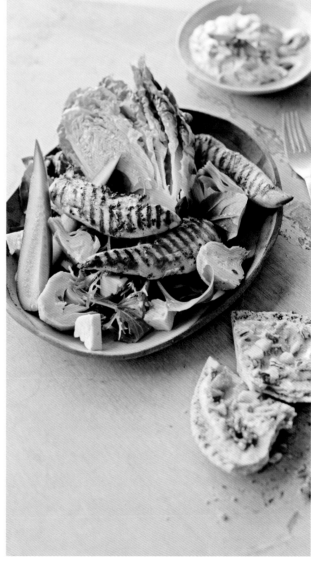

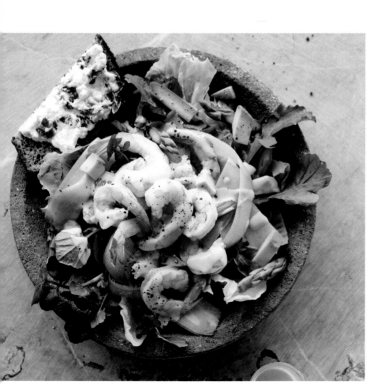

UNDERSTANDING THE DIET

Our research shows that the Low-carb Diet can help control blood glucose levels, improve blood fats and make weight loss easier, especially if you have pre-diabetes or type 2 diabetes. This diet isn't about saying *no* to carbohydrates, it's about choosing the right types and amounts – up to 70 grams of high-fibre, low-GI carbohydrates each day.

If you're taking medication that may have an impact on nutrient absorption or if you have a history of nutrient deficiencies, see your dietitian as you may need to take a supplement.

The Low-carb Diet is nutritionally complete and focuses on whole foods, with the majority of its kilojoules coming from healthy unsaturated fats and lean protein foods. Its carbohydrate foods are high in fibre and low-GI, and include foods high in resistant starch (see pages 31–32) for bowel health. The greatest benefits can be enjoyed by overweight or obese people with pre-diabetes or type 2 diabetes, but the diet can also help all adults who've struggled with their weight for various reasons, including those with insulin resistance. (Please note: low-carbohydrate diets are not suitable for children and pregnant women.)

How is this diet different from other diets?

This diet offers a way to reduce your intake of carbs while maintaining complete nutrition. To do this, we've sorted foods into groups based on the nutrients they provide (see the table opposite), and assigned them units based on their kilojoule value (anything lower than 0.5 of a unit is considered negligible). As fruits contain fructose, a carbohydrate, we recommend a low intake and have placed them in the carbohydrate 'extras' category (many of the nutrients fruits provide are also found in vegetables). Dairy contains the carbohydrate lactose, so we have reduced portions but have allowed for almond and soy alternatives. As dairy also provides calcium, we suggest reduced-fat or skim varieties, as the lower the dairy fat the higher the calcium concentration. If you choose alternative dairy or have a history of osteoporosis, you may need additional calcium – speak to your healthcare team.

Check with your healthcare team
If you have diabetes and are on insulin, we strongly advise discussing the diet with your endocrinologist or GP. They may need to review and monitor your medications, particularly before week 8.

Carbohydrate 'extras', for long-term maintenance

To improve the flexibility of the diet, we've devised a guide to acceptable **carbohydrate 'extras'**. Our studies found that the Low-carb Diet produced substantial weight loss and optimised health benefits. But some people were better at maintaining the diet *over the longer term* when they could consume slightly more carbs – 70 grams of high-fibre, low-GI carbohydrates each day, rather than 50 grams. So after six weeks on the diet, or as you start to achieve your health and weight goals, we've included optional carbohydrate 'extras' in the meal plans and some of the recipes to enable you to slightly increase your carbohydrate intake by 20 grams each day. Alternatively, you can make your own choice of extra carbs by using the quick-reference table on page 65.

There are four energy levels to choose from, offering 6000–9000 kJ per day, that cater for most individual's needs. Generally, levels 1 and 2 are suitable for women, while levels 3 and 4 are suitable for men.

Food groups for the diet	Level 1 (6000 kJ/day)	Level 2 (7000 kJ/day)	Level 3 (8000 kJ/day)	Level 4 (9000 kJ/day)	Key nutrients provided
Breads, cereals, legumes, starchy vegetables	1.5 units	1.5 units	1.5 units	1.5 units	Slow-release, low-GI, carbohydrates, folate, fibre and B-group vitamins.
Lean meat, fish, poultry, eggs, tofu	1 unit at lunch, 1.5 units at dinner	1 unit at lunch, 2 units at dinner	1 unit at lunch, 2.5 units at dinner	1.5 units at lunch, 2.5 units at dinner	Protein, zinc and vitamin B12. Red meats are highest in iron, fish in omega-3 fatty acids and pork in thiamin.
Dairy	3 units	3 units	3.5 units	4 units	Protein, calcium, vitamin B12 and zinc. Dairy (except most cheeses) also contains carbohydrates.
Low–moderate carb vegetables	At least 5 units	At least 5 units	At least 5 units	At least 5 units	Minimal carbohydrates, and plenty of fibre, folate, vitamins A, B6 and C, magnesium, beta-carotene and antioxidants.
Healthy fats	10 units	11 units	14 units	15 units	Vitamins A, E and K, antioxidants and omega-3 and omega-6 fats.
Indulgences	**2 units per week**	**2 units per week**	**2 units per week**	**2 units per week**	Limited beneficial nutrients. Most contain added sugars, alcohol and/or saturated fats.
Carbohydrate extras (Weeks 7+)	**2 extras per day**	**2 extras per day**	**2 extras per day**	**2 extras per day**	**Carbohydrates (see page 65). They also contribute vitamins and minerals as they come from your core food units.**

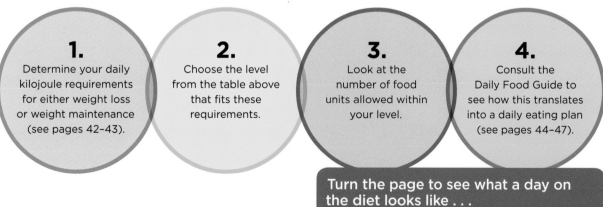

To choose which level is right for you . . .

1.
Determine your daily kilojoule requirements for either weight loss or weight maintenance (see pages 42–43).

2.
Choose the level from the table above that fits these requirements.

3.
Look at the number of food units allowed within your level.

4.
Consult the Daily Food Guide to see how this translates into a daily eating plan (see pages 44–47).

Turn the page to see what a day on the diet looks like . . .

One day on the diet

Putting it all together can seem daunting, so here's an overview of what one day following the level 1, 6000 kJ diet in the first six weeks might look like. After week 6, you can add two carbohydrate 'extras' if you wish (see page 65), to bring your carbohydrate intake up to 70 g per day.

BREAKFAST

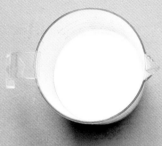

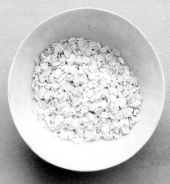

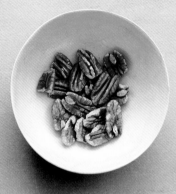

100 ml skim milk
(0.5 unit dairy)

30 g high-fibre, low-GI cereal
(1 unit breads, cereals, legumes,
starchy vegetables)

20 g (9) pecans
(2 units healthy fats)

LUNCH

40 g chopped avocado (2 units healthy fats)

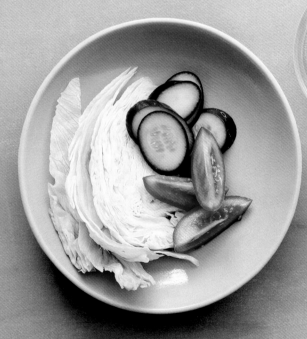

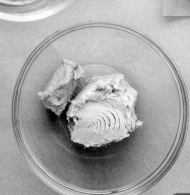

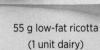

55 g low-fat ricotta
(1 unit dairy)

225 g low-carbohydrate salad
(1½ cups) – chopped and tossed lettuce, tomato
and cucumber (1.5 units low-carbohydrate
vegetables)

100 g tuna in spring water
(1 unit lean meat, fish, poultry, eggs, tofu)

**WEEKS 7+
CARB EXTRAS**

Add 40 g chickpeas
to the salad for
1 carb extra

DINNER

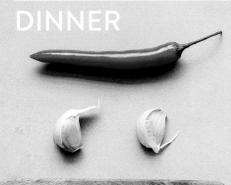

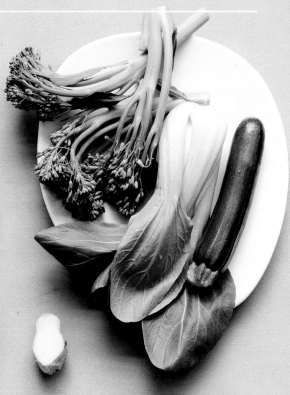

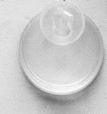

2 teaspoons olive oil
(2 units healthy fats)

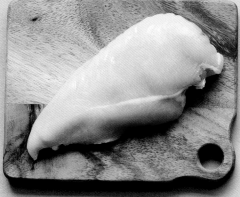

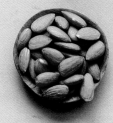

150 g (raw weight) lean chicken breast
(1.5 units lean meat, fish, poultry, eggs, tofu)

40 g raw unsalted almonds
(4 units healthy fats)

2 cups mixed low-carbohydrate vegetables
(you can use a mix of zucchini/broccolini/bok choy
or anything else from the low-carb vegetable list,
see pages 54–55), with basil, ginger, chilli and garlic
(3 units low-carbohydrate vegetables)

SNACK

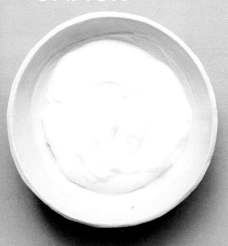

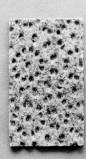

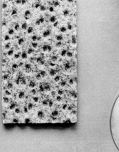

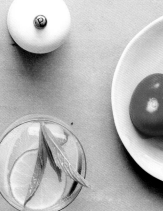

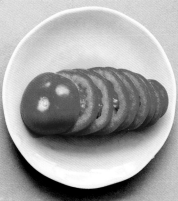

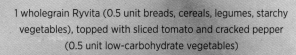

150 g low-fat Greek-style yoghurt
(1.5 units dairy)

1 wholegrain Ryvita (0.5 unit breads, cereals, legumes, starchy
vegetables), topped with sliced tomato and cracked pepper
(0.5 unit low-carbohydrate vegetables)

> **WEEKS 7+
> CARB EXTRAS**
>
> Add 200 g
> strawberries for
> 1 carb extra

Determining your daily kilojoule requirements

The following calculation was used in our scientific trial (see pages 18–19) to personalise the diet to each participant's energy needs. It estimates your daily kilojoule requirements to maintain normal body function (digestion, breathing, and so on) and keep your weight stable. This is known as your basal metabolic rate (BMR). To determine your BMR, use the appropriate formula from the table below. (If instead you'd prefer to use an online calculator, see Appendix B.)

Formulas for calculating your basal metabolic rate →

| Age (years) | BMR equation | |
	Women	Men
18–29	(62 x weight in kilograms) + 2036	(63 x weight in kilograms) + 2896
30–59	(34 x weight in kilograms) + 3538	(48 x weight in kilograms) + 3653
60 and over	(38 x weight in kilograms) + 2755	(49 x weight in kilograms) + 2459

Note: There are a few different methods for calculating BMR. We've used the Schofield equation.

Once you've determined your BMR, you need to multiply it by an activity factor from the table below to estimate your total daily kilojoule requirements.

Activity factors for determining your total daily kilojoule requirements →

| Activity level | Description | Activity factor | |
		Women	Men
Sedentary	Very physically inactive (work and leisure)	1.3	1.3
Lightly active	Daily activity of walking or intense exercise once or twice a week and a sedentary job	1.5	1.6
Moderately active	Intense exercise lasting 20–45 minutes at least three times a week or an active job with a lot of daily walking	1.6	1.7
Very active	Intense exercise lasting at least one hour each day or a heavy, physical job	1.9	2.1
Extremely active	Daily intense activity (i.e. nonstop training, e.g. an athlete in training) or a highly demanding physical job (e.g. armed forces)	2.2	2.4

If you're a healthy weight, there's no need to reduce your energy intake, so the number you're left with now is your daily requirement and you can use this to choose the level from the table on page 39.

If you need to lose weight, calculate your daily kilojoule requirement as follows. To reduce your weight by about 0.5 kilograms each week, you'll need to reduce your energy intake by 2000 kJ per day. Once you've calculated your total daily kilojoule requirements above, subtract 2000 from this number to determine how many kilojoules to eat each day to achieve weight loss and therefore which of the four levels to choose.

To reduce your weight by about 1 kilogram each week, you'll need to reduce your energy intake by 4000 kJ per day. Calculate your total daily kilojoule requirements as above and subtract 4000 from this number. The answer will tell you how many kilojoules to eat each day to achieve this weight loss and therefore which of the four levels to choose.

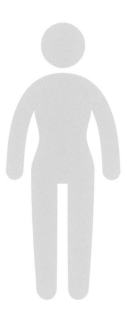

How it works in practice

Silvia is 58 years old and weighs 87 kilograms. She works part time as an office assistant and looks after her grandchildren two days a week. Silvia goes for a walk most days. This makes her activity factor 1.5. She chooses the appropriate formula from the table opposite and calculates her BMR like this:

BMR = (34 x weight in kilograms) + 3538
    = (34 x 87) + 3538
    = 6496 kJ per day

To calculate her total daily kilojoule requirements, Sylvia will multiply her BMR by her activity factor:

Total daily energy requirement   =   6496 x 1.5
                                 =   9744 kJ per day

This is the amount of energy Sylvia needs to maintain her current weight.

Sylvia is overweight and would like to start by losing about 0.5 kilogram a week. She'll therefore reduce her estimated total daily kilojoule intake by 2000 kJ per day:

Total dieting energy requirement   = 9744 – 2000
                                   = 7744 kJ per day

Sylvia rounds this down to the nearest thousand, 7000 kJ per day, and will therefore start on level 2. If she's feeling too hungry or losing weight too rapidly, Sylvia can move to level 3 (8000 kJ). If she's not losing weight, she can drop down to level 1 (6000 kJ).

Our clinical experience has shown that if your calculated energy requirements are greater than 9000 kJ a day, even by 2000–3000 kJ, following the level 4 diet will still result in significant health benefits.

Maintenance in the longer term

Sylvia reaches her weight-loss goal after 6 weeks, and her health has improved significantly. She decides she's enjoying the diet but would like to eat some fruit each day. As she's now on maintenance, she can have up to 70 grams carbohydrates each day, instead of the standard 50 grams. To add another carbohydrate serve, she uses the carbohydrate exchange table on page 65 to select a fruit portion.

See how you progress – if your chosen level isn't working, you can move between levels until you start to see the changes you desire. Many people hit a weight-loss plateau after an initial drop in weight. If this happens, you can simply switch to a lower level until you reach your target. Your dietitian and exercise physiologist can also help you overcome a weight plateau.

THE DAILY FOOD GUIDE

Once you've identified the level that's right for you and the food units it includes (see page 39), you can use the core lists of foods for each category on the following pages to choose what you want to include in your day. As long as the total units consumed tallies with the units required for your level, you can be flexible with when and how you consume these.

For example, if you're on the 6000 kJ level, you'll need to consume 1.5 units from the 'Breads, cereals, legumes, starchy vegetables' group each day. You could have 30 g suitable cereal for breakfast (1 unit), and then 50 g sweet potato at dinnertime (0.5 unit) OR you could opt to have a bigger breakfast (45 g cereal = 1.5 units) and then no more from this food group that day.

If you're on levels 2–4, you can use this base plan and add the extra allowances your plan provides. For example, if you're on a level 3 plan, you can have 0.5 serve more from the 'Dairy' group each day than the base (level 1) plan. You can choose how you'd like to do this: you may want to have an extra 10 g cheese or an extra 50 g yoghurt, for example.

The best way to enjoy flexibility within the eating plan is to understand the foods it includes, start from the basics and add new ones as you build confidence. Before the trial began, many participants thought they'd feel deprived, but once they started the Low-carb Diet, most reported no feelings of missing out. On the contrary, they said that having a narrow selection of foods to choose from helped them regain control of their eating habits. The remarkable improvements in their health was also a powerful motivator.

Easing in

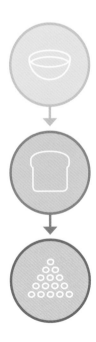

To eliminate temptation, start with the core lists of foods in the Daily Food Guide (see following pages) until you adapt to the style of eating, especially if it's drastically different from your usual intake. Once you're familiar with the foods from the daily guide, which usually takes about two weeks, you can start swapping foods within the same group that contain the same nutrients and energy. For example, if you don't feel like cereal for breakfast, you could swap the 30 g breakfast cereal with one 35 g slice of wholegrain bread, or 80 g red kidney beans. This gives you flexibility with your food choices but ensures that you stay within the nutrient targets of the diet.

When looking at the foods selected and the meal plans provided, remember that they've been designed so that each food group provides different key nutrients. By making sure you eat each food in the type and amount specified, you can be sure you'll be gaining the full benefit of the Low-carb Diet.

If you want to get started quickly, or you don't wish to follow the meal plans, you can just work your way through the recipes. They've all been developed to align with the key principles of the program, and each recipe gives an indication of the units it uses within the plan. They offer plenty of variety, and use herbs, spices and nuts to create taste and texture sensations.

YOUR DAILY FOOD GUIDE FOR LEVEL 1 (6000 kJ)

The following pages give examples of the types and quantities of foods that can make up your daily intake of units on the diet.

Breads, cereals, legumes, starchy vegetables

1.5 units per day

Choose from:

1 UNIT HIGH-SOLUBLE-FIBRE, LOW-GI CEREAL

30 g suitable breakfast cereals (e.g. All-Bran, All-Bran Fibre Toppers, All-Bran Wheat Flakes, Goodness Superfoods Heart, Goodness Superfoods Digestive, Hi-Bran Weet-Bix, untoasted natural muesli, unprocessed rolled oats)

1 UNIT BREADS

35 g multigrain bread
1 thin slice fruit bread
½ wholemeal pita bread (e.g. Mountain Bread wrap)
½ small wholemeal scone (25 g)
3 Ryvitas or 4 rye Cruskits
4 x 9 Grains Vita-Weats

1 UNIT LEGUMES

160 g cooked, drained lentils
80 g cooked, drained chickpeas or red kidney beans
100 g cooked, drained cannellini beans or four-bean mix

1 UNIT LOW-GI, HIGH-STARCH VEGETABLES

20 g raw or 40 g cooked quinoa or couscous
100 g sweet potato
70 g corn
100 g green peas or broad beans
200 g pumpkin

1 UNIT GRAINS

15 g wholemeal plain or self-raising flour, cornflour, rice flour, arrowroot or green banana flour
⅓ cup cooked rice

To increase the amount of resistant starch in your diet, you could exchange your allocated 30 grams of high-fibre, low-GI cereal and your allocated 1 crispbread with one of the items listed in the table on page 32.

Dairy

3 units per day

Choose from:

1 UNIT DAIRY

200 ml skim milk or low-fat, calcium-enriched soy or almond milk
100 g low-fat Greek-style yoghurt or low-fat, lactose-free soy yoghurt
20 g cheddar, parmesan, Swiss or feta cheese
55 g ricotta or cottage cheese
25 g mozzarella or bocconcini cheese, or low-fat cream cheese

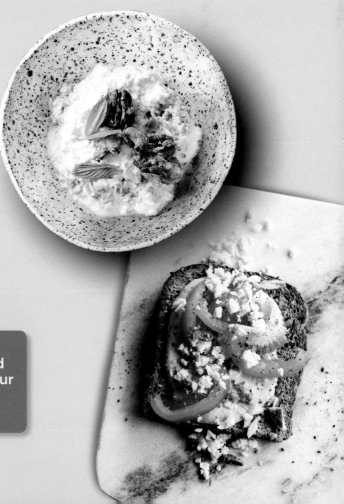

YOUR DAILY FOOD GUIDE FOR LEVEL 1 (6000 kJ)

Lean meat, fish, poultry, eggs, tofu

2.5 units per day

For lunch, choose from:

1 UNIT LEAN MEAT, FISH, POULTRY, EGGS, TOFU

100 g (cooked weight) lean meat or fish: tinned or fresh fish or seafood, chicken, turkey, pork, beef, lamb

2 eggs (50 g/½ unit each)

100 g tofu

We recommend fish for lunch at least twice a week.

> **If you wish to have an egg for breakfast, just have 50 g less meat at lunchtime to account for this.**

For dinner, choose from:

1.5 UNITS LEAN MEAT, FISH, POULTRY, EGGS, TOFU

150 g (raw weight) lean meat or fish: chicken, turkey, pork, beef, lamb, fish or seafood

3 eggs (50 g/½ unit each)

150 g silken tofu

We recommend fish for dinner at least twice a week and red meat no more than three times a week.

> **Depending on your food preferences, you may not wish to eat red meat, fish or chicken – or not every day. Legumes are an excellent source of protein for vegetarians or vegans, although they are higher in carbohydrates than their animal-based counterparts, so keep this in mind when planning your daily intake. 1 unit of legumes is as follows:**
>
> - 160 g cooked, drained lentils (provides 15 g carbs and 11 g protein)
> - 80 g cooked, drained chickpeas or red kidney beans (provides 12 g carbs and 6 g protein)
> - 100 g cooked, drained cannellini beans or four-bean mix (provides 13 g carbs and 6 g protein).

Low and moderate carbohydrate vegetables

At least 5 units per day

Choose from:

1 UNIT LOW-CARBOHYDRATE VEGETABLES (AT LEAST 3 UNITS OF THESE PER DAY)

½ cup (75 g) cooked vegetables

1 cup (150 g) salad vegetables

Low-carbohydrate vegetables: *lettuce, broccoli, broccolini, spinach, artichoke (high in resistant starch), bok choy, asparagus, bean sprouts, cucumber, mushrooms, tomato, zucchini, kale, rocket, garlic, chilli, fresh herbs and spices.*

1 UNIT MODERATE-CARBOHYDRATE VEGETABLES (UP TO 2 UNITS OF THESE PER DAY)

½ cup (75 g) cooked vegetables

1 cup (150 g) salad vegetables

Moderate-carbohydrate vegetables: *cauliflower, celery, green beans, capsicum (all colours), brussels sprouts, cabbage, spring onion, snow peas, carrot, eggplant, onion, leek, parsnip, swede, bamboo shoots, fennel, turnip and radish.*

> **Strawberries are a very low-carb fruit and can be substituted for a moderate-carb vegetable if you wish (100 g = 1 unit).**

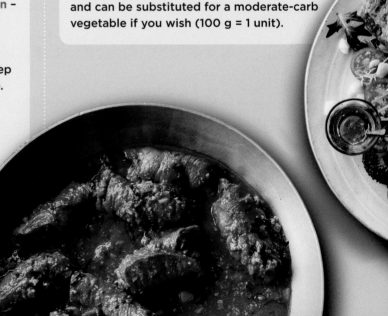

Healthy fats

10 units a day

Choose from:

1 UNIT HEALTHY FATS

5 g (1 teaspoon) olive, grapeseed or sunflower oil
5 g (1 teaspoon) tahini (sesame butter)
20 g avocado
20 g (1 tablespoon) hummus
5 g (1 teaspoon) olive oil or canola or Nuttelex margarine
10 g nuts (almonds, cashews, pecans or walnuts)

> **Nuts are a primary source of healthy fats in the Low-carb Diet. We encourage you to eat at least 60 g (6 units) of nuts each day.**

Indulgence foods

2 units per week

Choose from:

1 UNIT INDULGENCE FOOD

Any food or drink providing approximately 450 kJ – e.g. 150 ml wine, 20 g chocolate, 40 g store-bought low-fat dips, 10 Arnotts shapes, 1 x 20 g packet of chips, 10 Pringles, ½ slice of pizza or ¼ bucket (35 g) hot chips.

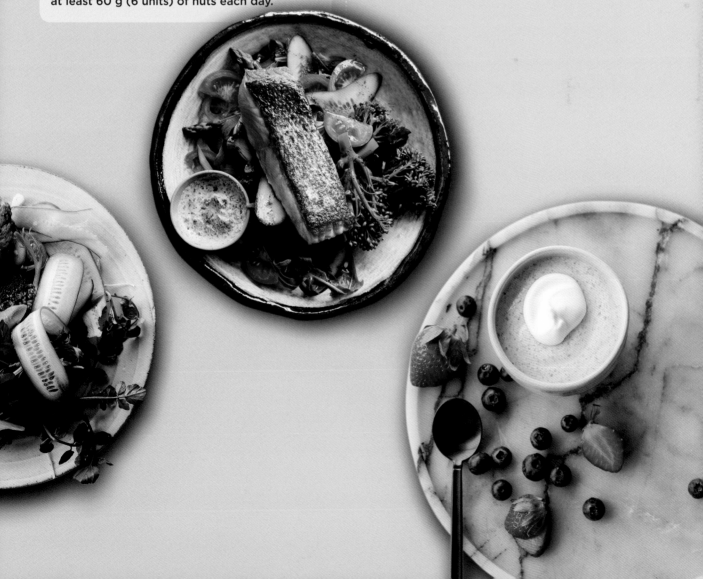

Daily units: **2.5** lean meat, fish, poultry, eggs, tofu | **1.5** breads, cereals, legumes, starchy vegetables | **3** dairy | **at least 5** mod–low-carb vegetables (**>3** low-carb vegetables) | **10** healthy fats

WEEK 1

> If you're having an egg for breakfast, reduce your lunch portion of lean meat, fish, etc, by 50 g to reach your daily target of 2.5 units for this category

> We've given you the breakdown of units here in Week 1 so you can see how the calculations work. These all add up to your total daily allowance for each da

	Monday	Tuesday	Wednesday	Thursday	Friday	Saturday	Sunday
Breakfast	1 boiled egg*, mashed with 20 g avocado and 20 g feta, served on a slice of mixed grain toast • 0.5 lean meat, fish, poultry, eggs, tofu • 1 breads, cereals, legumes, starchy veg • 1 dairy • 1 healthy fat	Nut and oat granola with orange zest (see page 123) • 1 breads, cereals, legumes, starchy veg • 1 dairy • 2 healthy fats	Overnight oats with sweet spiced nuts (see page 124) • 1 breads, cereals, legumes, starchy veg • 1 dairy • 1 healthy fat	Vanilla and chia seed oat smoothie shots (see page 127) • 1 breads, cereals, legumes, starchy veg • 1 dairy • 1.5 healthy fats	Nut and oat granola with orange zest (see page 123) • 1 breads, cereals, legumes, starchy veg • 1 dairy • 2 healthy fats	Baked ricotta with pesto and avocado toast (see page 114) • 1 breads, cereals, legumes, starchy veg • 1.5 dairy • 0.5 low-carb veg • 3 healthy fats	Mozzarella and pesto bruschetta (see page 119) • 1 breads, cereals, legumes, starchy veg • 1 dairy • 1 low-carb veg • 2 healthy fats
Lunch	Prawn no-rice paper rolls (see page 143) • 1 lean meat, fish, poultry, eggs, tofu • 1 dairy • 2 low-carb veg • 2 healthy fats	Quick tuna salad for one (page 153) • 1 lean meat, fish, poultry, eggs, tofu • 1 dairy • 2 low-carb veg • 2 healthy fats	Smoked chicken slaw with creamy avocado dressing (see page 153) • 1 lean meat, fish, poultry, eggs, tofu • 1 dairy • 1.5 low-carb veg • 0.5 mod-carb veg • 2 healthy fats	Tandoori chicken with grilled vegetable salad (see page 149) • 1 lean meat, fish, poultry, eggs, tofu • 0.5 breads, cereals, legumes, starchy veg • 1 dairy • 2.5 low-carb veg • 2.5 healthy fats	Chicken and asparagus salad (see page 154) • 1 lean meat, fish, poultry, eggs, tofu • 0.5 dairy • 2 low-carb veg • 3 healthy fats	Warm mushroom salad with poached eggs (see page 162) • 1 lean meat, fish, poultry, eggs, tofu • 0.5 breads, cereals, legumes, starchy veg • 0.5 dairy • 2 low-carb veg • 1 mod-carb veg • 3 healthy fats	Salmon and broccoli pesto wraps (see page 145) • 1 lean meat, fish, poultry, eggs, tofu • 0.5 breads, cereals, legumes, starchy veg • 1 dairy • 2 low-carb veg • 2 healthy fats
Dinner	Barbecued fillet steaks with stuffed mushrooms (see page 229) • 1.5 lean meat, fish, poultry, eggs, tofu • 3 low-carb veg • 4 healthy fats	Crisp-skin blue-eye trevalla with steamed Asian greens (see page 175) • 1.5 lean meat, fish, poultry, eggs, tofu • 3 low-carb veg • 0.5 mod-carb veg • 3 healthy fats	Sesame-crusted tofu with stir-fried Asian greens (see page 244) • 1.5 lean meat, fish, poultry, eggs, tofu • 3 low-carb veg • 3 healthy fats	Lamb cutlets with chargrilled vegetables and mint pesto (see page 241) • 1.5 lean meat, fish, poultry, eggs, tofu • 0.5 dairy • 2.5 low-carb veg • 1 mod-carb veg • 3 healthy fats	Baked snapper with gremolata and roasted vegetables (see page 180) • 1.5 lean meat, fish, poultry, eggs, tofu • 3 low-carb veg • 1 mod-carb veg • 4 healthy fats	Baked fish with thyme and fennel-seed crust (see page 197) • 1.5 lean meat, fish, poultry, eggs, tofu • 2 low-carb veg • 1 mod-carb veg • 3 healthy fats	Roast chicken with Brussels sprouts, artichokes and olives (see page 214) • 1.5 lean meat, fish, poultry, eggs, tofu • 2 low-carb veg • 1 mod-carb veg • 4 healthy fats
Snacks	100 g low-fat Greek-style yoghurt 1 wholegrain Ryvita with ¼ medium tomato, sliced 30 g raw almonds • 0.5 breads, cereals, legumes, starchy veg • 1 dairy • 0.5 low-carb veg • 3 healthy fats	100 g low-fat Greek-style yoghurt 1 wholegrain Ryvita topped with ¼ medium tomato, sliced 30 g pecans • 0.5 breads, cereals, legumes, starchy veg • 1 dairy • 0.5 low-carb veg • 3 healthy fats	100 g low-fat Greek-style yoghurt 75 g low-carb vegetable sticks (e.g. celery and cucumber) with 60 g avocado Spiced baked ricotta with almonds (see page 263) • 0.5 breads, cereals, legumes, starchy veg • 1 dairy • 1.5 low-carb veg • 4 healthy fats	30 g raw almonds Cucumber slices spread with 30 g cottage cheese • 0.5 dairy • 0.5 low-carb veg • 3 healthy fats	1 Ryvita wholegrain crispbread, topped with 10 g avocado and 2 slices of tomato Baked orange blossom custards (see page 271) • 0.5 lean meat, fish, poultry, eggs, tofu • 1 breads, cereals, legumes, starchy veg • 1 dairy • 1 healthy fat	Coffee yoghurt with nut sprinkle (see page 268) • 1 dairy • 1 healthy fat	Zucchini and avocado 'fries' (see page 260) • 1 low-carb veg • 1 dairy • 2 healthy fats

> These snacks are part of the overall diet plan. You can have these between meals or with a meal, depending on how hungry you are.

SHOPPING LIST See page 81 for a list of pantry items

QUANTITY	ITEM
....	limes
....	lemons
....	orange
....	asparagus
....	avocado
....	basil
....	baby bok choy
....	bean sprouts
....	broccolini
....	broccoli
....	brussels sprouts
....	carrots (and baby carrots)
....	chilli (small red)
....	choy sum
....	Lebanese cucumber
....	kale
....	cos lettuce
....	mixed salad leaves (mesclun, baby rocket, rocket, baby spinach)
....	radicchio
....	eggplant
....	baby fennel
....	green beans
....	leek
....	mushrooms (large field, fresh shiitake, button, portobello and oyster)
....	red cabbage
....	red capsicum
....	snow peas
....	tomatoes

QUANTITY	ITEM
....	cherry tomatoes
....	zucchini
....	mint
....	Vietnamese mint
....	flat-leaf parsley
....	thyme
....	firm tofu
....	sirloin/New York steaks
....	French-trimmed lamb cutlets
....	chicken (tenderloins, thigh cutlets, breast fillets)
....	smoked chicken breast fillet
....	king prawns
....	white fish fillets (rockling, blue-eye trevalla, pink snapper or barramundi)
....	mixed grain bread
....	mountain bread (or Herman Brot bread)
....	wholemeal pita bread

WEEK 2

	Monday	Tuesday	Wednesday	Thursday	Friday	Saturday	Sunday
Breakfast	Hummus and tomato toast with spiced nuts (see page 120)	Overnight oats with sweet spiced nuts (see page 124) 20 g pecans or raw almonds	Porridge with cinnamon nut crumble (see page 117)	Nut and oat granola with orange zest (see page 123)	Overnight oats with sweet spiced nuts (see page 124) 20 g raw almonds	Ricotta toast and sweet spiced nuts (see page 128) 25 g pecans	Mushrooms with feta croutons (see page 131)
Lunch	Nori omelette rolls with smoked salmon (see page 139)	Mushroom and spiced chicken 'burgers' (see page 140)	Green gazpacho with prawns and herbed ricotta toast (see page 167)	Quick tuna salad for one (page 153)	Tuna and bocconcini lettuce cups (see page 135)	Thai chicken soup with greens (see page 171) ½ slice mixed grain toast and 20 g cheese	Polenta-crusted chicken and avocado salad (see page 150)
Dinner	Moroccan tofu with grilled spiced-nut mushrooms (see page 252)	Portuguese chicken with cucumber and fennel salad (see page 213)	Spice-rubbed steaks with sautéed mushrooms (see page 225)	Crisp-skin salmon with herb and cashew 'butter' (see page 184)	Mediterranean vegetable and fish bake (see page 194) 50 g low-fat Greek-style yoghurt	Veal and mushroom involtini with crunchy Italian salad (see page 230)	Sesame-crusted tofu with stir-fried Asian greens (see page 244)
Snacks	100 g low-fat Greek-style yoghurt with a sprinkle of cinnamon	100 g low-fat Greek-style yoghurt with a sprinkle of cinnamon 1 wholegrain Ryvita topped with 40 g avocado and 4 slices of cucumber	75 g low-carb vegetable sticks (e.g. celery and cucumber) 100 g raita (see page 264) 10 g hummus	100 g low-fat Greek-style yoghurt 2 wholegrain Vita-Weats spread with 1 tablespoon of avocado 20 g raw almonds	10 g Sweet spiced nut clusters (see page 259)	20 g Sweet spiced nut clusters (see page 259) Indian-spiced kale chips with raita (see page 264)	Baked orange blossom custards (see page 271) 20 g Sweet spiced nut clusters (see page 259)

SHOPPING LIST See page 81 for a list of pantry items

QUANTITY	ITEM
....	lemons
....	oranges
....	asparagus
....	avocado
....	baby bok choy
....	baby fennel bulb
....	bean sprouts
....	broccolini
....	curly kale
....	eggplant (slender Japanese)
....	green capsicum
....	iceberg lettuce
....	kale
....	Lebanese cucumbers
....	mushrooms (mixed, button, large field, portobello, oyster, fresh shiitake)
....	onion
....	red capsicum
....	red chillies (small and long)
....	snow peas
....	spring onion
....	salad leaves (rocket, baby spinach)
....	radicchio
....	watercress
....	witlof
....	telegraph cucumber
....	tomatoes (including grape or cherry)
....	zucchini
....	basil

QUANTITY	ITEM
....	bay leaves
....	chives
....	coriander
....	dill
....	flat-leaf parsley
....	kaffir lime leaves
....	lemon thyme
....	lemongrass
....	mint
....	Thai basil
....	thyme
....	firm tofu
....	chicken (breast fillets and pieces)
....	veal steaks
....	scotch fillet steaks
....	king prawns
....	firm white fish fillets (snapper, blue-eye trevalla or other)
....	salmon fillets
....	smoked salmon
....	four-bean mix
....	hummus
....	mixed grain bread
....	wholemeal pita bread

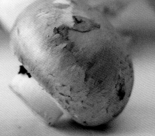

WEEK 3

	Monday	Tuesday	Wednesday	Thursday	Friday	Saturday	Sunday
Breakfast	Avocado and ricotta smash toast (see page 128)	Overnight oats with sweet spiced nuts (see page 124) 25 g pecans	1 boiled egg*, smashed together with 40 g avocado and 20 g feta, served on a slice of mixed grain toast	Porridge with cinnamon nut crumble (see page 117)	Baked ricotta with pesto and avocado toast (see page 114) 25 g pecans	Mozzarella and pesto bruschetta (see page 119)	Mushrooms with feta croutons (see page 131)
Lunch	Chicken salad with tzatziki (see page 146)	Chicken and asparagus salad (see page 154)	Cucumber and salmon 'sandwiches' (see page 136)	Prawn no-rice paper rolls (see page 143)	Salmon and cauliflower 'tabbouleh' with crispbreads (see page 161)	Smoked chicken slaw with creamy avocado dressing (see page 153)	Salmon and broccoli pesto wraps (see page 145)
Dinner	Hummus-crusted chicken with roasted cauliflower and haloumi salad (see page 206)	Thai fish cakes with broccoli salad (see page 176)	Vegetable fried 'rice' with tofu and egg (see page 248)	Madras beef curry with cauliflower and broccoli 'rice' (see page 226)	Tofu and turmeric 'scramble' with steamed greens (see page 253)	Biryani-style lamb with spinach and mint salad (see page 237)	Lemon oregano roast chicken with rocket and tahini salad (see page 205)
Snacks	1 wholegrain Ryvita topped with 2 slices of tomato and a sprinkle of pepper 20 g pecans	100 g low-fat Greek-style yoghurt 1 wholegrain Ryvita topped with 10 g low-fat cheddar cheese and 2 slices of tomato	100 g low-fat Greek-style yoghurt 40 g raw unsalted almonds	Greek-style crispbread (see page 256) 25 g pecans	Tomato, bocconcini, and basil skewers: 8 cherry tomatoes, 40 g bocconcini cheese and ½ cup fresh basil, threaded alternately onto skewers	Spiced baked ricotta with almonds (see page 263) 10 g Sweet spiced nut clusters (see page 259)	Berry yoghurt jellies (see page 272) 25 g Sweet spiced nut clusters (see page 259)

*If you're having an egg for breakfast, reduce your lunch portion of lean meat, fish, etc by 50 g to reach your daily target of 2.5 units of lean meat, fish, poultry, eggs, tofu.

SHOPPING LIST See page 81 for a list of pantry items

QUANTITY	ITEM
....	lemons
....	limes
....	asparagus
....	avocado
....	baby bok choy
....	bean sprouts
....	broccoli
....	broccolini
....	brussels sprouts
....	carrot
....	cauliflower
....	choy sum
....	cauliflower
....	frisee lettuce
....	green beans
....	kale
....	Lebanese cucumber
....	lettuce (cos, baby cos)
....	mushrooms (button, flat, portobello)
....	onion
....	radishes
....	red cabbage
....	red chilli (small)
....	red onion
....	salad leaves (baby rocket, baby spinach, rocket)
....	snow peas
....	spinach
....	spring onions

QUANTITY	ITEM
....	tomatoes (including cherry or grape)
....	water chestnuts
....	watercress
....	zucchini
....	basil
....	coriander (leaves, roots and stems)
....	dill
....	flat-leaf parsley
....	fresh bay leaves
....	kaffir lime leaves
....	lemon thyme
....	mint
....	thyme
....	Vietnamese mint leaves
....	firm tofu
....	silken tofu
....	chicken breast (fillets and tenderloins)
....	smoked chicken breast fillet
....	beef rump steaks
....	lamb leg steaks or backstraps
....	king prawns
....	firm white fish fillets (snapper, blue-eye trevalla or other)
....	haloumi
....	hummus
....	mixed grain bread
....	mountain bread (or Herman Brot bread)

All these vegetables and salad ingredients contain low amounts of carbohydrates (less than 3 grams per serve) and can be enjoyed in generous quantities on this diet (150 g raw, 75 g cooked = 1 unit). **These get the green light!**

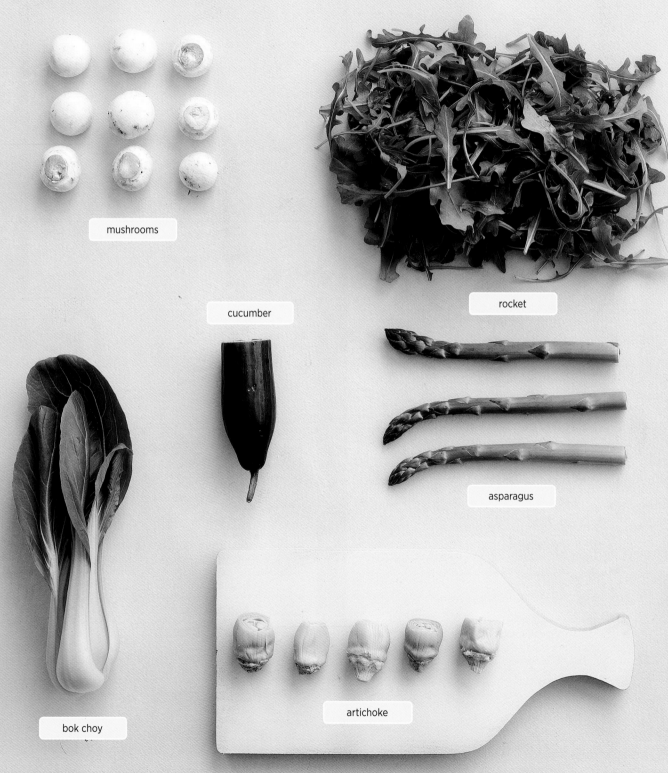

mushrooms

rocket

cucumber

asparagus

bok choy

artichoke

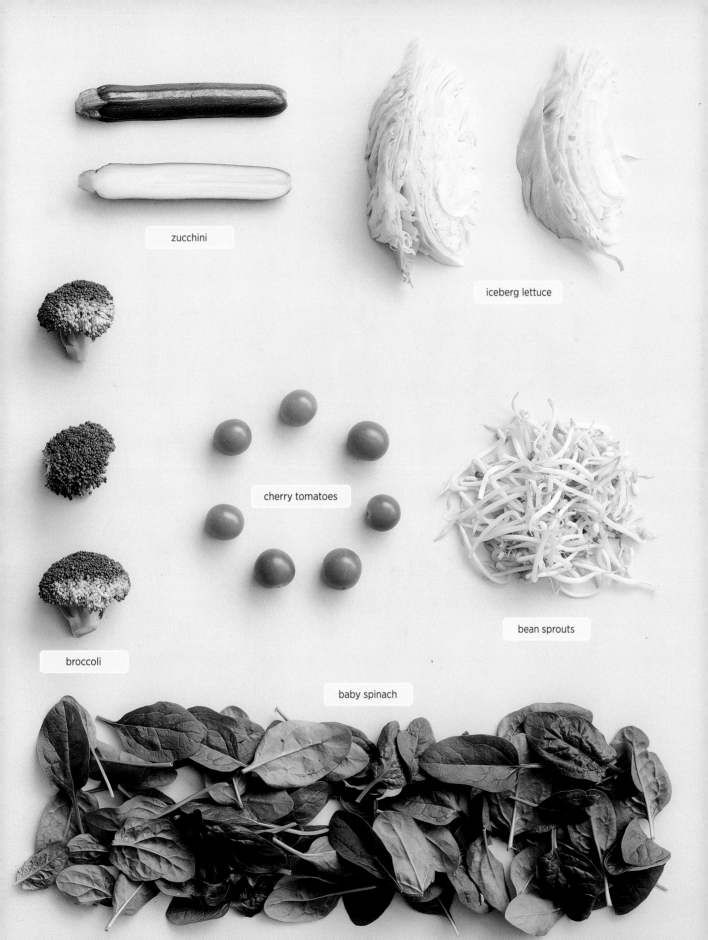

zucchini

iceberg lettuce

broccoli

cherry tomatoes

bean sprouts

baby spinach

WEEK 4

	Monday	Tuesday	Wednesday	Thursday	Friday	Saturday	Sunday
Breakfast	Nut and oat granola with orange zest (see page 123)	Overnight oats with sweet spiced nuts (see page 124)	Baked ricotta with pesto and avocado toast (see page 114)	Hummus and tomato toast with spiced nuts (see page 120)	Nut and oat granola with orange zest (see page 123)	Ricotta toast and sweet spiced nuts (see page 128)	Hummus and tomato toast with spiced nuts (see page 120)
Lunch	Nori omelette rolls with smoked salmon (see page 139)	Prawn cocktail salad with buttermilk and yoghurt dressing (see page 158)	Tuna 'pasta' salad with almond and tomato pesto (see page 164)	Thai chicken soup with greens (see page 171)	Spiced chicken broth with bok choy (see page 165)	Warm mushroom salad with poached eggs (see page 162)	Chicken salad with tzatziki (see page 146)
Dinner	Lemongrass and chilli beef with zucchini 'noodles' (see page 222)	Salmon with macadamia and watercress pesto (see page 191)	Orange and mustard roasted pork fillet (see page 219)	Herb fish skewers with cauliflower and almond puree (see page 188)	Chargrilled Cajun chicken and broccolini with salad (see page 203)	Chermoula prawns with cauliflower mash (see page 195)	Mini herb and chilli lamb roasts with roasted vegetables (see page 238)
Snacks	100 g low-fat Greek-style yoghurt 5 g Sweet spiced nut clusters (see page 259)	1 small carrot and celery sticks with 50 g raita (see page 264) 60 g hummus 20 g pecans	15 g raw almonds 50 g low-fat Greek-style yoghurt	100 g low-fat Greek-style yoghurt 1 wholegrain Ryvita with ½ a tomato, 25 g mozzarella and a sprinkle of dried or fresh basil 40 g raw unsalted almonds	150 g low-fat Greek-style yoghurt with a sprinkle of cinnamon 20 g raw unsalted almonds	150 g low-fat Greek-style yoghurt 40 g raw unsalted almonds	Zucchini and avocado 'fries' (see page 260)

SHOPPING LIST See page 81 for a list of pantry items

QUANTITY	ITEM
....	lemons
....	limes
....	oranges
....	avocado
....	asparagus
....	baby bok choy
....	bean sprouts
....	broccoli
....	broccolini
....	brussels sprouts
....	cabbage
....	carrots (including baby)
....	cauliflower
....	celery
....	green beans
....	kale
....	Lebanese cucumbers
....	leek
....	lettuce (iceberg, green oak, baby cos, lambs lettuce or frisee)
....	mushrooms (button, oyster, portobello)
....	onion
....	red chilli (small)
....	salad leaves (mesclun, rocket, baby rocket, baby spinach)
....	snow peas
....	tomatoes (including cherry tomatoes)
....	watercress
....	zucchini

QUANTITY	ITEM
....	basil
....	coriander
....	dill
....	mint
....	flat-leaf parsley
....	kaffir lime leaves
....	lemongrass
....	lemon thyme
....	rosemary
....	Thai basil leaves
....	thyme
....	chicken breast (fillets and tenderloins)
....	pork fillet
....	lamb rump
....	rump steaks
....	king prawns
....	firm white fish fillets (snapper, blue-eye trevalla or other)
....	salmon fillets
....	smoked salmon
....	hummus
....	mixed grain bread
....	semi-dried tomatoes
....	wholemeal pita bread

WEEK 5

	Monday	Tuesday	Wednesday	Thursday	Friday	Saturday	Sunday
Breakfast	Porridge with cinnamon nut crumble (see page 117)	Mushrooms with feta croutons (see page 131) 25 g pecans	Nut and oat granola with orange zest (see page 123)	Overnight oats with sweet spiced nuts (see page 124)	Vanilla and chia seed oat smoothie shots (see page 127) 10 g pecans	Mozzarella and pesto bruschetta (see page 119)	Avocado and ricotta smash toast (see page 128)
Lunch	Mushroom and spiced chicken 'burgers' (see page 140)	Cucumber and salmon 'sandwiches' (see page 136)	Easy chicken salad for one (see page 153)	Prawn no-rice paper rolls (see page 143)	Salmon and cauliflower 'tabbouleh' with crispbreads (see page 161)	Smoked chicken slaw with creamy avocado dressing (see page 153)	Green gazpacho with prawns and herbed ricotta toast (see page 167)
Dinner	Roasted salmon with vegetable parcels and pistou (see page 193)	Mushroom, tofu and miso 'noodle' stir-fry (see page 251)	Thai beef and 'fried rice' lettuce wraps (see page 234)	Moroccan tofu with grilled spiced-nut mushrooms (see page 252)	Turkey and lemon meatballs with 'spaghetti' Napolitana (see page 210)	Barbecued fillet steaks with stuffed mushrooms (see page 229)	Chicken tikka skewers with Indian summer salad (see page 209)
Snacks	1 wholegrain Ryvita or 2 wholegrain Vita-Weats topped with 20 g avocado and mint leaves 50 g raita (see page 264) with cherry tomatoes and cucumber sticks 25 g pecans	Coffee yoghurt with nut sprinkle (see page 268) 10 g Sweet spiced nut clusters (see page 259)	100 g low-fat Greek-style yoghurt 2 wholegrain Vita-Weats spread with 2 tablespoons avocado 30 g pecans	Indian-spiced kale chips with raita (see page 264) 1 wholegrain Ryvita topped with 2 slices of tomato and a sprinkle of pepper 25 g raw unsalted almonds	Zucchini and avocado 'fries' (see page 260)	100 g low-fat Greek-style yoghurt with a sprinkle of cinnamon ¼ baked wholemeal pita bread topped with 40 g homemade guacamole	Berry yoghurt jellies (see page 272) 20 g raw unsalted almonds

SHOPPING LIST See page 81 for a list of pantry items

QUANTITY	ITEM
....	lemons
....	limes
....	oranges
....	asparagus
....	avocado
....	baby bok choy
....	baby fennel bulb
....	bean sprouts
....	broccoli
....	broccolini
....	carrot
....	cauliflower
....	cucumber (Lebanese and telegraph)
....	curly kale
....	radicchio
....	green beans
....	green cabbage
....	green capsicum
....	lettuce (cos, iceberg)
....	salad leaves (rocket, baby rocket, baby spinach)
....	mushrooms (button, field, flat, portobello)
....	onion
....	red cabbage
....	red capsicum
....	spring onions
....	spinach
....	tomatoes (including cherry and mixed baby tomatoes)

QUANTITY	ITEM
....	zucchini
....	basil
....	chives
....	coriander
....	flat-leaf parsley
....	lemon thyme
....	mint
....	thyme
....	Vietnamese mint leaves
....	firm tofu
....	chicken breast fillets
....	smoked chicken breast fillets
....	lean minced turkey
....	lean minced beef
....	sirloin/New York steaks
....	king prawns
....	salmon (centre-cut)
....	hummus
....	mixed grain bread

WEEK 6

	Monday	Tuesday	Wednesday	Thursday	Friday	Saturday	Sunday
Breakfast	1 boiled egg*, smashed together with 40 g avocado and 20 g feta, served on a slice of mixed grain toast	Overnight oats with sweet spiced nuts (see page 124)	Porridge with cinnamon nut crumble (see page 117)	Overnight oats with sweet spiced nuts (see page 124)	Nut and oat granola with orange zest (see page 123)	Porridge with cinnamon nut crumble (see page 117)	Hummus and tomato toast with spiced nuts (see page 120)
Lunch	Roasted tomato, capsicum and fish soup (see page 168) ½ slice mixed grain wholemeal toast with 40 g cheddar cheese	Salmon and broccoli pesto wraps (see page 145)	Quick tuna salad for one (see page 153)	Chicken and asparagus salad (see page 154)	Prawn cocktail salad with buttermilk and yoghurt dressing (see page 158)	Tuna and bocconcini lettuce cups (see page 135)	Salmon and cauliflower 'tabbouleh' with crispbreads (see page 161)
Dinner	Crisp-skin blue-eye trevalla with steamed Asian greens (see page 175)	Hoisin-marinated tofu and eggplant with cashew satay sauce (see page 247)	Roasted salmon with vegetable parcels and pistou (see page 193)	Mu shu pork stir-fry with cauliflower 'rice' (see page 217)	Spiced salmon fillets with cauliflower 'couscous' (see page 183)	Spice-rubbed steaks with sautéed mushrooms (see page 225)	Roast chicken with Brussels sprouts, artichokes and olives (see page 214)
Snacks	1 stick celery filled with 2 tablespoons avocado, topped with fresh coriander	100 g low-fat Greek-style yoghurt 35 g Sweet spiced nut clusters (see page 259)	50 g raita (see page 264) with low-carb vegetable sticks (e.g. celery and cucumber) 40 g raw unsalted almonds	Greek-style crispbread (see page 256) 50 g low-fat Greek-style yoghurt 25 g pecans	Berry yoghurt jellies (see page 272) 30 g Sweet spiced nut clusters (see page 259)	50g low-fat Greek-style yoghurt 15 g Sweet spiced nut clusters (see page 259)	Indian-spiced kale chips with raita (see page 264) plus an extra 50 g raita (see page 264) with steamed asparagus spears 1 stick celery filled with 1 tablespoon avocado

*If you're having an egg for breakfast, reduce your lunch portion of lean meat, fish, etc by 50 g to reach your daily target of 2.5 units of lean meat, fish, poultry, eggs, tofu.

SHOPPING LIST See page 81 for a list of pantry items

QUANTITY	ITEM
....	lemons
....	limes
....	oranges
....	avocado
....	asparagus
....	baby fennel bulb
....	baby bok choy
....	bean sprouts
....	broccoli
....	broccolini
....	brussels sprouts
....	carrot
....	cauliflower
....	Chinese cabbage (wombok)
....	celery
....	choy sum
....	cucumber
....	curly kale
....	eggplant (slender Japanese)
....	green beans
....	iceberg lettuce
....	Lebanese cucumbers
....	mixed Asian baby salad greens (including tatsoi, mizuna, watercress, red oakleaf lettuce and coral lettuce)
....	mushrooms (mixed and fresh shiitake or oyster)
....	red capsicum
....	salad leaves (baby rocket, rocket, baby spinach)

QUANTITY	ITEM
....	snow peas
....	spinach
....	spring onion
....	tomatoes (including cherry and mixed baby tomatoes)
....	watercress
....	basil
....	coriander
....	flat-leaf parsley
....	firm tofu
....	chicken (tenderloins and thigh cutlets)
....	scotch fillet steaks
....	pork fillets
....	king or tiger prawns
....	salmon (fillets and centre-cut)
....	white fish fillets (including blue-eye trevalla and flathead, whiting or monkfish)
....	hummus
....	four-bean mix
....	mixed grain bread
....	mountain bread (or Herman Brot bread)

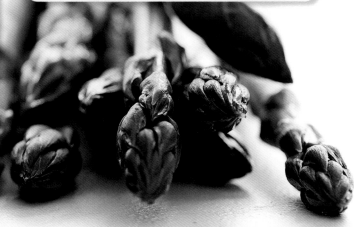

These vegetables and salad ingredients contain moderate amounts of carbohydrates (3–5 grams per serve) and can be enjoyed in moderation on this diet (150 g raw, 75 g cooked = 1 unit).

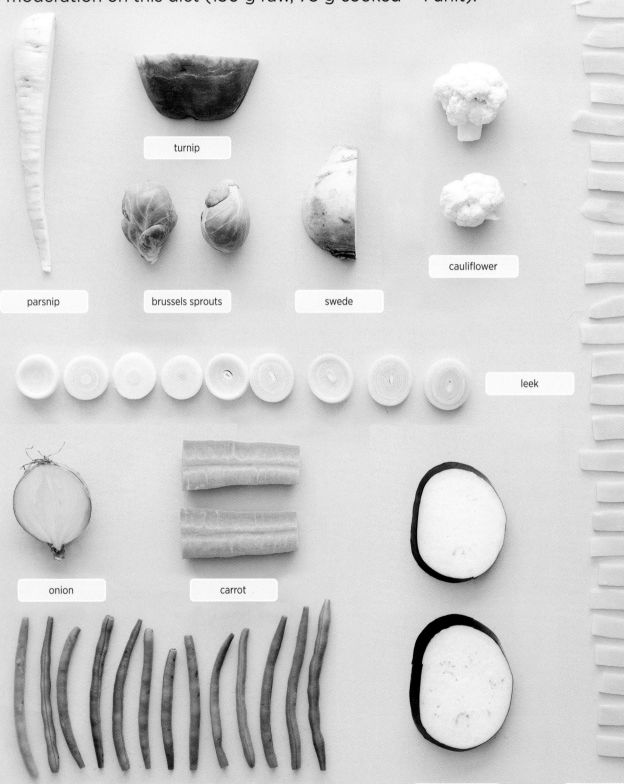

turnip

cauliflower

parsnip

brussels sprouts

swede

leek

onion

carrot

green beans

eggplant

bamboo shoots

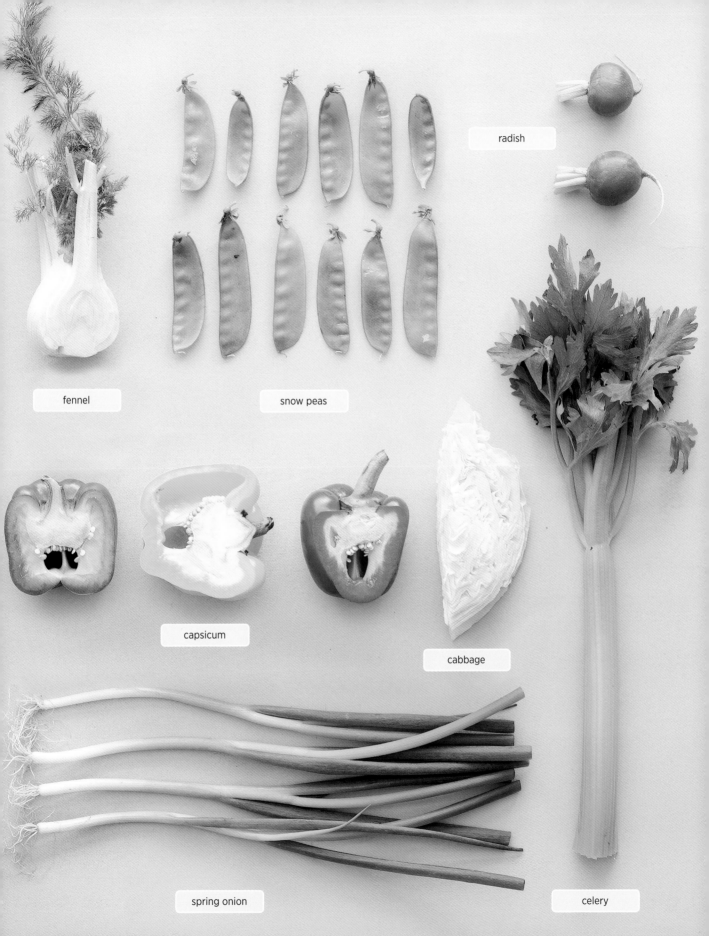

radish

fennel

snow peas

capsicum

cabbage

spring onion

celery

Carbohydrate extras from week 7

After 6 weeks on the diet, you might want to increase your intake of carbs slightly to give you more flexibility. The foods here all provide 5–10 grams of carbohydrates per serve, **so you can choose to add two of these per day to give an extra 20 grams of carbohydrates each day**. This will increase your daily energy intake by 500 kJ. The meal plans from Week 7 onwards include suggested options for carb extras.

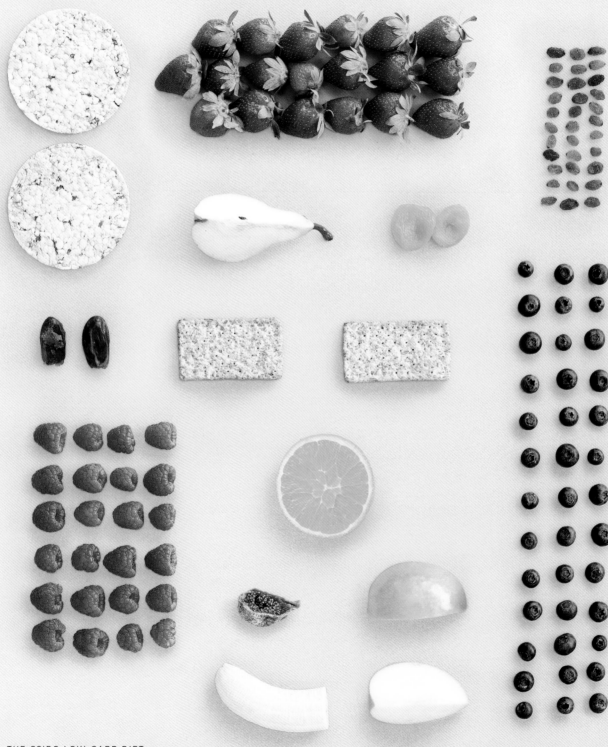

These foods are all on the core list in the Daily Food Guide (see pages 44–47), but here we're featuring them as extras, so you can easily increase your carb intake without having to work out how it affects the units (their unit serves in grams do differ). Remember, adding these extra carbs is optional, and you can do it on any level from Week 7 onwards.

Carbohydrate foods	Serving size
Mixed dried fruit	10 g
Dried figs	1 fig (20 g)
Fresh figs	2 figs
Dried apricots	20 g
Fresh apricots	2 medium
Sultanas	10 g
Dried dates	2 dates
Kiwifruit	2 small
Oranges	100 g
Cherries	60 g
Strawberries	200 g
Blueberries, frozen or fresh	60 g
Sultanas	10 g
Raspberries, frozen or fresh	100 g
Bananas	40 g
Apples	50 g
Pears	50 g
Vita-Weats, regular	2 biscuits (12 g)
Corn cakes/thins, multigrain	2 cakes (11 g)
Rice crackers (e.g. Sakata, Fantastic)	5 crackers (8 g)
Lentils, drained	80 g
Lentils, dried	15 g
Chickpeas, drained	40 g
Red kidney beans, drained	40 g
Four-bean mix, drained	40 g
Cannellini beans, drained	50 g
Mountain bread (wheat, rye and barley varieties)	½ regular rectangle
Fruit loaf	½ regular slice
Scone, wholemeal (commercial)	½ small scone (20 g)
Tortilla, corn	½ small
Wholegrain bread	½ regular slice
Low-fat yoghurt (Greek-style)	75 g
Reduced-fat evaporated milk (e.g. Carnation)	100 ml
Skim milk	100 ml
Green peas	120 g (¾ cup) (cooked weight)
Sweet potato	50 g (cooked weight)
Corn kernels	40 g or 2 tablespoons kernels (cooked weight), or ½ small ear (cooked)

Daily units

2.5 lean meat, fish, poultry, eggs, tofu | **1.5** breads, cereals, legumes, starchy vegetables | **3** dairy |
at least 5 mod–low-carb vegetables (**>3** low-carb vegetables) | **10** healthy fats

Carbohydrate 'extras' are shown in red from Week 7 onwards – these are optional.

WEEK 7

	Monday	Tuesday	Wednesday	Thursday	Friday	Saturday	Sunday
Breakfast	Porridge with cinnamon nut crumble (see page 117)	30 g All-Bran with 100 ml skim milk, topped with 50 g low-fat Greek-style yoghurt and 25 g pecans 60 g blueberries	Vanilla and chia seed oat smoothie shots (see page 127) 60 g blueberries	1 boiled egg*, smashed together with 20 g avocado and 20 g feta, served on a slice of mixed grain toast	Mozzarella and pesto bruschetta (see page 119)	Hummus and tomato toast with spiced nuts (see page 120)	Baked ricotta with pesto and avocado toast (see page 114) 50 g low-fat Greek-style yoghurt
Lunch	Nori omelette rolls with smoked salmon (see page 139)	Chicken and asparagus salad (see page 154) ¼ tortilla or pita bread	Polenta-crusted chicken and avocado salad (see page 150) 40 g corn kernels	Smoked chicken slaw with creamy avocado dressing (see page 153) ½ medium orange (100 g)	Tandoori chicken with grilled vegetable salad (see page 149) with raita (see page 264) ¼ cup cooked quinoa	Thai chicken soup with greens (see page 171) ½ slice mixed grain toast	Warm mushroom salad with poached eggs (see page 162)
Dinner	Moroccan tofu with grilled spiced-nut mushrooms (see page 252) 80 g cooked lentils	Lamb cutlets with chargrilled vegetables and mint pesto (see page 241)	Chermoula prawns with cauliflower mash (see page 195)	Sesame-crusted tofu with stir-fried Asian greens (see page 244) ¼ cup cooked quinoa	Ginger-soy beef skewers with zucchini 'noodle' salad (see page 233)	Fish tagine with watercress, coriander and radish salad (see page 179) 50 g cannellini beans	Baked fish with thyme and fennel-seed crust (see page 197) 50 g steamed sweet potato
Snacks	150 g low-fat Greek-style yoghurt with a sprinkle of cinnamon 200 g strawberries	Spinach, basil and almond dip (see page 267) 20 g pecans	Berry yoghurt jellies (see page 272) 1 tablespoon Sweet spiced nut clusters (see page 259) 35 g raw unsalted almonds	Grilled swiss cheese and tomato toast fingers (see page 259) 40 g pecans	100 g low-fat Greek-style yoghurt 30 g Sweet spiced nut clusters (see page 259) 2 fresh or baked figs with 1 tablespoon ricotta	100 g low-fat Greek-style yoghurt Caprese crispbread (see page 256) 40 g raw unsalted almonds	Coffee yoghurt with nut sprinkle (see page 268) ½ medium apple (50 g)

*If you're having an egg for breakfast, reduce your lunch portion of lean meat, fish, etc by 50 g to reach your daily target of 2.5 units of lean meat, fish, poultry, eggs, tofu.

SHOPPING LIST See page 81 for a list of pantry items

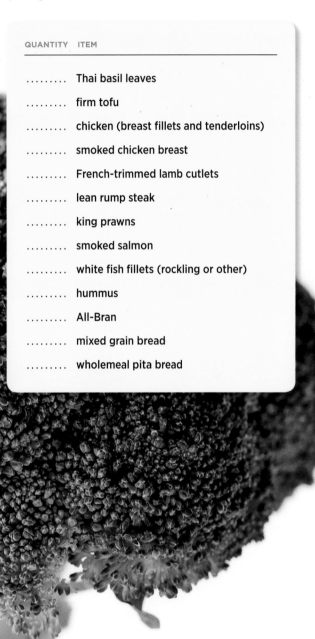

QUANTITY	ITEM
....	apples
....	blueberries
....	figs (baked or fresh)
....	strawberries
....	oranges
....	baby bok choy
....	baby radishes
....	bean sprouts
....	broccoli
....	broccolini
....	brussels sprouts
....	carrot (including baby)
....	corn
....	cos lettuce
....	eggplant
....	kale
....	leek
....	salad leaves (mesclun, rocket, spinach)
....	mushrooms (field, oyster, fresh shiitake, button, portobello)
....	red cabbage
....	red capsicum
....	snow peas
....	tomato
....	zucchini
....	basil
....	coriander
....	dill
....	kaffir lime leaves

QUANTITY	ITEM
....	Thai basil leaves
....	firm tofu
....	chicken (breast fillets and tenderloins)
....	smoked chicken breast
....	French-trimmed lamb cutlets
....	lean rump steak
....	king prawns
....	smoked salmon
....	white fish fillets (rockling or other)
....	hummus
....	All-Bran
....	mixed grain bread
....	wholemeal pita bread

WEEK 8

	Monday	Tuesday	Wednesday	Thursday	Friday	Saturday	Sunday
Breakfast	Mozzarella and pesto bruschetta (see page 119)	Overnight oats with sweet spiced nuts (see page 124) 60 g blueberries	Vanilla and chia seed oat smoothie shots (see page 127) 200 g strawberries	1 boiled egg*, smashed together with 30 g avocado and 20 g feta, served on a slice of mixed grain toast	Porridge with cinnamon nut crumble (see page 117)	Nut and oat granola with orange zest (see page 123)	Avocado and ricotta smash toast (see page 128)
Lunch	Greek salad with fennel and prawns (see page 157)	Cucumber and salmon 'sandwiches' (see page 136)	Prawn no-rice paper rolls (see page 143)	Tuna 'pasta' salad with almond and tomato pesto (see page 164)	Smoked chicken slaw with creamy avocado dressing (see page 153)	Salmon and broccoli pesto wraps (see page 145)	Chicken salad with tzatziki (see page 146)
Dinner	Hummus-crusted chicken with roasted cauliflower and haloumi salad (see page 206) 120 g steamed butternut pumpkin	Mediterranean vegetable and fish bake (see page 194)	Turkey larb with 'noodle' salad (see page 204) 120 g steamed green peas	Crisp-skin salmon with herb and cashew 'butter' (see page 184) 50 g cannellini beans	Biryani-style lamb with spinach and mint salad (see page 237) 80 g cooked lentils	Hoisin-marinated tofu and eggplant with cashew satay sauce (see page 247) 100 g baby corn spears	Lemon oregano roast chicken with rocket and tahini salad (see page 205)
Snacks	50 g raita (see page 264) with low-carb vegetable sticks (e.g. cucumber, celery) ½ small banana (40 g)	50 g low-fat Greek-style yoghurt 20 g Sweet spiced nut clusters (see page 259) 2 fresh figs	Spinach, basil and almond dip (see page 267) with low-carb vegetable sticks (e.g. cucumber, celery) 45 g Sweet spiced nut clusters (see page 259)	Coffee yoghurt with nut sprinkle (see page 268) 1 extra teaspoon of pecans 2 kiwifruit	Spiced baked ricotta with almonds (see page 263) 60 g blueberries 10 g pecans	100 g low-fat Greek-style yoghurt 25 g Sweet spiced nut clusters (see page 259) 60 g blueberries	Berry yoghurt jellies (see page 272) 5 plain rice crackers with 2 teaspoons hummus

*If you're having an egg for breakfast, reduce your lunch portion of lean meat, fish, etc by 50 g to reach your daily target of 2.5 units of lean meat, fish, poultry, eggs, tofu.

SHOPPING LIST See page 81 for a list of pantry items

QUANTITY	ITEM
....	bananas
....	blueberries
....	fresh figs
....	kiwifruit
....	oranges
....	strawberries
....	asparagus
....	avocado
....	baby bok choy
....	baby corn spears
....	baby fennel bulb
....	baby radishes
....	bean sprouts
....	broccoli
....	broccolini
....	butternut pumpkin
....	carrot
....	cauliflower
....	celery
....	chilli (long red)
....	Chinese cabbage (wombok)
....	cos lettuce
....	cucumber (including telegraph and Lebanese)
....	eggplant (including slender Japanese)
....	green cabbage
....	green peas
....	kale
....	mushrooms (button, flat)
....	mixed Asian baby salad greens (including tatsoi, mizuna, watercress, red oakleaf lettuce and coral lettuce)
....	onion

QUANTITY	ITEM
....	red cabbage
....	red capsicum
....	salad leaves (baby spinach, rocket, baby rocket, frisee, mesclun)
....	spring onion
....	tomatoes (including mixed cherry and baby roma tomatoes)
....	watercress
....	zucchini
....	basil
....	coriander
....	kaffir lime leaves
....	flat-leaf parsley
....	lemongrass
....	mint
....	oregano
....	thyme
....	Vietnamese mint leaves
....	firm tofu
....	chicken breast (fillets and tenderloins)
....	smoked chicken breast fillets
....	lamb leg steaks or backstraps
....	lean minced turkey
....	white fish fillets (blue-eye trevalla or other)
....	king prawns
....	salmon fillets
....	haloumi
....	hummus
....	mixed grain bread
....	mountain bread (or Herman Brot bread)
....	semi-dried tomatoes
....	wholemeal pita bread

WEEK 9

	Monday	Tuesday	Wednesday	Thursday	Friday	Saturday	Sunday
Breakfast	Nut and oat granola with orange zest (see page 123) 100 g raspberries	Overnight oats with sweet spiced nuts (see page 124) 60 g blueberries	Nut and oat granola with orange zest (see page 123) 60 g blueberries	Hummus and tomato toast with spiced nuts (see page 120)	Vanilla and chia seed oat smoothie shots (see page 127) 60 g blueberries	1 boiled egg*, smashed together with 20 g avocado and 20 g feta, served on a slice of mixed grain toast 25 g pecans 2 kiwifruit	Baked ricotta with pesto and avocado toast (see page 114) 15 g pecans
Lunch	Spiced chicken broth with bok choy (see page 165) ½ slice mixed grain bread, toasted	Quick tuna salad for one (page 153) with 20 g avocado 60 g four bean mix	Prawn no-rice paper rolls (see page 143)	Polenta-crusted chicken and avocado salad (see page 150)	Mushroom and spiced chicken 'burgers' (see page 140) 100 g mixed berries	Thai chicken soup with greens (see page 171)	Salmon and cauliflower 'tabbouleh' with crispbreads (see page 161) 80 g cooked lentils
Dinner	Chargrilled Cajun chicken and broccolini with salad (see page 203)	Thai beef and 'fried rice' lettuce wraps (see page 234)	Asian-glazed salmon with stir-fried greens (see page 187) 50 g steamed broad beans	Baked snapper with gremolata and roasted vegetables (see page 180) 50 g steamed sweet potato	Roasted salmon with vegetable parcels and pistou (see page 193)	Veal and mushroom involtini with crunchy Italian salad (see page 230) ¼ cup cooked quinoa	Tofu and turmeric 'scramble' with steamed greens (see page 253) 50 g steamed sweet potato
Snacks	150 g low-fat Greek-style yoghurt with a sprinkle of cinnamon 20 g raw unsalted almonds	Grilled Swiss cheese and tomato toast fingers (see page 259) 40 g pecans	Zucchini and avocado 'fries' (see page 260) 1 wholegrain Ryvita topped with 1 tablespoon avocado and 2 slices tomato	Coffee yoghurt with nut sprinkle (see page 268) 200 g strawberries	Spinach, basil and almond dip (see page 267) with low-carb vegetable sticks (e.g. celery, cucumber) 35 g pecans	20 g Sweet spiced nut clusters (see page 259) Indian-spiced kale chips with raita (see page 264) 1 wholegrain Ryvita with 20 g cheddar cheese and 2 slices tomato	Zucchini and avocado 'fries' (see page 260)

*If you're having an egg for breakfast, reduce your lunch portion of lean meat, fish, etc by 50 g to reach your daily target of 2.5 units of lean meat, fish, poultry, eggs, tofu.

SHOPPING LIST See page 81 for a list of pantry items

QUANTITY	ITEM
....	blueberries
....	kiwifruit
....	lemons
....	limes
....	mixed berries
....	oranges
....	raspberries
....	strawberries
....	asparagus
....	avocado
....	baby bok choy
....	baby fennel bulb
....	baby radishes
....	bean sprouts
....	broad beans
....	broccoli
....	broccolini
....	cauliflower
....	celery
....	chilli (small red)
....	choy sum
....	cucumber
....	green beans
....	kale (including curly)
....	Lebanese cucumber
....	lettuce (cos, baby cos, green oak)
....	mushrooms (button, oyster, portobello)
....	onion (including red)
....	salad leaves (rocket, baby rocket, baby spinach)

QUANTITY	ITEM
....	radicchio
....	witlof
....	red capsicum
....	snow peas
....	spring onion
....	spinach
....	sweet potato
....	tomato (including cherry and mixed baby tomatoes)
....	watercress
....	zucchini
....	basil
....	coriander
....	flat-leaf parsley
....	lemongrass
....	kaffir lime leaves
....	mint
....	Thai basil
....	thyme
....	Vietnamese mint
....	firm tofu
....	silken tofu
....	chicken breast (fillets and tenderloins)
....	lean minced beef
....	veal steaks
....	king prawns
....	pink snapper or barramundi fillets
....	salmon (fillets and centre-cut)
....	hummus
....	mixed grain bread

Herbs

Using herbs in your cooking is an excellent way to add flavour and interest. Some herbs naturally partner with some foods – such as basil and tomatoes, parsley and fish, and lamb and rosemary – but in general you can't go wrong by adding a handful of fresh herbs or a pinch of dried herbs to liven up a dish.

Fresh herbs can be expensive, and knowing how to store them properly will help you get the most out of them. Keep parsley and coriander in a glass filled with 1–2 cms of water. Cover the leaves with a plastic bag and store in the fridge. Some herbs (thyme, mint, chives, sage, oregano and dill) like to be kept damp and cool. Wrap the ends in damp paper towel, then store in a sealed plastic bag or container in the fridge. Basil, however, needs to kept dry or the leaves will bruise and wilt, so wrap the ends in dry paper towel, then store in a sealed plastic bag or container in the fridge.

Dried herbs are a convenient alternative to fresh, and so stock up your pantry and you'll always have some flavour on hand.

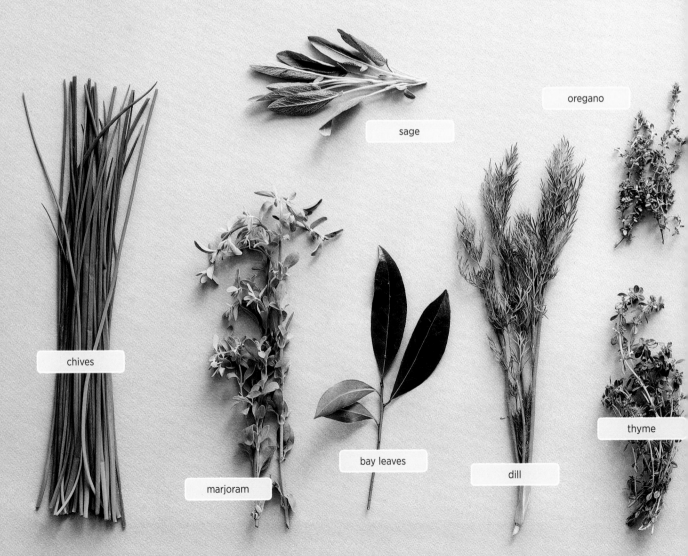

sage

oregano

chives

marjoram

bay leaves

dill

thyme

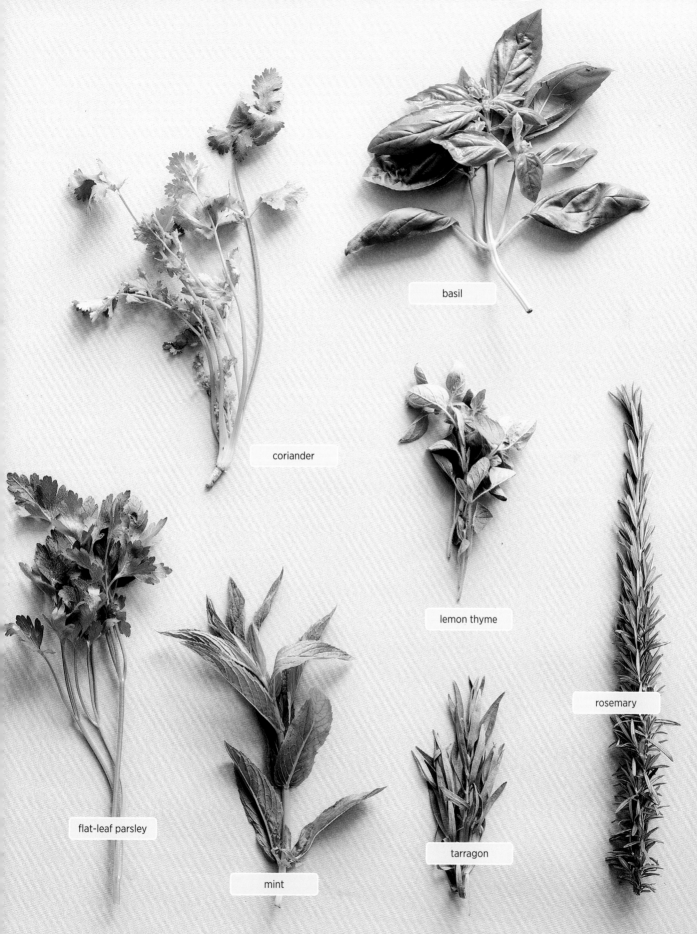

basil

coriander

lemon thyme

rosemary

flat-leaf parsley

mint

tarragon

WEEK 10

	Monday	Tuesday	Wednesday	Thursday	Friday	Saturday	Sunday
Breakfast	Overnight oats with sweet spiced nuts (see page 124) 60 g blueberries	Nut and oat granola with orange zest (see page 123) 60 g blueberries	Vanilla and chia seed oat smoothie shots (see page 127) 60 g blueberries	Nut and oat granola with orange zest (see page 123) 100 g raspberries	Vanilla and chia seed oat smoothie shots (see page 127)	Hummus and tomato toast with spiced nuts (see page 120)	Avocado and ricotta smash toast (see page 128)
Lunch	Prawn no-rice paper rolls (see page 143)	Green gazpacho with prawns and herbed ricotta toast (see page 167)	Polenta-crusted chicken and avocado salad (see page 150) 60 g chickpeas	Chicken and asparagus salad (see page 154) ¼ cup cooked quinoa	Tuna and bocconcini lettuce cups (see page 135)	Greek salad with fennel and prawns (see page 157)	Roasted tomato, capsicum and fish soup (see page 168) Grilled swiss cheese and tomato toast fingers (see page 259)
Dinner	Crisp-skin blue-eye trevalla with steamed Asian greens (see page 175)	Spice-rubbed steaks with sautéed mushrooms (see page 225) ¼ cup cooked quinoa	Sesame-crusted tofu with stir-fried Asian greens (see page 244)	Mu shu pork stir-fry with cauliflower 'rice' (see page 217)	Ginger-soy beef skewers with zucchini 'noodle' salad (see page 233) 50 g cannellini beans	Herb fish skewers with cauliflower and almond puree (see page 188) 50 g cannellini beans	Chicken tikka skewers with Indian summer salad (see page 209) 50 g chickpeas
Snacks	Caprese crispbread (see page 256) 25 g pecans 200 g strawberries	Indian-spiced kale chips with raita (see page 264)	Baked orange blossom custards (see page 271) 20 g Sweet spiced nut clusters (see page 259)	Greek-style crispbread (see page 256) 25 g avocado mixed with 10 g feta, spread onto celery sticks	Zucchini and avocado 'fries' (see page 260) 2 pitted dates	100 g low-fat Greek-style yoghurt 2 teaspoons mixed seeds 100 g raspberries	Caprese crispbread (see page 256) 30 g pecans 10 g dried cranberries

SHOPPING LIST
See page 81 for a list of pantry items

QUANTITY	ITEM
....	blueberries
....	cranberries
....	lemons
....	limes
....	oranges
....	dates
....	raspberries
....	strawberries
....	asparagus
....	avocado
....	baby bok choy
....	baby fennel bulb
....	bean sprouts
....	broccolini
....	cabbage (red, green)
....	carrot
....	cauliflower
....	celery
....	chilli (small red)
....	choy sum
....	cucumber (Lebanese, telegraph)
....	curly kale
....	eggplant (slender)
....	green capsicum
....	lettuce (cos, baby cos, iceberg)
....	mushrooms (mixed, flat, fresh shiitake, oyster)
....	onion
....	red capsicum

QUANTITY	ITEM
....	salad leaves (baby spinach, rocket, mixed)
....	snow peas
....	spring onion
....	tomatoes (including cherry)
....	watercress
....	zucchini
....	basil
....	chives
....	coriander
....	flat-leaf parsley
....	lemon thyme
....	mint
....	oregano
....	Vietnamese mint leaves
....	firm tofu
....	chicken breast (fillets and tenderloins)
....	pork fillets
....	lean rump steaks
....	scotch fillet steaks
....	firm white fish fillets (snapper, blue-eye trevalla or other)
....	white fish fillets (flathead, whiting or monkfish)
....	king prawns
....	four-bean mix
....	hummus
....	mixed grain bread
....	wholemeal pita bread

WEEK 11

	Monday	Tuesday	Wednesday	Thursday	Friday	Saturday	Sunday
Breakfast	Mozzarella and pesto bruschetta (see page 119) 10 g pecans	Nut and oat granola with orange zest (see page 123) 10 g dried cranberries	Avocado and ricotta smash toast (see page 128)	1 boiled egg*, smashed together with 20 g avocado and 20 g feta, served on a slice of mixed grain toast	Baked ricotta with pesto and avocado toast (see page 114)	Mushrooms with feta croutons (see page 131) 25 g pecans	Ricotta toast and sweet spiced nuts (see page 128)
Lunch	Spiced chicken broth with bok choy (see page 165)	Prawn cocktail salad with buttermilk and yoghurt dressing (see page 158)	Warm mushroom salad with poached eggs (see page 162)	Mushroom and spiced chicken 'burgers' (see page 140)	Tuna 'pasta' salad with almond and tomato pesto (see page 164)	Cucumber and salmon 'sandwiches' (see page 136)	Warm mushroom salad with poached eggs (see page 162) 40 g kidney beans
Dinner	Turkey and lemon meatballs with 'spaghetti' Napolitana (see page 210) 40 g corn kernels	Thai fish cakes with broccoli salad (see page 176) ¼ cup cooked rice	Lemongrass and chilli beef with zucchini 'noodles' (see page 222) ½ cup baby corn	Portuguese chicken with cucumber and fennel salad (see page 213) 50 g steamed sweet potato	Orange and mustard roasted pork fillet (see page 219) ¼ cup cooked quinoa	Mushroom, tofu and miso 'noodle' stir-fry (see page 251) 120 g steamed green peas	Aromatic steamed fish with vegetable stir-fry (see page 198)
Snacks	Zucchini and avocado 'fries' (see page 260) ½ medium orange (100 g)	Indian-spiced kale chips with raita (see page 264) 20 g pecans	100 g low-fat Greek-style yoghurt 20 g almonds 60 g blueberries	Spinach, basil and almond dip (see page 267) 30 g pecans 2 fresh apricots	50 g low-fat Greek-style yoghurt 15 g pecans 100 g raspberries	Coffee yoghurt with nut sprinkle (see page 268) plus an extra 10 g Sweet spiced nut clusters (see page 259) 60 g blueberries	150 g low-fat Greek-style yoghurt 35 g raw unsalted almonds 2 fresh figs

*If you're having an egg for breakfast, reduce your lunch portion of lean meat, fish, etc by 50 g to reach your daily target of 2.5 units of lean meat, fish, poultry, eggs, tofu.

SHOPPING LIST See page 81 for a list of pantry items

QUANTITY	ITEM
....	blueberries
....	cranberries
....	lemons
....	limes
....	oranges
....	dates
....	raspberries
....	strawberries
....	asparagus
....	avocado
....	baby bok choy
....	baby fennel bulb
....	bean sprouts
....	broccolini
....	cabbage (red, green)
....	carrot
....	cauliflower
....	celery
....	chilli (small red)
....	choy sum
....	cucumber (Lebanese, telegraph)
....	curly kale
....	eggplant (slender)
....	green capsicum
....	lettuce (cos, baby cos, iceberg)
....	mushrooms (mixed, flat, fresh shiitake, oyster)
....	onion
....	red capsicum

QUANTITY	ITEM
....	salad leaves (baby spinach, rocket, mixed)
....	snow peas
....	spring onion
....	tomatoes (including cherry)
....	watercress
....	zucchini
....	basil
....	chives
....	coriander
....	flat-leaf parsley
....	lemon thyme
....	mint
....	oregano
....	Vietnamese mint leaves
....	firm tofu
....	chicken breast (fillets and tenderloins)
....	pork fillets
....	lean rump steaks
....	scotch fillet steaks
....	firm white fish fillets (snapper, blue-eye trevalla or other)
....	white fish fillets (flathead, whiting or monkfish)
....	king prawns
....	four-bean mix
....	hummus
....	mixed grain bread
....	wholemeal pita bread

WEEK 12

	Monday	Tuesday	Wednesday	Thursday	Friday	Saturday	Sunday
Breakfast	Porridge with cinnamon nut crumble (see page 117) 200 g strawberries	Mushrooms with feta croutons (see page 131)	Vanilla and chia seed oat smoothie shots (see page 127) 10 g mixed seeds 100 g raspberries	Overnight oats with sweet spiced nuts (see page 124) 60 g blueberries	Vanilla and chia seed oat smoothie shots (see page 127) 50 g grated apple and a sprinkle of cinnamon	Hummus and tomato toast with spiced nuts (see page 120)	Overnight oats with sweet spiced nuts (see page 124)
Lunch	Chicken and asparagus salad (see page 154)	Tandoori chicken with grilled vegetable salad (see page 149)	Prawn no-rice paper rolls (see page 143)	Smoked chicken slaw with creamy avocado dressing (see page 153)	Roasted tomato, capsicum and fish soup (see page 168) ½ slice mixed grain wholemeal toast with 20 g cheddar cheese	Salmon and cauliflower 'tabbouleh' with crispbreads (see page 161)	Nori omelette rolls with smoked salmon (see page 139) ½ medium orange (100 g)
Dinner	Salmon with macadamia and watercress pesto (see page 191) 120 g steamed green peas	Madras beef curry with cauliflower and broccoli 'rice' (see page 226)	Vegetable fried 'rice' with tofu and egg (see page 248) 40 g chickpeas	Spiced salmon fillets with cauliflower 'couscous' (see page 183)	Fish tagine with watercress, coriander and radish salad (see page 179)	Mini herb and chilli lamb roasts with roasted vegetables (see page 238) 50 g steamed sweet potato	Turkey larb with 'noodle' salad (see page 204)
Snacks	Caprese crispbread (see page 256) 25 g pecans	Coffee yoghurt with nut sprinkle (see page 268) 20 g pecans 1 small banana (80g)	Greek-style crispbread (see page 256) 40 g raw unsalted almonds	Grilled Swiss cheese and tomato toast fingers (see page 259) 40 g almonds 2 kiwifruit	Berry yoghurt jellies (see page 272) 25 g pecans 60 g blueberries	Baked orange blossom custards (see page 271) 100 g watermelon 50 g tzatziki with low-carb vegetable sticks (e.g. cucumber and celery) 10 g pecans	Zucchini and avocado 'fries' (see page 260) 20 g pecans 2 fresh figs

SHOPPING LIST See page 81 for a list of pantry items

QUANTITY	ITEM
....	banana
....	blueberries
....	fresh figs
....	kiwifruit
....	lemons
....	limes
....	oranges
....	strawberries
....	watermelon
....	asparagus
....	avocado
....	baby bok choy
....	baby fennel bulb
....	bean sprouts
....	broccoli
....	broccolini
....	brussels sprouts
....	cabbage (including red and green)
....	carrots (including baby carrots)
....	cauliflower
....	celery
....	chilli (small red, long red)
....	cucumber
....	green beans
....	green peas
....	kale
....	Lebanese cucumbers
....	lettuce (cos, lamb's lettuce or frisee)
....	mushrooms (portobello, button)
....	onion (including red)
....	radishes

QUANTITY	ITEM
....	red capsicum
....	salad leaves (baby spinach, baby rocket, rocket, mixed salad leaves)
....	sweet potato
....	tomatoes (including cherry or grape)
....	watercress
....	zucchini
....	basil
....	coriander (leaves, roots and stems)
....	dill
....	flat-leaf parsley
....	kaffir lime leaves
....	lemon thyme
....	lemongrass
....	mint
....	Thai basil leaves
....	thyme
....	Vietnamese mint
....	firm tofu
....	chicken (breast fillets and tenderloins)
....	lean minced turkey
....	beef rump steak
....	lamb rump
....	king prawns
....	salmon fillets
....	smoked salmon
....	firm white fish fillets (snapper, blue-eye trevalla or other)
....	white fish fillets (flathead, whiting or monkfish)
....	mixed grain bread
....	hummus
....	wholemeal pita bread

PUTTING IT INTO PRACTICE AT HOME

Change needn't be daunting. You'll find you can do it if you formulate a plan, break it down into small and achievable steps, and start by looking at what you already do well. No one diet fits all, but our research has helped us identify a low-carbohydrate eating plan that's flexible enough to benefit many people, including those with type 2 diabetes.

Being focused is crucial for success, no matter what your target. If your environment and mind aren't prepared, you'll find it harder to stay on track. These four steps could help you get started:

1. Prepare yourself

To set yourself up for success you must be willing to make lifestyle changes. If you can't get over it seeming like a chore, you'll never get there. How ready are you to change? If it feels like you're stalling in your decision, it can help to seek guidance from professionals. Having a network of supporters, such as family and friends, who give you confidence in managing your health is another huge first step. Let your friends and family know you're starting a program of exercise and carefully considered meal plans, and ask them to help you stick to it.

2. Prepare your pantry

Have a look in your pantry, freezer and fridge. If they're crammed full of foods that aren't part of the Low-carb Diet, give them away. Make room at eye level for the foods you need each day. This will help you avoid the temptation to eat foods that aren't a core part of the program.

3. Prepare your kitchen

To make the meals in this book, you'll often need to have the right equipment handy. Have a look at the recipes, then go through your kitchen and decide which utensils you'll be most likely to use to prepare them. These might include spoon and cup measures, scales, grater, wok, spiraliser, colander and saucepans. Make sure you can get to them easily.

4. Spice it up

Sticking to a few core foods might seem boring and bland at first, so get creative and make sure you have some herbs and spices handy. Try the spice rubs, herb crusts and dukkahs in the recipe section, or make a list of your favourite combinations and try them. If you make the rubs up in advance, they're great when you're in a rush and don't have time to cook a full recipe. Simply rub into your meat then pan-fry lightly in a little of your oil allowance. Throw in your vegies and you're set.

Understanding your hunger and appetite

It's easy to confuse hunger with appetite, but hunger is the physiological need for food, while appetite is the psychological desire to eat. The body regulates hunger, signalling the need to eat with growling in the stomach or lower blood glucose levels, and it's usually relieved by eating a small amount of food. Appetite, however, is a conditioned response to food that can make you eat until you feel completely stuffed. Is there a particular food you feel you just can't resist, no matter how full you are? That desire is appetite.

Hunger can be the worst side effect of dieting,

and with many eating plans is one of the main reasons people feel crankier and eventually give up. One of the best things about a low-carbohydrate diet is that it reduces feelings of hunger and/or the desire to eat and increases feelings of fullness in comparison with a high-carbohydrate diet.

Studies have demonstrated that both pure protein and fat provide a greater feeling of fullness and reduce feelings of hunger more than a similar kilojoule load of carbohydrates. They not only make us eat less in that particular meal, but also consume fewer kilojoules in our next meal. This is because they slow down the process by which food leaves the stomach. As we've seen, the energy it takes to digest, absorb and store protein in the body – the thermic effect of food (see page 28) – is higher than that for either carbohydrate or fat, which means a higher-protein diet may burn slightly more energy.

Your appetite toolkit

Use these tips to manage your appetite and hunger:

1. Be aware of what you're eating
Use a food diary (on paper or in an app) to track your hunger and fullness levels. It will help you identify if your appetite is a response to boredom or if you're actually physiologically hungry.

2. Prepare daily snacks and meals in advance
Keep your pantry stocked with a variety of healthy snacks; stock the freezer with a few ready-made meals that fit the plan as an emergency meal; and when shopping, make sure you're not hungry, use a shopping list, don't buy in bulk and only buy food that's part of your eating plan.

3. Keep moving and stay hydrated
One way to distract yourself from responding to your appetite is to do some exercise, even if only for 10 minutes. And don't forget to drink some water when you start to feel your stomach growling.

4. Eat until you feel comfortably full, not stuffed
If you're really craving a particular food, first eat your planned meal, then allow yourself a small portion of that food – but don't do this every day.

Keeping your pantry well-stocked with these items means you will always have what you need to create delicious homecooked meals.

wholegrain crispbreads
(Ryvita, Vita-Weats)
plain rice crackers
polenta
rice
quinoa
raw (natural) rolled oats
salt-reduced tomato paste
salt-reduced tomato passata
tinned tuna in springwater
tinned salmon
reduced-salt stock
light coconut-flavoured
evaporated milk
tinned lentils
tinned beans
almonds (raw, flaked)
walnuts
pecans
macadamias
sesame seeds
sunflower seed kernels
raw unsalted cashew butter
tahini

olives
marinated artichoke hearts
natural vanilla bean paste
stevia granules
unsweetened cocoa powder

SAUCES & CONDIMENTS
olive oil spray
extra virgin olive oil
sesame oil
wholegrain mustard
Dijon mustard
dry white wine
Shaoxing rice wine or
dry sherry
red wine vinegar
white wine vinegar
white balsamic vinegar
salt-reduced soy sauce
Worcestershire sauce
oyster sauce
fish sauce
hoisin sauce
Tabasco sauce (optional)

HERBS & SPICES
Moroccan seasoning
mixed spice
ground cinnamon
ground cumin
ground coriander
ground turmeric
ground cloves
ground cardamom
ground allspice
fennel seeds
sumac
garam masala
hot paprika
sweet smoked paprika
black pepper
bay leaves
chilli powder
dried chilli flakes
dried oregano
dried thyme
nutmeg
fresh or dried curry leaves

FRIDGE
garlic
ginger
eggs
buttermilk
skim milk
low-fat Greek-style yoghurt
mozzarella
low-fat fresh ricotta
low-fat cottage cheese
low-fat cheddar
salt-reduced low-fat feta
Swiss cheese
grated parmesan
low-fat cream cheese

Eating out low-carb style

It used to be said that being on a diet meant eating plain, boring meals and staying at home to avoid temptation. This is no longer the case. It's far easier these days to walk into a restaurant and specify what you'd like. Try these simple strategies, be confident and stay strong.

Make good choices

- When eating out, build your meal around the low-carbohydrate plan. Go for vegetables and lean protein foods – lean red meat, poultry or fish – and avoid carbohydrate-rich foods such as bread, pasta, rice, noodles and chips.
- Ask for a serve of salad or tasty seasonal vegetables instead of chips or potato.
- Choose grilled, steamed, poached or baked options rather than fried or deep-fried foods.
- Look for meals that use herbs and spices to create flavour, rather than those that rely on carbohydrates and sugary or creamy dressings or sauces.
- Ask for sauces and dressings on the side so you can limit the amount you add to your meal.
- Share a range of dishes – order steamed or stir-fried vegetables, salads and grilled meats.
- Don't be afraid to ask for changes to meals, but be specific – good chefs can cater for any meal plan.
- Use the table below for good and bad options in different cuisines.

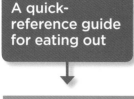

A quick-reference guide for eating out

Cuisine	Try	Avoid
Greek	Grilled fish and meat Fresh salads and simply cooked vegetables Tzatziki	Saganaki Spanakopita Moussaka Baklava
Italian	Ratatouille Salads with a little olive oil and lemon juice Vegetable-based dishes with meat on the side Zucchini-ribbon 'pasta' (if available) with napolitana sauce	Pasta Pizza Bread
Japanese	Sashimi Salads with vegetables	Noodles Rice
Spanish and Mexican	Grilled meat with salsa Salad dressed in olive oil and lemon Tomato and beef-based chilli con carne Guacamole	Corn-based breads (tortillas, tacos, corn chips) Too many beans
Vietnamese and Thai	Grilled and dry-fried protein foods such as chicken and beef Fresh seafood Fresh salad ingredients flavoured with herbs, chilli and citrus Cold rolls – roll your own and ask for extra lettuce instead of rice paper Grilled and steamed greens flavoured with ginger or garlic Stir-fried lean meat and seasonal vegetables with minimal sauce	High-sugar dressings Vermicelli noodles Rice and rice paper Coconut milk sauces
Sandwich and salad bar	Salads of low-carb vegetables Lettuce as a wrap	Breads beyond your daily allowance
Modern Australian and pub-style meals	Grilled or baked lean steak or chicken breast Salads and roast vegetables	Chips and mashed potato Deep-fried foods Bread rolls

Special occasions

Religious or seasonal festivals that involve food, such as Christmas, Passover or the end of Ramadan, can be some of the hardest occasions when you're trying to stick to a new eating plan, as can parties. This is the case whether you're at home or out. Try these tips to stay on track.

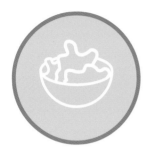

Organise what to take

Ask what they're having, and if it's not something you can eat, offer to take a dish. Use the list of allowed foods and recipes from this book to prepare a dish or two to share. You could:

- Take a garden salad, roasted greens, cold meat such as turkey, fresh seafood including prawns and oysters.
- Contribute to the barbecue with lean beef steaks, lamb fillet or fish wrapped in foil.
- Try taking a frittata slice and salad.
- Take a plate of vegetables from the 'low-carb' list (see pages 62–63) and a salsa for snacks.

Plan well when you're the host

- Be organised. Decide in advance the dishes you'll prepare, and choose some that can be made ahead of time to reduce stress on the day.
- Make time for exercise. Plan a walk for after a big Christmas lunch. You might even get some people to join you.
- Watch your portions. Take a small amount of each dish and aim to take up two-thirds of the plate with low-carbohydrate vegetables and the remaining third with lean protein.

On the day

- Drink soda water with a squeeze of fresh lemon or lime, or mint and strawberry rather than alcohol.
- Reduce snacking by staying away from cheese platters and other similar temptations.
- Remember your goals – it's easier to keep on track when you have your motivations in mind.
- Remind yourself that indulging every now and then won't derail all your plans – so don't feel guilty if you slip off the program from time to time.

Staying motivated

When you start a new eating plan, you might feel yourself in danger of lapse or relapse. These might sound like the same thing, but when we talk about a relapse, we mean either making a conscious decision to return to or slipping back into old habits. By lapse, on the other hand, we mean a one-off or short-term return to old habits. When losing weight or starting a new way of eating, lapses are common and to be expected.

Studies suggest that a dietary lapse can result in a food intake in one sitting of 4200 kJ to 14,280 kJ. That's 70–238 per cent of your daily intake!

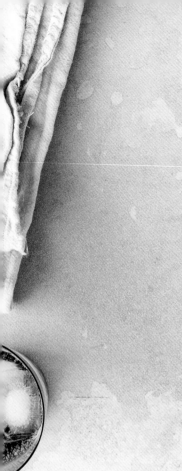

During these lapses, a few people in our trials consumed high-fat or sugary foods that were not part of the eating plan, while others consumed higher portions of the allowed foods.

Learning from your lapses is important. The main thing to remember is not to treat a lapse as a total dietary collapse. One single incident does not destroy all your efforts. It's when you don't learn from your lapses that they become a problem.

The first step in preventing a lapse is to identify your triggers or high-risk situations. These could be job problems, conflicts with family members, illness or depression. Once you know what causes you to lose control, you can take steps to avoid the same reaction next time. You might promise yourself, for example, that when you feel like a lapse, you'll reward yourself with activities and outings rather that food or drinks.

The three most common 'clusters' of situations that result in a dietary lapse are:

1.
social mealtime situations
At a restaurant, bar or family member's home, because tempting foods are around and people offer you food.

2.
emotional situations
At home or at work, usually when you're alone, because you eat for comfort in response to feelings of anger, stress, anxiety or depression.

3.
boring situations
Anywhere, when you're relaxing, waiting, on a long drive or between activities, to distract yourself and relieve the boredom.

Overcoming a lapse takes time and often support from friends and family, but also kindness from yourself. Some people find it helpful to seek the support of a counsellor.

Deal with saboteurs

- Remind friends, family and colleagues that this isn't just a diet, but a lifestyle plan to improve your health and wellbeing. This will stop them inadvertently acting as saboteurs.
- Seek support. Let the people close to you know that their encouragement is meaningful to you and will help you succeed.
- Show your friends and family that a low-carbohydrate diet doesn't mean missing out – you can still dine out and choose tasty meals that suit the eating plan and meet your health goals.
- Host a low-carbohydrate meal at your house. Perhaps provide a few dishes using recipes from this book, and use them as an opportunity to show how tasty low-carbohydrate recipes can be.
- Remember your goals and your progress. It's worth saying no to some things, in the knowledge you'll feel much better in the long run because your health will improve. Your friends and family should respect this.

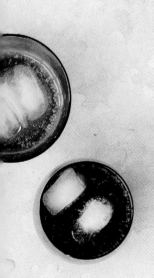

Consider your approach

Over the years we've identified two types of people who undergo weight loss – regainers and maintainers. The characteristics of each are summarised below. If you want to be a maintainer, bear these characteristics in mind as you embark on your weight-loss journey.

Regainers

- More commonly reported all-or-nothing thinking.
- Were far more likely to indulge in comfort eating or in avoidance eating to distract themselves from unpleasant thoughts and moods.
- Exercised less frequently and less vigorously than maintainers.
- Ate an average of 4.6 extra snacks a day.
- Reported that the effort involved in weight maintenance wasn't worthwhile.

Maintainers

- Persisted with the new diet and exercise plans until they established new patterns.
- Frequently monitored their weight and/or shape.
- Responded quickly to counteract any detected weight gain by reducing food intake or making an effort to increase activity levels.
- Set non-weight-related goals, such as improved appearance, health or self-esteem.
- After successful weight loss remained vigilant about their weight, particularly with regard to food intake.
- Engaged in high levels of physical activity – from more than 30 minutes three times a week to one hour a day of moderate-intensity activity.
- Reported that the benefits of successful weight maintenance outweighed the substantial effort involved.
- Were aware that they needed to remain conscious of the quantity and type of food they consumed as well as the level of activity necessary to stay at their reduced weight.

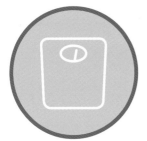

Weighing in

Some people find that weighing themselves motivates them in their quest to improve their health, but others find it quite confronting. A growing body of evidence now suggests that a daily weigh-in can maintain your motivation to stick to a healthy lifestyle, resulting in greater weight loss. In one particular study, those who weighed themselves daily showed greater self-control and a lower tendency to overeat than those who weighed in once a week.

We recommended that you monitor your progress regularly, perhaps by weighing yourself daily, perhaps weekly, according to your personal preference. Or you might prefer to measure your waist circumference rather than step on the scales. But don't get lost in the numbers and panic if your weight goes up slightly now and then – our weight can fluctuate across the week. What's important is the long-term trend.

PART 4

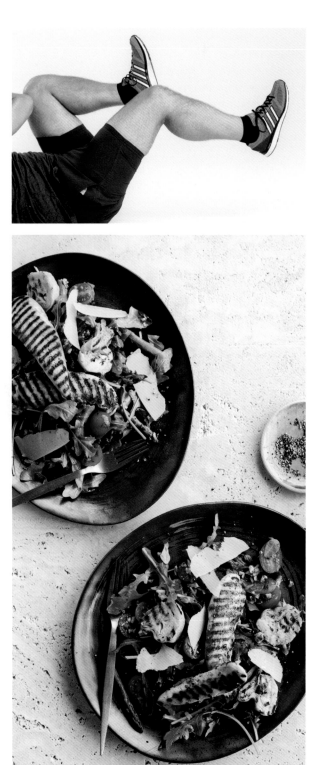

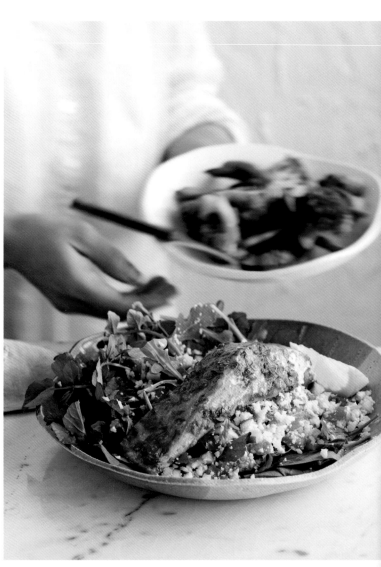

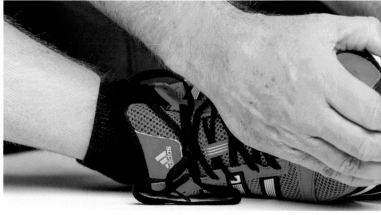

The CSIRO Exercise Plan

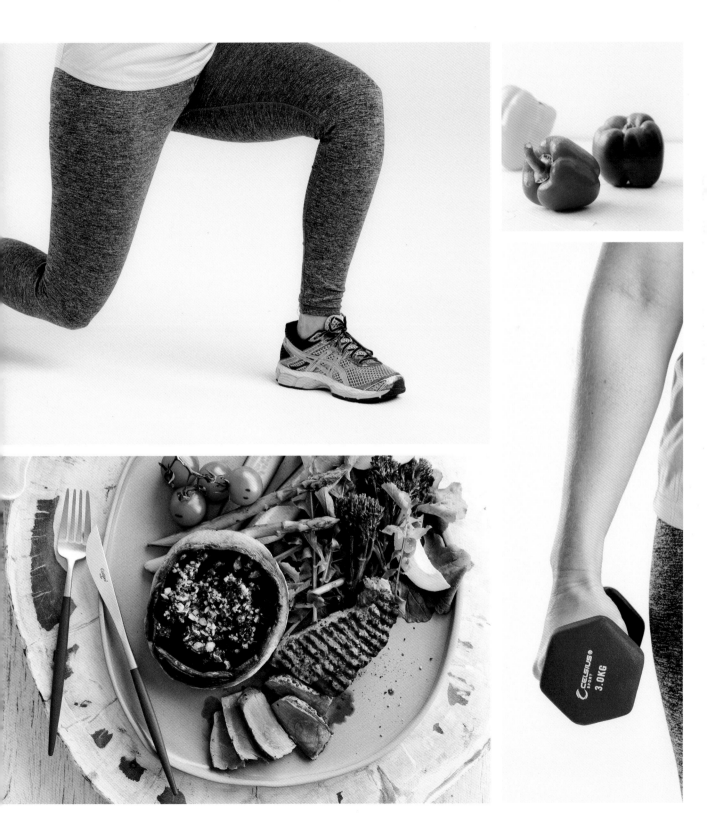

WHY WE NEED TO EXERCISE

Changing your diet is all very well, but regular physical activity is just as important a part of any lifestyle program aimed at improving health. A high level of physical activity is one of the main factors in successful weight control. Increased physical activity has also been associated with numerous health benefits, including enhanced control of blood glucose and diabetes; reduced risk of cardiovascular disease and premature death; lower blood pressure and blood fat levels; and reduced rates of some forms of cancer, depression and osteoporosis, regardless of whether you lose weight.

The main types of exercise

There are many different forms of exercise training, but the three common categories are:

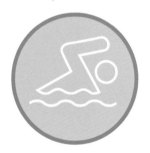

1. Aerobic exercise

Also known as endurance exercise or cardiorespiratory fitness training (cardio), aerobic exercise involves sustained activities that use large muscle groups and are rhythmic in nature, such as walking, swimming and cycling. The 'aerobic' part of the name simply means that it uses oxygen to generate energy; in other words, it's a form of exercise that relies on the heart and lungs to increase their work rate and provide a continual release of energy to fuel the activity.

Australian Government guidelines recommend that we participate in at least 150 minutes of moderate-intensity aerobic exercise per week, spread over at least three days, with no more than two consecutive days between sessions. Additional benefit can be obtained by exercising for a longer period and/or at a higher (vigorous) intensity.

Moderate-intensity exercise (e.g. brisk walking) noticeably increases your heart rate. Vigorous-intensity exercise (e.g. jogging) requires a large amount of effort; it substantially increases your heart rate and causes rapid breathing.

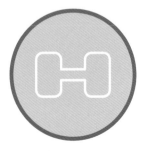

2. Resistance training

Also known as strength training, resistance training is a form of anaerobic exercise (i.e. not relying on oxygen). It consists of shorter, more intense activities that promote increases in strength, speed, power and muscle mass. These activities typically involve overloading the muscles with some kind of weight. They're only sustainable for between a few seconds up to a minute or two, as they need to use immediately available but limited stores of energy. This type of activity can result in an accumulation of lactic acid, which causes muscles to fatigue.

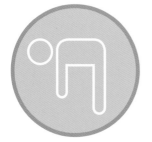

Resistance training activities should be done with a level of resistance that is adequate to reach the onset of muscle fatigue (i.e. reach a point where the activity can no longer be performed without having a brief rest). Exercise guidelines recommend at least two sessions of resistance training per week on non-consecutive days. Each session should involve two or three sets (groups of repetitions) of eight to ten different exercises that provide a whole-body workout – upper body, core and lower body, such as those provided in this book (pages 94–103). Exercises can be performed using your own body weight to provide resistance (e.g. push-ups, or squats and lunges) or using appropriate equipment (e.g. resistance bands or dumbbells) to overload the muscle.

3. Flexibility training

Also commonly referred to as stretching, flexibility training involves stretching or repeated movement through a joint's complete range of motion. Flexibility activities should complement aerobic and resistance training activities, but not be used as a substitute.

These types of exercise all produce different health outcomes, but participating in all three will generally provide the best overall mix of health benefits. While **aerobic exercise** improves fitness, which independently reduces the risk of premature death, **resistance training** increases muscle mass (or slows age-related loss of muscle mass), which enhances strength and metabolism, helps stabilise blood glucose and increases bone strength. **Flexibility activities** can increase or prevent the loss of joint range of motion, which makes the other types of exercise easier to pursue and improves general quality of life.

You'll find that over time, as you become fitter and/or stronger, the activities will become easier to perform. To continue to improve and benefit fully from the exercise program, it's important to increase the difficulty of the activity gradually. For aerobic exercise, this may mean moving faster or walking further, or progressing from a brisk walk to slow jogging (if your knees and ankles are up to it), while for resistance training it might mean using a heavier weight or stronger resistance.

It's important to remember that regular physical activity is more beneficial than the occasional vigorous workout. It makes sense, therefore, to select exercise activities you can enjoy and that can be incorporated into your regular schedule, so that they become a long-term habit. Don't choose something you don't really like or you think is boring.

In addition to your structured exercise program, you should take every opportunity to reduce sedentary time (i.e. time spent sitting or lying down) throughout the day, and increase the amount of physical activity that's part of your daily routine. This includes incidental physical activity, such as walking upstairs rather than taking the lift or standing rather than sitting. Reducing sedentary time and increasing incidental physical activity both provide a health benefit, independent of formal planned exercise.

The exercise plan in the following pages prescribes separate aerobic and resistance training programs (see pages 92–93), as well as an array of flexibility activities (see pages 104–109) that can be incorporated into the cool-down phase of both types of session.

Before starting any new exercise program, it's a good idea to talk to your healthcare team, to check whether there's any physical issue you need to bear in mind. If you have diabetes, impaired health or limited mobility, we strongly advise that you consult your healthcare team to ensure it's safe to commence exercise. If you can exercise, you should, and you should make it part of your daily routine, because the long-term benefits will outweigh any short-term inconvenience. If you don't already have one on your healthcare team, you could also consult an accredited exercise physiologist to tailor an exercise program to your individual needs and abilities.

EXERCISING SAFELY AND STAYING MOTIVATED

Warm up and cool down

You should start every exercise session with a 5–10-minute warm-up. This reduces the risk of injury and prepares your body for exercise by raising your heart rate and increasing blood flow to your working muscles. A typical warm-up consists of gentle aerobic activities that involve the muscle groups and movements associated with the proposed exercise. This might be jogging on the spot or walking, for example. By the end of the warm-up, your heart rate should have increased noticeably and you may even be sweating lightly.

After your workout, you should do a 5–10-minute cool-down. This can consist of the flexibility exercises on pages 104–109. In each of these you should stretch to the point of tightness or slight discomfort and hold the stretch for 10–30 seconds. Never stretch the joint past its normal range or to the point of pain. Repeat each stretch two to four times on both sides of the body.

Set yourself targets

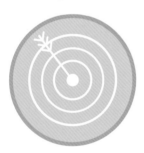

The best way to maintain your motivation to exercise is to set yourself achievable goals. These may be short-term goals that relate to a specific exercise session (e.g. walk 3 kilometres), or long-term goals that relate to an activity or event in which you may wish to take part (e.g. walk up a flight of stairs without needing to stop or compete in a fun run in a few months' time).

One simple method of determining how active you are each day is to record your daily step count using a pedometer. Basic pedometers are cheap, and most smartphones now record step counts too. Although any increase in your daily step count is likely to be beneficial, a common objective is to achieve 10,000 steps per day, which is generally considered to indicate that you're physically active. Regularly achieving 10,000 steps per day has been associated with a number of health benefits, including reduced body fat, lower blood pressure and improved insulin sensitivity.

A concerted effort or dedicated exercise session is usually required to reach 10,000 steps per day. The average Australian adult achieves less than 7500 steps per day, which is generally considered a low level of physical activity. Although the step-counting method provides a reasonable overall estimate of physical activity, it doesn't factor in the intensity of the activity or, depending on the pedometer, capture non-step-based activity such as cycling or swimming. A simple method you can use to gauge the relative intensity of an aerobic exercise session is to do the talk test. During moderate-intensity activity you'll still be able to talk comfortably but not sing. During vigorous-intensity activity, you won't be able to say more than a few words without needing to pause and take a breath. You can also use the 'Rating of perceived exertion' scale opposite.

YOU CAN TRAIN AT ANY AGE

It might seem impossible at the start, but the fact is that most people can do at least some form of exercise safely, as long as they take certain precautions, and they will derive a significant health benefit from doing so. It can be very helpful to have initial instruction and periodic supervision from an accredited exercise physiologist. This ensures you not only exercise safely and in the best way, but also stay motivated. The more you can make exercise part of your life, the greater the benefits will be for your weight management, blood glucose control, blood pressure, blood fats and cardiovascular disease risk.

If you're older, exercise and particularly resistance training can help protect you against declining bone density and muscle mass and strength. It's a valuable tool, therefore, for maintaining your independence and capacity to continue daily living activities for as long as possible, and to improve your ability to brace yourself or stay balanced, to prevent falls and injury.

Rating of perceived exertion of exercise session	
0	Rest
1	Very, very easy
2	Easy
3	Moderate
4	Somewhat hard
5	Hard
6	–
7	Very hard
8	–
9	–
10	Maximum

Source: C Foster et al., 'A new approach to monitoring exercise training', *Journal of Strength and Conditioning Research*, 2001, vol. 15, no. 1, pp. 109–15.

Monitor your progress

Another great motivator is keeping track of your exercise sessions and performance over time. This enables you to monitor your progress and gradually adjust the intensity of your workouts so you can continue to achieve maximum benefits. You can use a smartphone app for this or the training diary templates in Appendix C. Aerobic exercise can be monitored relatively simply by recording the type of exercise you do and the duration of the activity. For resistance training sessions, you should note the specific exercise, the resistance or weight used and the number of sets and repetitions completed.

For both aerobic exercise and resistance training sessions, you can keep track of the relative intensity of your workout (i.e. the overall difficulty of the entire exercise session) using a number from the table opposite. A moderate-intensity workout, which you should be aiming for as a minimum, corresponds to a rating of 3.

Sedentary Time

Research shows that independent of the overall amount of physical exercise you do, the amount of sedentary behavior and sitting time represents a distinct risk factor or diabetes and heart disease risk. Therefore, in addition to undertaking sufficient physical activity, it is important to reduce the amount of sitting time throughout the day. Some practical tips to reduce your sedentary time could include:

- Taking a walk every time you take a coffee break
- Stand up and move when you have a drink of water at work, or during the television advert break
- Wherever possible, stand up as opposed to sitting down, such as when talking on the phone
- Plan in some active time when you are usually sedentary
- Set time limits on sedentary behavior – such as limiting television to an hour in the evening or that you ban yourself from reading emails or using the internet for a certain period in the day. If you have a family, it's great for everyone to follow these limits.

YOUR WEEKLY AEROBIC EXERCISE PROGRAM

The exercise plan that accompanies the Low-carb Diet recommends participating in at least three sessions per week of aerobic exercise. At least initially, it might be easiest if this is brisk walking, but over time you might like to move on to jogging, cycling, rowing, aerobics and so on. Alternatively, you might find that a variety of aerobic activities is more fun and keeps you motivated.

The program builds up the duration of these aerobic exercise sessions progressively over several weeks. Ultimately, you should try to achieve at least 150 minutes of moderate-intensity or 75 minutes of vigorous-intensity aerobic exercise each week (or an equivalent combination of moderate- and vigorous-intensity aerobic exercise). You don't have to do your aerobic exercise all at once: if it suits you better, you can break it up into smaller 'snacks' of at least 10 minutes rather than doing one continuous block. This also allows you to vary your activities if you prefer.

Use the guide in the table below to help you build up stamina over the first eight weeks of the plan.

Increasing your moderate-intensity aerobic exercise sessions →

Week	Target time per session (minutes)
1	25–30
2	30–35
3	35–40
4	40–45
5	45–50
6	45–50
7	50–55
8+	55–60

With each aerobic exercise session, make sure you start with a warm-up and end with a cool-down (see pages 104–109).

Don't forget to monitor your progress using the training diary template (see Appendix C).

YOUR RESISTANCE TRAINING PROGRAM

We recommend at least two resistance training sessions per week on non-consecutive days. A specific selection of resistance training activities is provided on the following pages. In each session you should do eight to 10 of these exercises, including three to four upper-body exercises, three to four lower-body exercises and two core exercises.

While doing a resistance training exercise, it's important to consider the pace at which you perform each repetition. A general rule is to use a 2:1:2-second tempo. Using a biceps curl with a dumbbell as an example, this would mean taking 2 seconds to lift the dumbbell, holding the dumbbell at the top of the lift for 1 second, then taking 2 seconds to return the dumbbell to its start position. This will help you maximise the strength and muscle gain while minimising the risk of injury.

As the resistance training program is designed to fatigue the muscles you're working on, you should allow yourself a rest of 1–2 minutes between sets for recovery. You should perform two to three sets of each exercise during your workout.

Remember your breathing

Breathing technique is important in order to avoid a spike in blood pressure during the exercise. Never hold your breath during a resistance exercise repetition. You should aim to breathe out during the concentric phase, when the muscle is shortened under tension (e.g. lifting a dumbbell), or the effort phase; and breathe in during the eccentric phase, when the muscle is lengthened under tension (e.g. lowering the dumbbell), or the release phase.

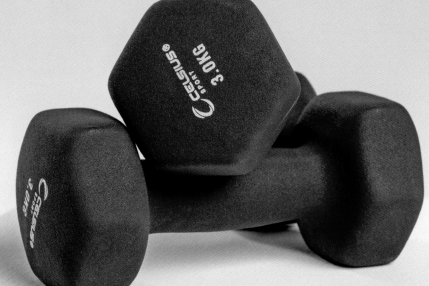

UPPER BODY

1.

Push-ups

For Triceps/chest **Weight** Body

Start position Kneel on the floor on your hands and knees then walk your hands forward until your knees, hips and shoulders are in a straight line. Keep your knees close together. Your arms should be straight (without locking your elbows) with your hands positioned under your shoulders, but slightly more than shoulder width apart, with your fingers pointing forwards.

1. Breathe in as you lower your body, pivoting from your knees, with your elbows pointing outwards slightly, until your chest is an inch or two above the floor (or as far down as you can).

2. Breathe out as you push your torso away from the ground until your arms are straight.

Easier variation Perform the exercise against a raised bench instead of the floor, using your feet as a pivot point.

Advanced Straighten your legs and use your toes as a pivot point.

2.

Triceps kickback

For Triceps **Weight** Dumbbell

Start position Kneel on the floor, supporting your weight on your knees and left hand (arm straight without locking your elbow). Take a dumbbell in your right hand and bend your right elbow to raise your upper arm so it's parallel to the floor. Your forearm should remain pointing down and the front end of the dumbbell should be pointing forward.

1. Breathe out and, keeping your right upper arm still and your elbow close to your torso, straighten your right arm behind you until your entire arm is parallel to the floor and the front end of the dumbbell points towards the floor.

2. Breathe in and slowly return the dumbbell to the start position, continue repetitions until you fatigue, then repeat the sequence with the dumbbell in your left hand. A complete left- and right-side series equals one set.

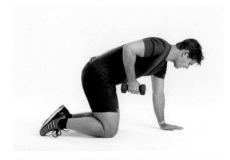

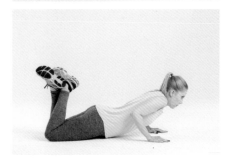

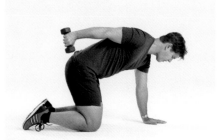

3.

Bench dips

For Triceps/deltoid (shoulder) **Weight** Body

Start position Position yourself with your back perpendicular to a bench, step or stable chair. Hold on to the edge of the bench, step or chair behind you with your arms fully extended and your hands slightly wider than shoulder width apart. Extend your legs in front of you with your heels on the floor and a slight bend in your knees.

1. Breathe in and slowly lower your body by bending at the elbows until the angle between your upper arm and forearm is approximately 90 degrees. Try to keep your elbows above your hands.

2. Breathe out and lift yourself back to the start position.

Advanced Place your feet up on a solid object in front of you, no higher than the bench, step or chair that your hands are on.

4.

Biceps curl

For Biceps **Weight** Dumbbell

Start position Stand with your feet shoulder width apart and your arms by your sides and a dumbbell in each hand. Your elbows should be close to your torso and your palms should be facing your thighs.

1. Breathe out and, holding your upper arm still, lift the dumbbell in your right hand as you turn your wrist so your palm is facing upwards. Continue to lift the dumbbell until it's at shoulder level. Avoid swinging your body to lift that weight. If you find you need to do this, decrease the weight until you become stronger.

2. Breathe in and slowly return the dumbbell to the start position. Repeat the movement on the left side. A complete left- and right-side sequence equals one repetition.

Note Brace your abdominal muscles and keep your tummy muscles tight throughout the exercise to maintain your exercise form and prevent injury. This is good advice for all these exercises.

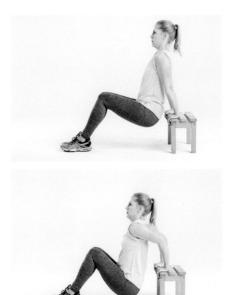

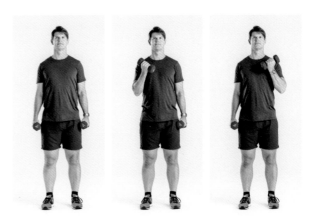

UPPER BODY

5.

Shoulder lateral raises

For Deltoid (shoulder) **Weight** Dumbbell

Start position Stand with your feet shoulder width apart and your arms by your sides and a dumbbell in each hand. Hold your elbows close to your torso, with your palms facing your thighs. Bend your elbows at a 90-degree angle, with your palms still facing inwards.

1. Breathe out and, keeping your torso still, lift your upper arms outwards and upwards while maintaining the 90-degree elbow bend. Do not allow your shoulders to rotate forward during the lift. Continue to lift until your arms are parallel to the floor and your palms are facing downwards.

2. Breathe in and slowly lower the dumbbells to the start position.

Variations This exercise can also be performed sitting down. To increase difficulty, perform the exercise with straight arms.

6.

Front dumbbell raise

For Deltoid (shoulder) **Weight** Dumbbell

Start position Stand with your feet shoulder width apart and your arms down in front of you, a slight bend in your elbows and a dumbbell in each hand. Your palms should be facing your thighs.

1. Breathe out and, keeping your torso still, raise your right arm out in front of you while maintaining a slight bend in your elbow. Continue to lift until your arm is parallel to the floor and the dumbbell is at shoulder height.

2. Breathe in and slowly lower the dumbbell to the start position while simultaneously lifting the left dumbbell. A complete left- and right-side sequence equals one repetition.

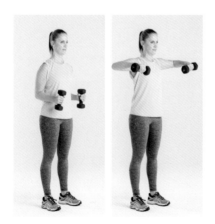

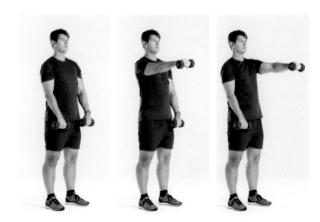

7.
Dumbbell upright row

For Trapezius **Weight** Dumbbell

Start position Stand with your feet shoulder width apart and your arms down in front of you and a dumbbell in each hand. Your palms should be facing your thighs.

1. Breathe out and, keeping your torso still, bend your elbows out to the sides to lift both dumbbells until they nearly touch your chin, keeping them close to your body throughout. At the top of the lift, your elbows should remain higher than your hands.

2. Breathe in and slowly lower the dumbbells to the start position.

8.
One-dumbbell row

For Back **Weight** Dumbbell

Start position Stand with your feet shoulder width apart and your knees slightly bent, facing a bench, chair or low stable object. Hold a dumbbell in your right hand with your palm facing your thigh. Lean forward at the hips and place your left hand on the bench, chair or low stable object, allowing your right arm to hang straight down. Your back should be almost parallel to the floor.

1. Breathe out and, keeping your torso still, pull the dumbbell straight up to the side of your chest. Keep your upper arm close to your side throughout.

2. Breathe in and slowly lower the dumbbell to the start position. Continue repetitions until you fatigue, then repeat the sequence on the left side. A complete left- and right-side series equals one set.

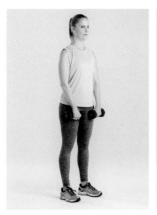
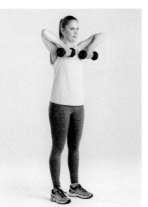
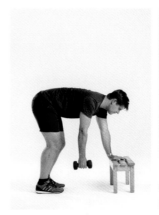
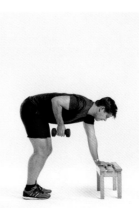

UPPER BODY

9.

Bent-over two-dumbbell row

For Back Weight Dumbbell

> **Caution: Do not try this exercise if you have back problems.**

Start position Stand with your feet shoulder width apart and your knees slightly bent. Bend forward at the hips so you're leaning over your feet. Hold a dumbbell in each hand with your palms facing each other and your arms straight down in front of you. Keep your head up facing forward.

1. Breathe out and, keeping your torso still, lift both dumbbells up to your sides without rotating them, squeezing your shoulder blades together.

2. Breathe in and slowly lower the dumbbells to the start position.

CORE

10.

Sit-ups

For Abdominals Weight Body

Start position Lie on your back with your knees bent at 90 degrees, your feet flat on the floor and your toes held under something that won't move (or have a partner hold your feet to the floor). Your arms should be by your sides, raised slightly off the floor and pointing towards your feet.

1. Breathe out and, keeping your feet and bottom on the floor and your arms parallel to the floor, lift your shoulder blades and torso as close as you can to your knees. Take care not to strain your neck forward as you rise.

2. Breathe in and slowly lower your torso and shoulder blades back to the floor.

Advanced 1 Keep your feet flat on the floor without having them anchored. Crossing your arms in front of your chest or placing your hands behind your head will progressively increase the difficulty.

Advanced 2 Hold a weight across your chest to further increase the difficulty and resistance.

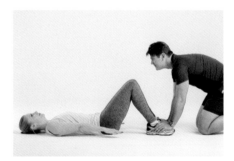

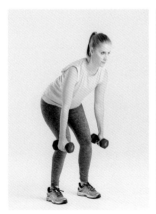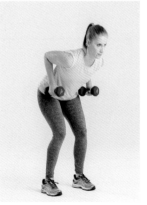

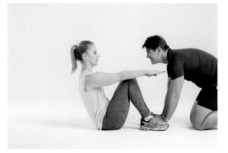

11.

Crunches

For Abdominals **Weight** Body

Start position Lie on your back with your knees bent at 90 degrees, your feet flat on the floor and your toes held under something that won't move (or have a partner hold your feet to the floor). Your arms should be crossed in front of your chest.

1. Breathe out and, keeping your feet and bottom on the floor and your arms crossed in front of your chest, lift your shoulder blades and torso towards the ceiling. Your shoulder blades should lift about 10 centimetres off the floor while your lower back remains in contact with the floor.

2. Breathe in and slowly lower your torso and shoulder blades back to the floor.

Advanced 1 Keep your feet flat on the floor without having them anchored. Placing your hands behind your head or stretching your arms behind your head will progressively increase the difficulty.

Advanced 2 Hold a weight across your chest to further increase the difficulty and resistance.

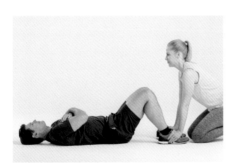

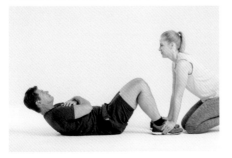

12.

Bicycle crunches

For Abdominals **Weight** Body

Start position Lie on your back with your hands behind your head and your elbows out to the sides. Bend your thighs and knees at 90 degrees so that your lower legs are parallel with the floor. Lift your shoulder blades into the crunch position.

1. Breathe out and, as if riding a bike, kick towards your toes with your left leg while bringing your right knee towards your head. As your right knee comes up, bring your left elbow across to meet it while crunching your abdomen on the left.

2. Breathe in and kick with the right leg while bringing up your left knee to meet your right elbow, crunching your abdomen on the right. Continue the cycling motion in this way. A complete left- and right-side sequence equals one repetition.

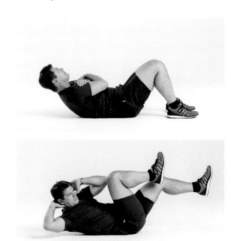

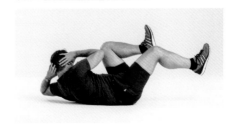

CORE

13.

Dumbbell side bend

For Abdominal obliques (side abdominals)
Weight Dumbbell

Start position Stand upright with your feet shoulder width apart, your left hand on your hip and your right hand by your side holding a dumbbell, with your palm facing your thigh.

1. Breathe in and bend sideways to the right at the waist as far as possible. Be careful not to bend forwards or backwards.

2. Pause for 1 second then breathe out and return to the start position. Continue repetitions until you fatigue, then repeat the sequence on the left side, with the dumbbell in your left hand. A complete left- and right-side series equals one set.

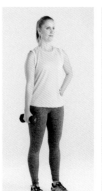
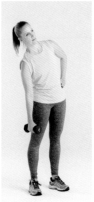

14.

Plank

For Abdominals **Weight** Body

Start position Position your body with your tummy facing downwards, resting your weight on your knees. Your upper arms should be pointing straight down, your elbows shoulder width apart and bent at 90 degrees, and your forearms flat with your hands in a loose fist and touching to make in an inverted 'V'. You should be looking at the floor just in front of your hands, and your weight should be supported entirely on your knees with your knees, hips and shoulders in a straight line.

1. Breathing in and out steadily, keep your body straight and hold this position for at least 10 seconds. Keep your back straight throughout this exercise and avoid sticking your buttocks in the air (i.e. no Sydney Harbour Bridges).

Intermediate Rest your weight on your toes and elbows.

Advanced Increase the length of time you hold the plank position.

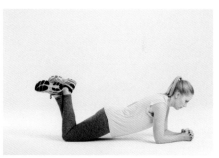

Advanced

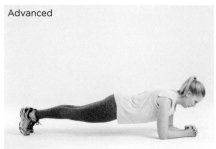

15.

Arm and leg raises

For Lower back **Weight** Body

Start position Lie on your tummy with your head up, your arms fully extended in front of you and your legs straight, with your feet together and toes pointed.

1. Breathe out while simultaneously raising your right arm and left leg off the floor. Hold this position for at least 10 seconds, breathing in and out steadily.

2. Lower your arm and leg back to the floor and repeat with the opposite arm and leg. A complete left- and right-side sequence equals one set.

Advanced 1 Increase the length of time you hold the raised position.

Advanced 2 Raise both arms and legs simultaneously (Superman position).

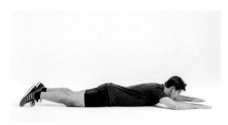

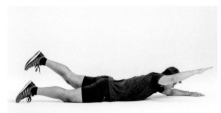

Advanced

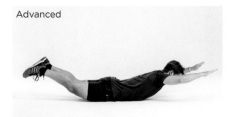

LOWER BODY

16.

Squats

For Quads/glutes **Weight** Body or dumbbells

Start position Stand with your feet shoulder width apart. If using your body weight, place your hands behind your head with your elbows out. If using dumbbells (advanced), hold one in each hand by your side, with your palms facing your thighs.

1. Breathe in while bending your knees and hips so you're sitting back, keeping your weight on your heels. Keep your head and chest high, and your buttocks out during the movement. Squat as low as you can, ideally until your thighs are parallel to the floor or beyond. Avoid leaning so far forward that your knees go over the front of your toes.

2. Breathe out and return to the start position.

Advanced Hold a dumbbell in each hand to increase the difficulty and resistance. Keep your arms straight down throughout.

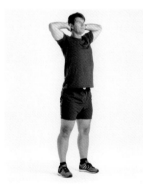
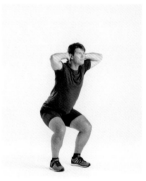

Advanced

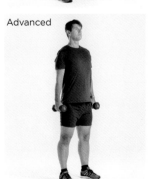

Advanced

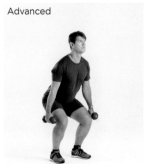

LOWER BODY

17.
Forward lunge

For Quads/glutes **Weight** Body or dumbbells

Start position Stand with your feet shoulder width apart. If using your body weight, place your hands on your hips. If using dumbbells (advanced), hold one in each hand by your side, with your palms facing your thighs.

1. Breathe in and, maintaining an upright posture, take a large step forward with your left foot. Drop your hips until your right knee gets close to the floor without touching it. Your left knee should bend to approximately 90 degrees and shouldn't go past your toes (take a slightly larger step to avoid this if required). If you're holding dumbbells, keep your arms straight down throughout.

2. Breathe out and push up from your left foot, returning it to the start position. Repeat the movement with your right foot stepping forward. A complete left- and right-side sequence equals one repetition.

Advanced Hold a dumbbell in each hand to increase the difficulty and resistance.

18.
Reverse lunge

For Quads/glutes **Weight** Body or dumbbells

Start position Stand with your feet shoulder width apart. If using your body weight, place your hands on your hips. If using dumbbells (advanced), hold one in each hand by your side, with your palms facing your thighs.

1. Breathe in and, maintaining an upright posture, take a large step backward with your right foot. Drop your hips until your right knee gets close to the floor without touching it. Your front knee should bend to approximately 90 degrees and shouldn't go past your toes (take a slightly larger step to avoid this if required). If you're holding dumbbells, keep your arms straight down throughout.

2. Breathe out and push up from your right foot, returning it to the start position. Repeat the movement with your left foot stepping backward. A complete left- and right-side sequence equals one repetition.

Advanced Hold a dumbbell in each hand to increase the difficulty and resistance.

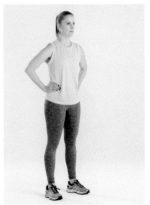 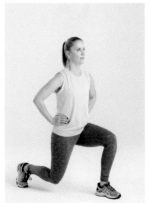 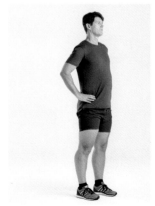 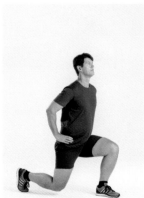

19.

Glute kickbacks

For Glutes **Weight** Body

Start position Position yourself on the floor with your knees bent at 90 degrees, your hips in line with your knees, your back straight and your arms straight down. Your hands should be on the floor under your shoulders, shoulder width apart with your fingers pointing forwards, and your head should be facing the floor.

1. Breathe out and lift your right leg, maintaining the 90-degree knee bend, until your thigh is parallel with the floor.

2. Breathe in and return the leg to the start position. Repeat the movement with the left leg. A complete left- and right-side sequence equals one repetition.

20.

Calf raises

For Calves **Weight** Body or dumbbells

Start position Stand with your feet shoulder width apart, supporting your weight on the balls of your feet. Your feet should be pointing straight ahead. If using your body weight, hang your arms by your sides. If you're having trouble balancing, support yourself by holding onto something solid such as a doorframe with one hand. If using dumbbells (advanced), hang your arms by your sides with a dumbbell in each hand and your palms facing your thighs. If you're having trouble balancing, use one dumbbell only and support yourself by holding onto a doorframe with your free hand.

1. Breathe out and raise your heels off the floor by contracting your calves.

2. Breathe in and slowly lower your heels until they contact the ground.

Advanced 1 Hold a dumbbell in each hand to increase the difficulty and resistance.

Advanced 2 To increase the range of motion, start with your toes and the balls of your feet on a sturdy wooden board 5–10 centimetres thick, and your heels hanging off and touching the ground.

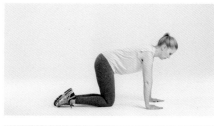

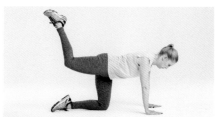

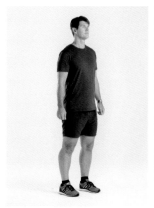

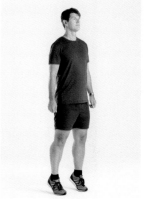

YOUR FLEXIBILITY EXERCISES

UPPER BODY

Chest

Stand side-on to a fixed vertical object, such as a wall or post, stretch your right arm straight out and place your palm flat against the object with your fingers pointing behind you. Turn your body away from the wall and feel the stretch in your chest. Repeat on the other side.

Triceps

Lift your right arm over and behind your head with your elbow bent and your hand above or on your back as if reaching down your spine. Use your left hand to push your right elbow down gently, extending the stretch. Repeat on the other side.

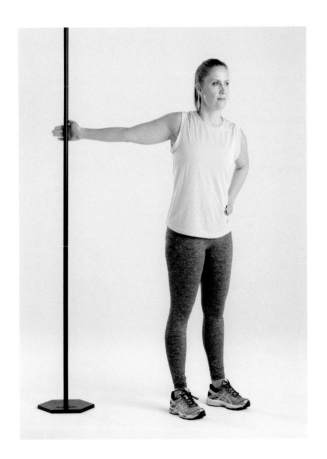

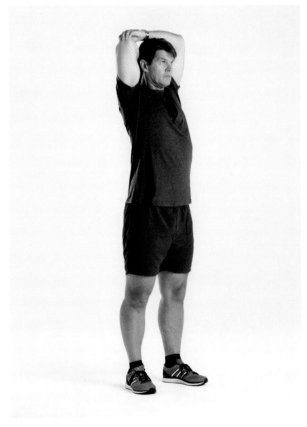

Biceps

In a standing position, stretch both arms straight out, then turn your wrists so your thumbs point upwards, pushing your arms back slightly. Repeat with your thumbs pointing downwards.

Shoulder

Stretch your left arm across your chest with your elbow slightly bent, and pull your elbow towards you with your right arm until you feel the stretch in the back of your shoulder. Repeat on the other side.

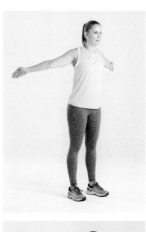

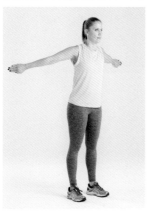

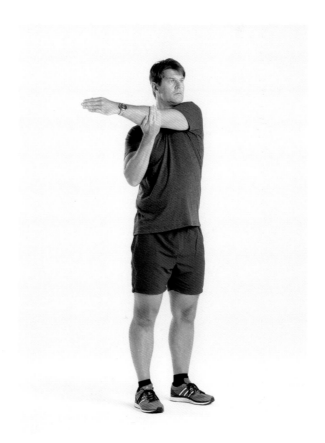

CORE

Upper back

Clasp your fingers together with your palms facing out and thumbs pointing down, round your shoulders and reach your hands forward to feel a gentle stretch in your upper back.

Lower back

Kneel on the floor on your hands and knees. Gradually arch your back like a cat, letting your head drop down, and feel a gentle stretch in your lower back.

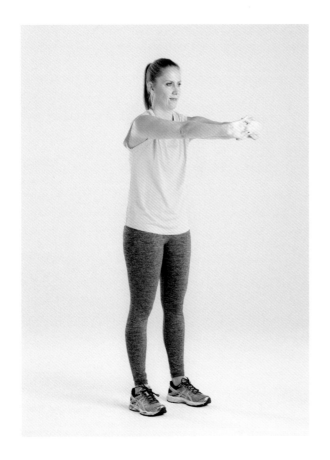

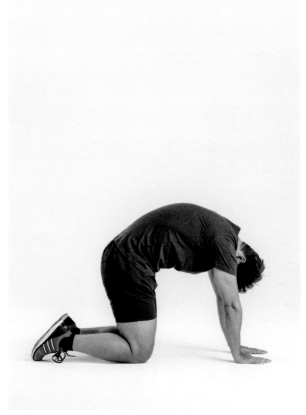

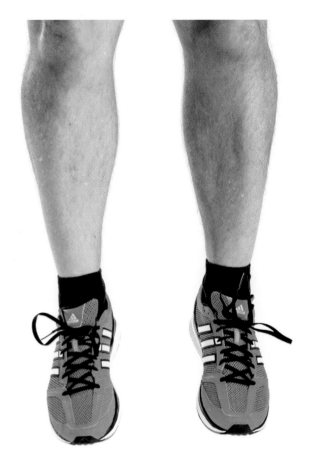

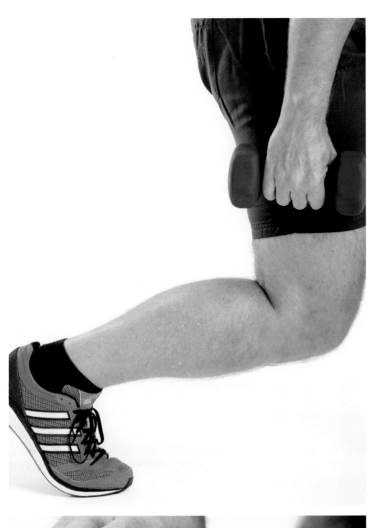

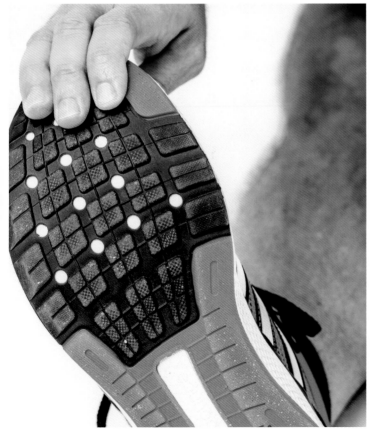

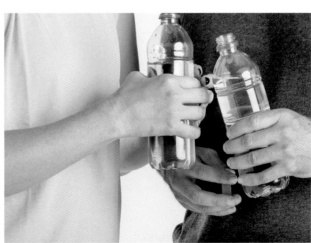

LOWER BODY

Quad

Lie on your left side, propping your head up with your left hand, with your left leg straight and your right leg bent at the knee so your foot is behind you. Grasp your right foot around the ankle with your right hand. During the hold, press your hips forward and pull your heel towards your buttocks to increase the stretch in your quadriceps. Repeat lying on your right side and stretching your left leg.

Calf

Stand with your hands on your hips and take a large step forward with your left foot. Keep your back foot on the floor and pointing forwards. Slowly transfer your weight forward onto your left foot and bend your left knee to feel the stretch in your right calf. Repeat on the other side to stretch your left calf. If necessary to maintain your balance, support yourself by holding on to a sturdy object.

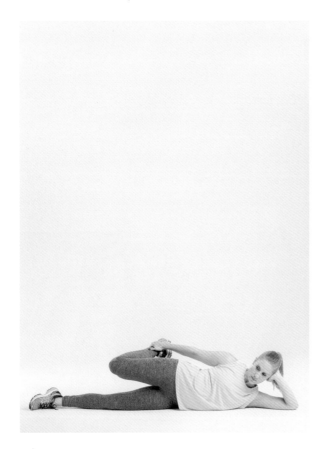

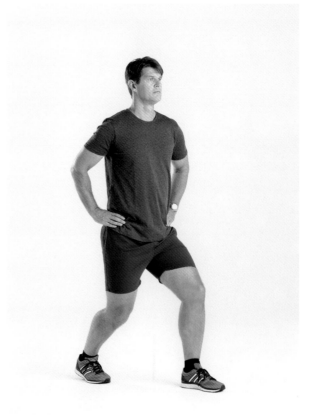

Hamstring

Lie on your back with your knees slightly bent. Lift your right leg, maintaining the slight bend in your knee, then grasp the back of your right thigh with both hands and pull it gently towards your chest, slowly straightening the knee until you feel a comfortable stretch in the back of the thigh. Repeat on the other side.

Glute

Lie on your back with both knees bent. Lift your right foot and cross it over your left leg so your right ankle is resting just above your left knee. Lift your left leg off the floor and grasp the back of your left thigh with both hands, pulling it gently towards you until you feel the stretch in your buttocks and outer thigh. Repeat on the other side.

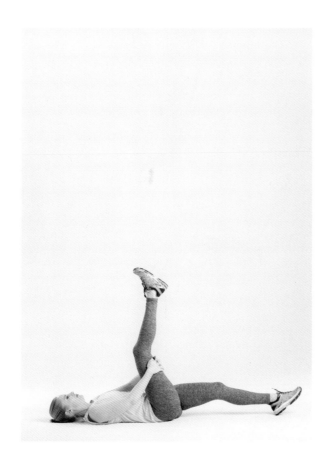

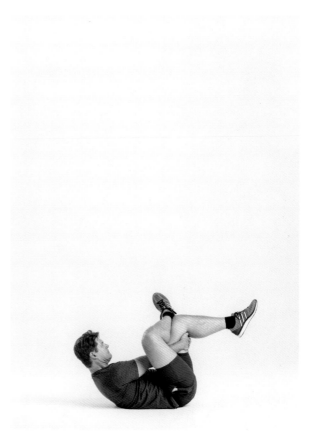

PART 5

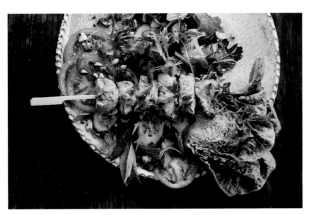

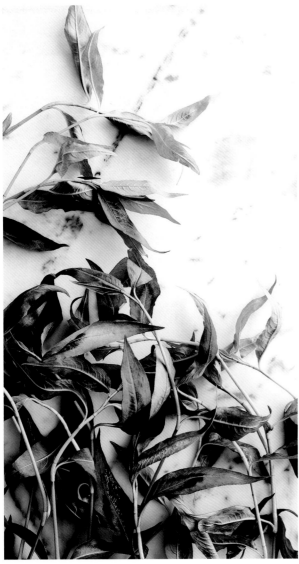

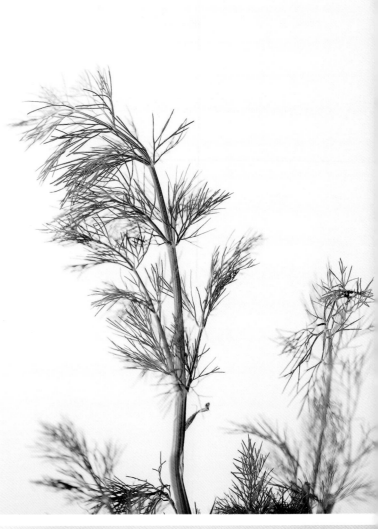

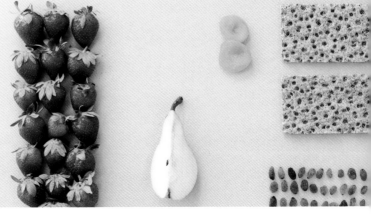

The CSIRO Low-carb Recipes

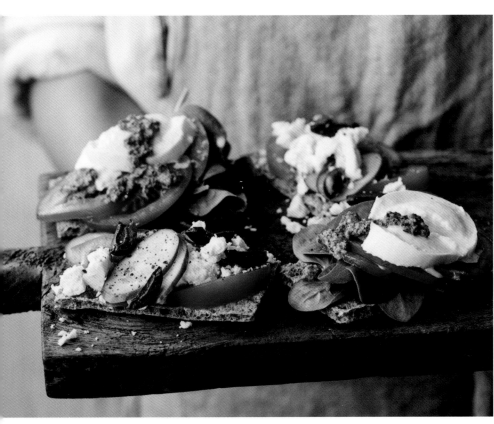

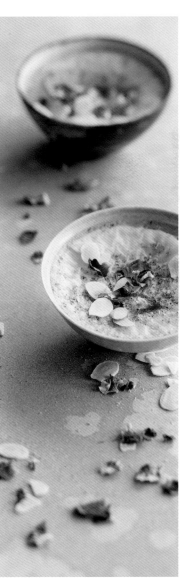

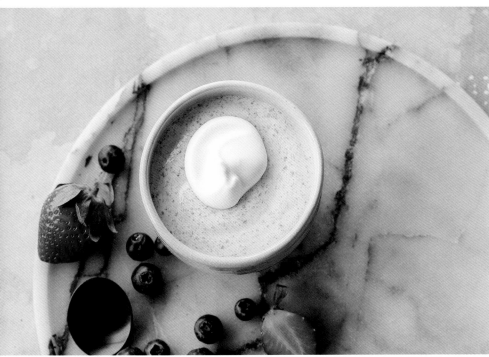

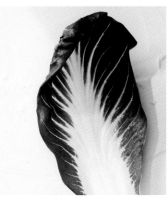

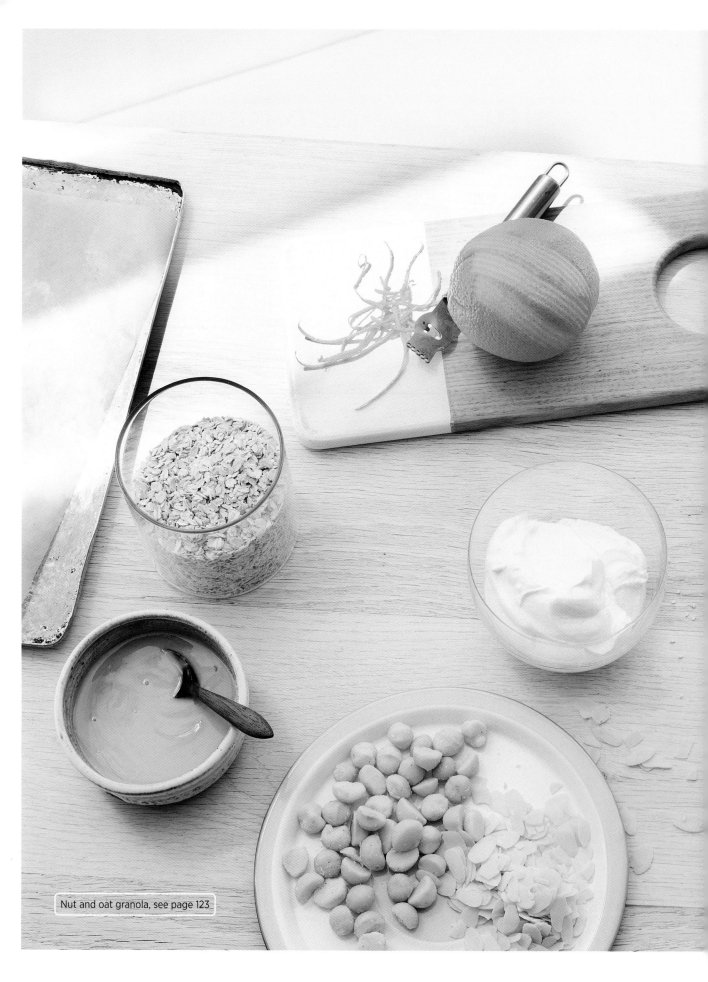

Nut and oat granola, see page 123

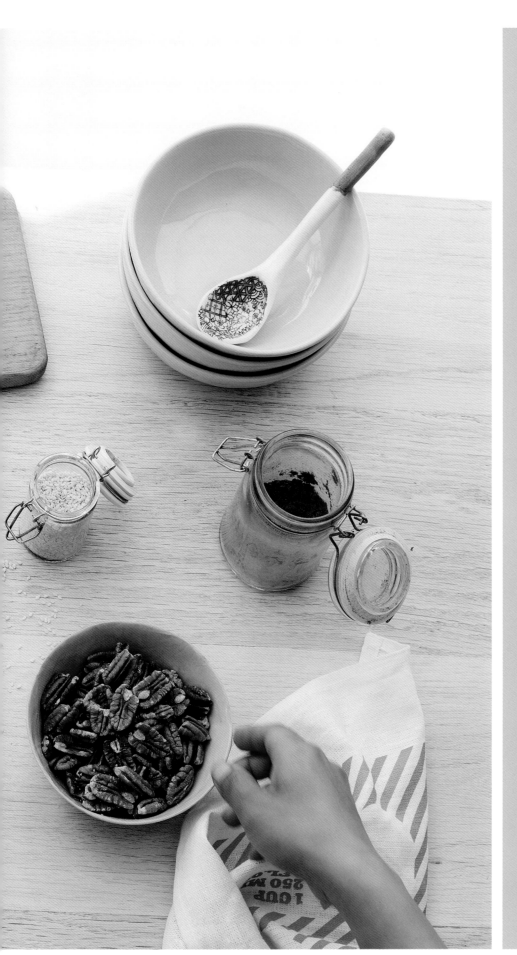

Breads, cereals, legumes,
starchy vegetables **1**
Dairy **1.5**
Low-carb vegetables **0.5**
Healthy fats **2**

---

220 g low-fat fresh ricotta
1½ teaspoons ground flaxseed, mixed
   with 1½ tablespoons water
1 teaspoon finely chopped thyme
4 x 35 g slices mixed grain bread
20 g avocado
100 g rocket leaves, trimmed

PESTO

1 tablespoon raw almonds
1¼ cups basil leaves
1 large clove garlic, crushed
1 tablespoon extra virgin olive oil
1½ tablespoons finely grated parmesan

Baked ricotta with pesto and avocado toast

15 G
CARB
PER
SERVE

🍴 **Serves 4**   🕐 **Preparation: 15 minutes, plus resting time**
🍲 **Cooking: 35 minutes**

To make the pesto, place the almonds, basil and garlic in a small food processor and process until finely chopped. With the motor running, drizzle in the olive oil, then season to taste with freshly ground black pepper and stir in the parmesan.

Preheat the oven to 180°C (160°C fan-forced). Line four cups of a muffin tin with paper cases.

Mix the ricotta, flaxseed mixture and thyme until well combined. Spoon one-quarter of the pesto into each paper case, then top each with one-quarter of the ricotta mixture and smooth the surface.

Bake for 30–35 minutes or until the ricotta is firm and light golden on top. Turn off the oven and leave to stand in the oven for 10 minutes, then remove from the tin.

Toast the bread, spread evenly with avocado and cut in half. Top with the rocket leaves. Gently turn the baked ricotta out of the paper cases, and serve 1 per person with a slice of avocado toast.

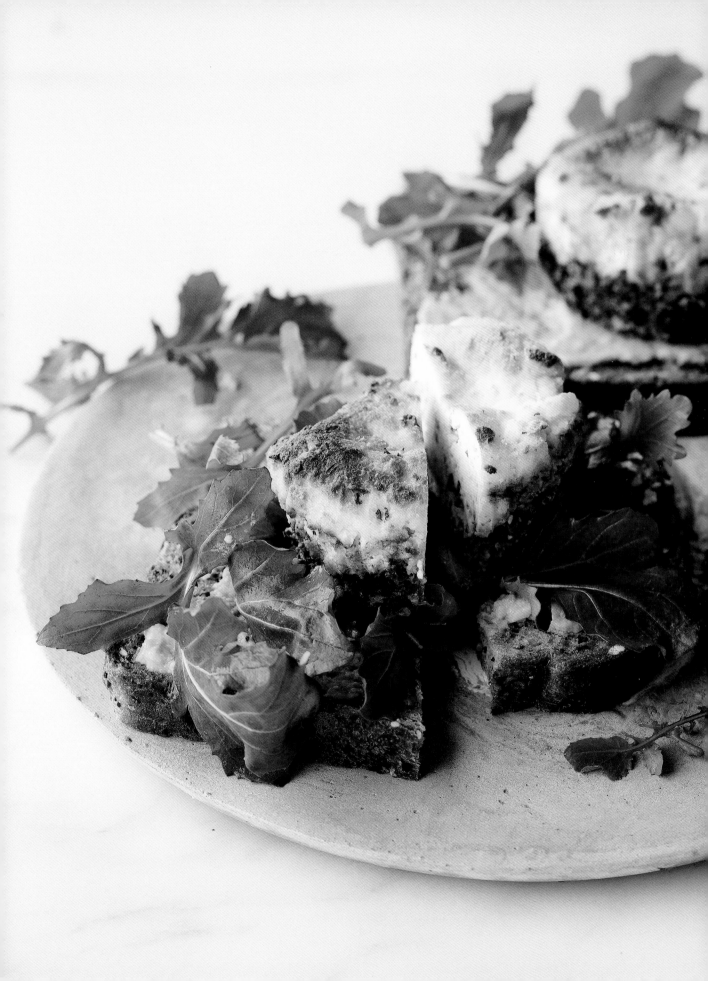

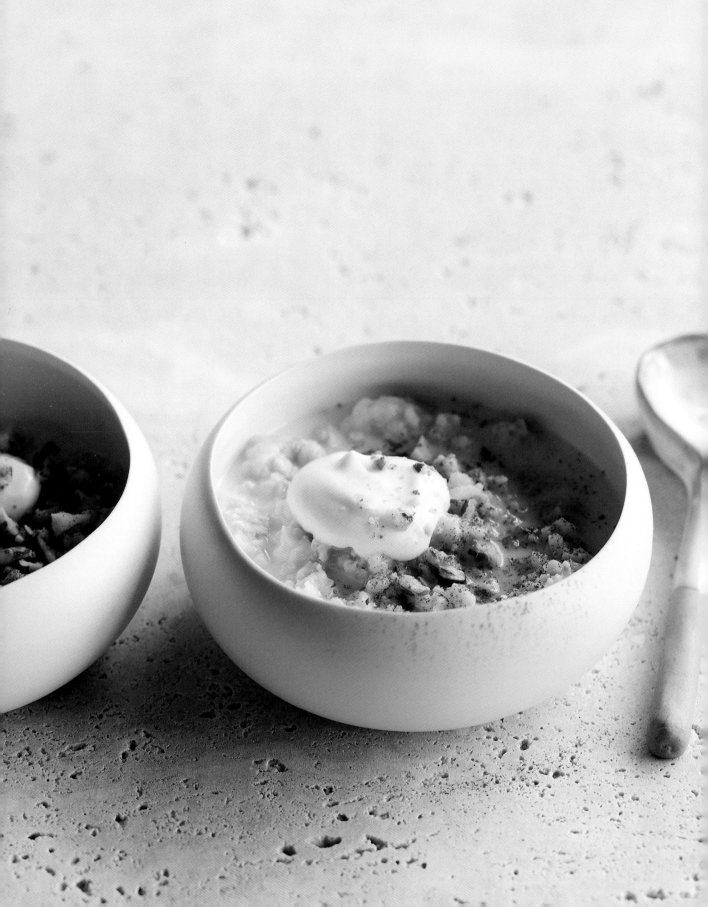

UNITS PER SERVE
Breads, cereals, legumes,
starchy vegetables **1**
Dairy **1**
Healthy fats **2**

1⅓ cups (120 g) raw (natural)
    rolled oats
2 cups (500 ml) skim milk
⅓ cup (95 g) low-fat
    Greek-style yoghurt

CINNAMON NUT CRUMBLE
30 g raw almonds
30 g pecans or walnuts
20 g macadamias
pinch of ground cinnamon, or to taste

Porridge with cinnamon nut crumble

🍴 **Serves 4**   🕐 **Preparation: 10 minutes, plus standing time**
〰 **Cooking: 15 minutes**

To make the cinnamon nut crumble, preheat the oven to
180°C (160°C fan-forced). Line a baking tray with baking paper.

Spread out the nuts on the prepared tray and roast for 6–8 minutes
or until light golden. Transfer to a mortar, sprinkle in the cinnamon
and coarsely crush with the pestle.

Place the oats in a heavy-based saucepan, add 1⅓ cups (330 ml)
cold water and stir well. Stir in 1¾ cups (435 ml) near-boiling water and
stir vigorously. Bring to the boil over medium heat, then cook, stirring
frequently, for 5 minutes or until the porridge is thickened and creamy.

Divide the porridge evenly among four bowls and serve each with
½ cup (125 ml) milk and 1 tablespoon yoghurt. Sprinkle the nut
crumble evenly over the top.

> **WEEKS 7–12 CARB EXTRAS**
>
> For an extra 10 g carbs per serve, add 240 g (60 g per person)
> blueberries.

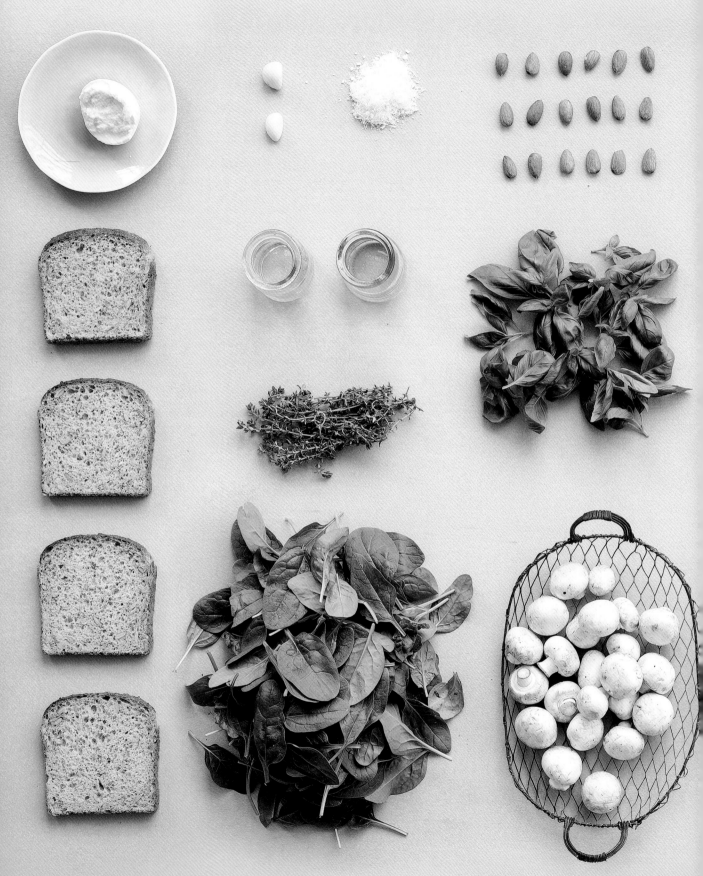

Mozzarella and pesto bruschetta

15 G
CARB
PER
SERVE

🍴 Serves 4   🕐 Preparation: 10 minutes   🍳 Cooking: 10 minutes

3 teaspoons olive oil
300 g button mushrooms, sliced
1 clove garlic, finely chopped
2 teaspoons chopped thyme
150 g baby spinach leaves, trimmed
4 × 35 g slices mixed grain bread
1 quantity Pesto (see page 114)
50 g mozzarella, torn

Heat the olive oil in a heavy-based non-stick frying pan over medium heat. Add the mushrooms and cook, stirring frequently, for 6 minutes, then add the garlic and thyme and cook for a further 2 minutes or until the mushrooms are golden and tender. Add the spinach and stir through just until wilted.

Toast the bread, then spread evenly with the pesto and top with the mushroom mixture and the mozzarella. Season to taste with freshly ground black pepper and serve.

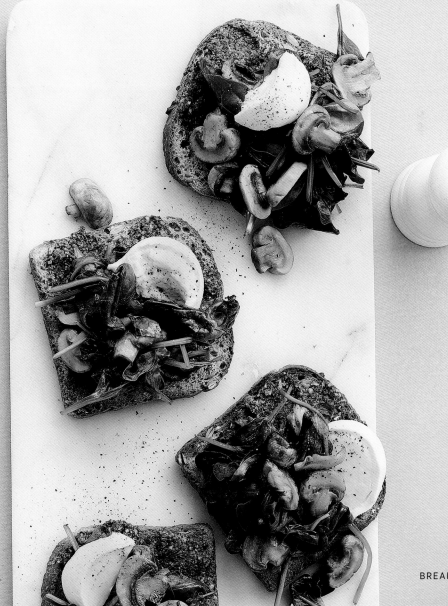

UNITS PER SERVE
Breads, cereals, legumes,
starchy vegetables **1**
Dairy **1**
Low-carb vegetables **0.5**
Healthy fats **2.5**

---

4 × 35 g slices mixed grain bread
40 g hummus
2 tomatoes, thickly sliced
80 g salt-reduced low-fat feta,
    sliced or crumbled

SPICED NUT SPRINKLE
40 g pecans or walnuts
40 g macadamias
large pinch of ground cumin, or to taste
large pinch of sweet paprika, or to taste

Hummus and tomato toast with spiced nuts

🍴 **Serves 4**   🕐 **Preparation: 10 minutes**   🌀 **Cooking: 10 minutes**

To make the spiced nut sprinkle, preheat the oven to 180°C (160°C fan-forced). Line a baking tray with baking paper.

Spread out the nuts on the prepared tray and roast for 6–8 minutes or until light golden. Transfer to a mortar, sprinkle in the cumin and paprika and coarsely crush with the pestle. Set aside.

Toast the bread, then spread evenly with the hummus and top with the tomato. Season to taste with freshly ground black pepper. Scatter with the feta and the nut sprinkle and serve.

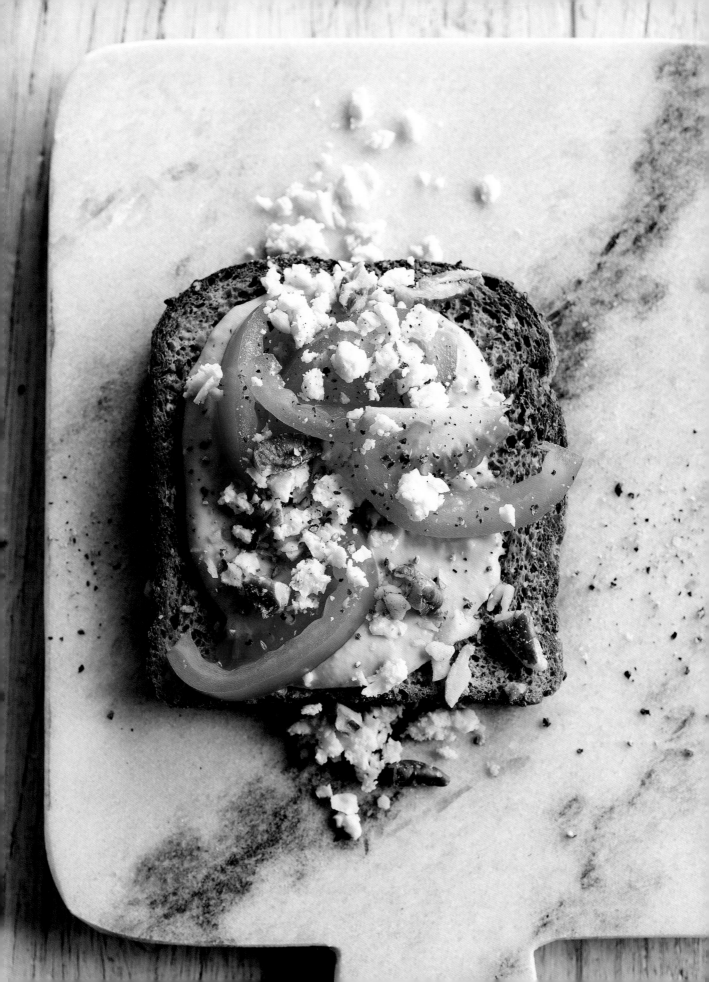

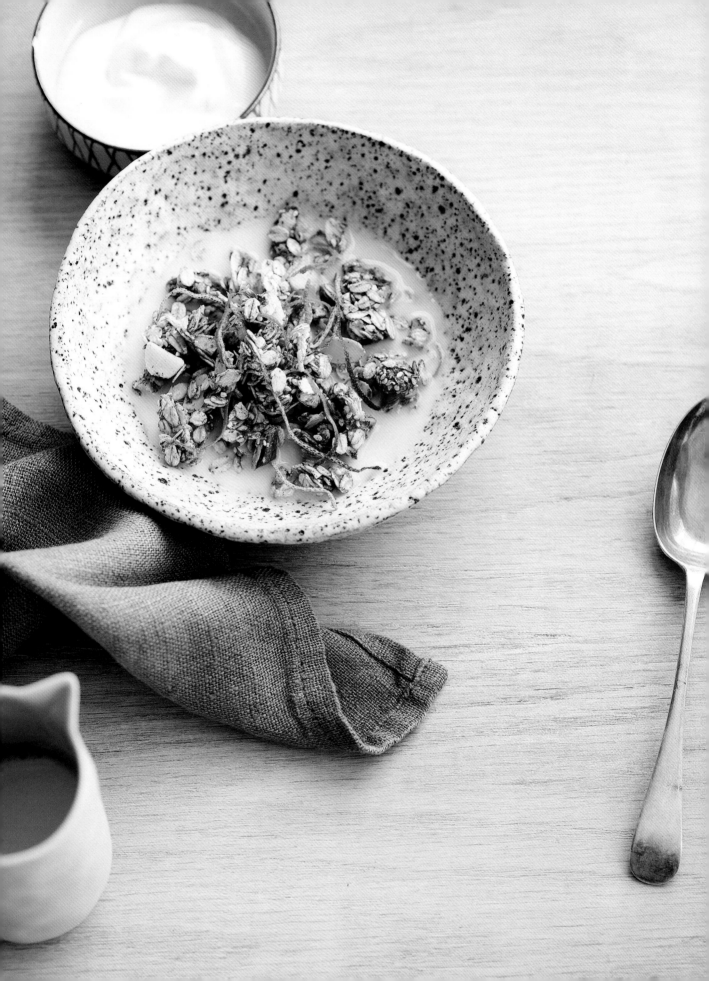

Nut and oat granola with orange zest

UNITS PER SERVE
Breads, cereals, legumes,
starchy vegetables **1**
Dairy **1**
Healthy fats **2**

🍴 Serves 8   🕐 Preparation: 15 minutes   ))) Cooking: 15 minutes

1 large egg white
pinch of cream of tartar
2 tablespoons tahini
2 teaspoons stevia granules
2 teaspoons mixed spice or
    ground cinnamon
20 g flaked almonds
30 g pecans or walnuts,
    roughly chopped
2 tablespoons macadamias,
    roughly chopped
1 tablespoon sesame seeds
1 teaspoon julienned orange zest,
    plus extra to serve
2½ cups (225 g) raw (natural)
    rolled oats
600 ml skim milk
320 g low-fat Greek-style yoghurt

Preheat the oven to 170°C (150°C fan-forced) and line two baking trays with baking paper.

Beat the egg white in a bowl with an electric mixer until frothy. Add the cream of tartar and beat until soft peaks form, then beat in the tahini, stevia granules and spice until combined. (The mixture will be thick but not airy.) Fold in the nuts, sesame seeds and orange zest. Add the oats and use your fingertips to gently rub them through the mixture until everything is coated.

Spread the mixture evenly over the prepared trays, keeping little clusters of mixture together for extra texture. Bake for 15 minutes, stirring gently after 10 minutes, or until it is just starting to smell toasted. The mixture will not brown very much but will start to feel dry. Remove from the oven and cool completely on the trays.

For each serving, place ½ cup (45 g) toasted muesli in a small bowl and add 75 ml milk. Serve with 40 g yoghurt and a sprinkling of extra orange zest.

Store the granola in an airtight container for 2–3 weeks.

> **WEEKS 7–12 CARB EXTRAS**
>
> For an extra 10 g carbs per serve, top with 100 g raspberries, 200 g strawberries or 60 g blueberries per person.

UNITS PER SERVE

Breads, cereals, legumes,
starchy vegetables **1**
Dairy **1**
Healthy fats **1**

1¼ cups (110 g) raw (natural)
   rolled oats
1 tablespoon sunflower seed kernels
½ teaspoon ground cardamom or
   mixed spice
300 ml skim milk
250 g low-fat Greek-style yoghurt
¼ cup (40 g) Sweet Spiced Nut Clusters
   (see page 259)
mint leaves (optional), to serve

Overnight oats with sweet spiced nuts

23 G CARB PER SERVE

🍴 **Serves 4**   🕐 **Preparation: 10 minutes, plus refrigerating time**
♨ **Cooking: nil**

Combine the oats, seeds, spice and milk in a medium bowl. Cover
and refrigerate for a minimum of 2 hours, or overnight.

Just before serving, stir in the yoghurt. Divide the oats evenly among
four bowls and top each serve with one-quarter of the nut clusters
and mint leaves, if using.

Store in an airtight container in the refrigerator for 2–3 days.

> **WEEKS 7–12 CARB EXTRAS**
>
> For an extra 10 g carbs per serve, top with 100 g raspberries,
> 200 g strawberries or 60 g blueberries per person.

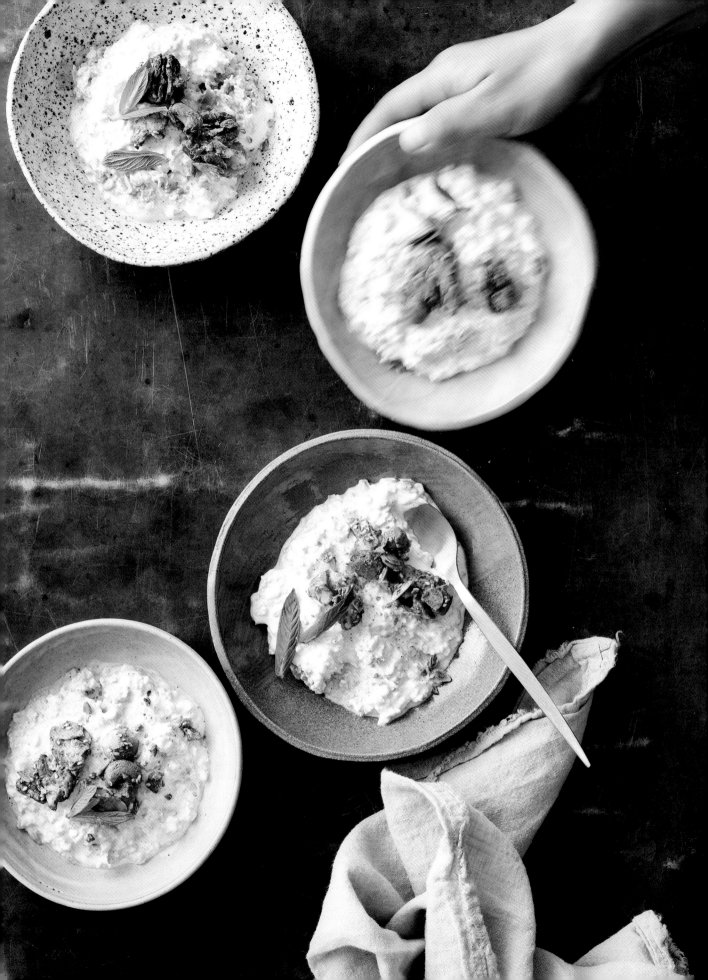

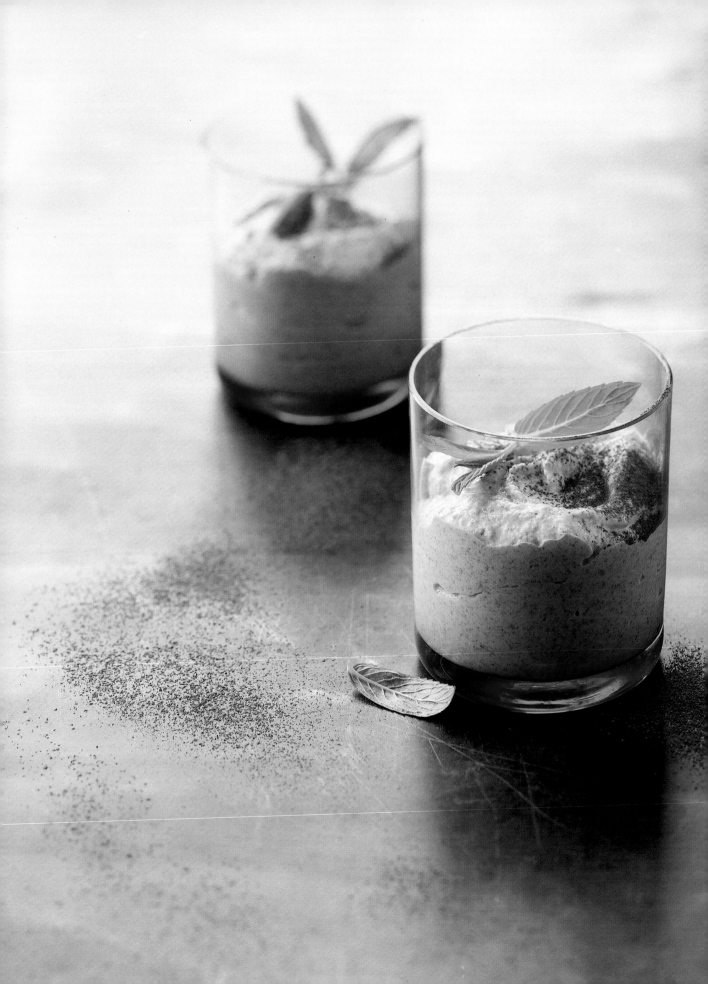

UNITS PER SERVE
Breads, cereals, legumes,
starchy vegetables **1**
Dairy **1**
Healthy fats **1.5**

1¼ cups (110 g) raw (natural)
    rolled oats
40 g raw almonds
1 tablespoon chia seeds
1 teaspoon natural vanilla bean paste
200 ml skim milk
300 g low-fat Greek-style yoghurt
ground cinnamon, for sprinkling
mint leaves (optional), to serve

Vanilla and chia seed oat smoothie shots

🍴 **Serves 4**   🕐 **Preparation: 10 minutes, plus refrigerating time**
〰 **Cooking: nil**

Combine the oats, almonds, chia seeds, vanilla and milk in a medium bowl. Cover and refrigerate for a minimum of 1 hour, or even overnight.

Spoon the oat mixture into a blender, add the yoghurt and blend until smooth. (Add a little cold water to thin the mixture, if desired.)

Pour into small serving glasses, sprinkle with cinnamon and scatter with mint leaves, if using. Serve immediately, with a spoon for scooping.

WEEKS 7–12 CARB EXTRAS

For an extra 10 g carbs per serve, add 240 g (60 g per person) blueberries to the blender.

Avocado and ricotta smash toast

16 G CARB PER SERVE

🍴 **Serves 4**   🕐 **Preparation: 15 minutes**
🍲 **Cooking: 15 minutes**

olive oil spray, for cooking
300 g flat mushrooms, stems trimmed, thickly sliced
200 g cherry tomatoes, halved
2 cloves garlic, thinly sliced
100 g baby spinach leaves
4 × 35 g slices mixed grain bread

AVOCADO AND RICOTTA SMASH

140 g avocado, chopped
220 g low-fat fresh ricotta, crumbled
small handful coriander leaves, roughly chopped
1 teaspoon lime juice, or to taste
3–4 drops Tabasco sauce (optional)

Lightly spray a large non-stick frying pan with olive oil and place over medium heat. Add the mushrooms and 1 tablespoon water and cook, covered, for 5 minutes or until the mushrooms start to lose their moisture, stirring occasionally. Remove the lid, add the tomatoes and garlic and cook, stirring occasionally, for 5 minutes or until the tomatoes start to collapse. Stir in the spinach and cook for 30 seconds or until the spinach is wilted.

Meanwhile, to make the avocado and ricotta smash, mash the avocado with a fork, leaving some texture. Gently mix in the ricotta, coriander, lime juice and Tabasco (if using). Season to taste with freshly ground black pepper.

Toast the bread and top with the avocado smash and mushroom mixture and serve immediately.

UNITS PER SERVE

Breads, cereals, legumes, starchy vegetables **1**
Dairy **1**
Low-carb vegetables **1**
Healthy fats **2**

Ricotta toast and sweet spiced nuts

15 G CARB PER SERVE

🍴 **Serves 4**   🕐 **Preparation: 5 minutes**
🍲 **Cooking: 2 minutes**

220 g low-fat fresh ricotta or cottage cheese
small handful mint leaves, shredded,
    plus extra leaves to serve
finely grated zest of ½ lemon
4 × 35 g slices mixed grain bread
¼ cup (40 g) Sweet Spiced Nut Clusters
    (see page 259)

Place the ricotta or cottage cheese, shredded mint and lemon zest in a bowl and mash together gently with a fork, retaining some texture in the cheese.

Toast the bread and top each piece with one-quarter of the minty ricotta.

Scatter evenly with the sweet spiced nuts and a few extra mint leaves and serve.

UNITS PER SERVE

Breads, cereals, legumes, starchy vegetables **1**
Dairy **1**
Healthy fats **1**

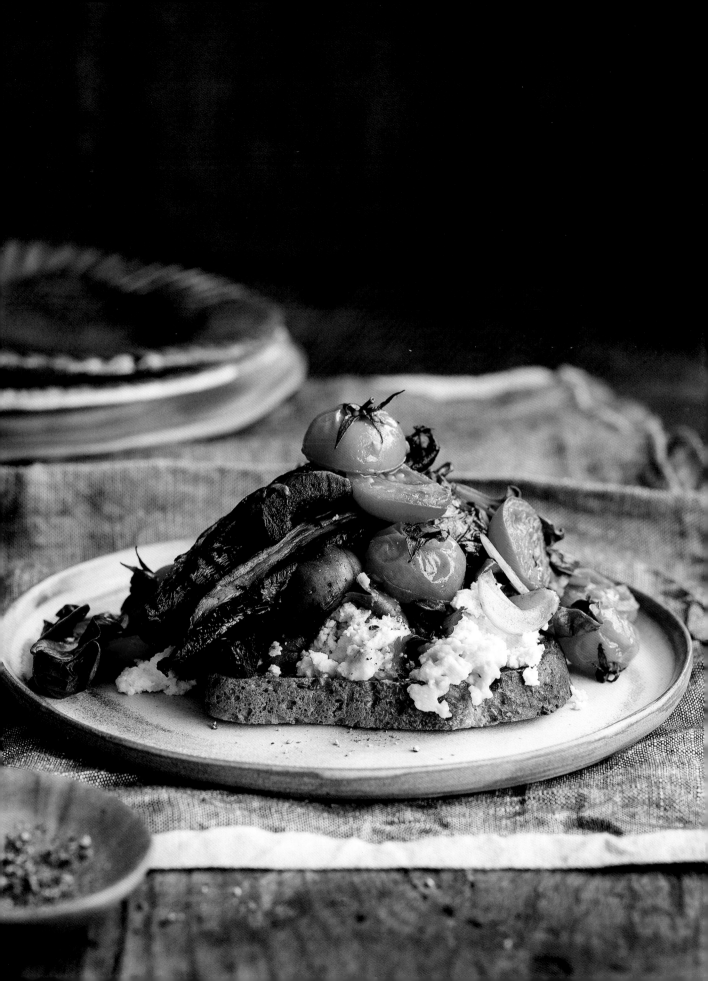

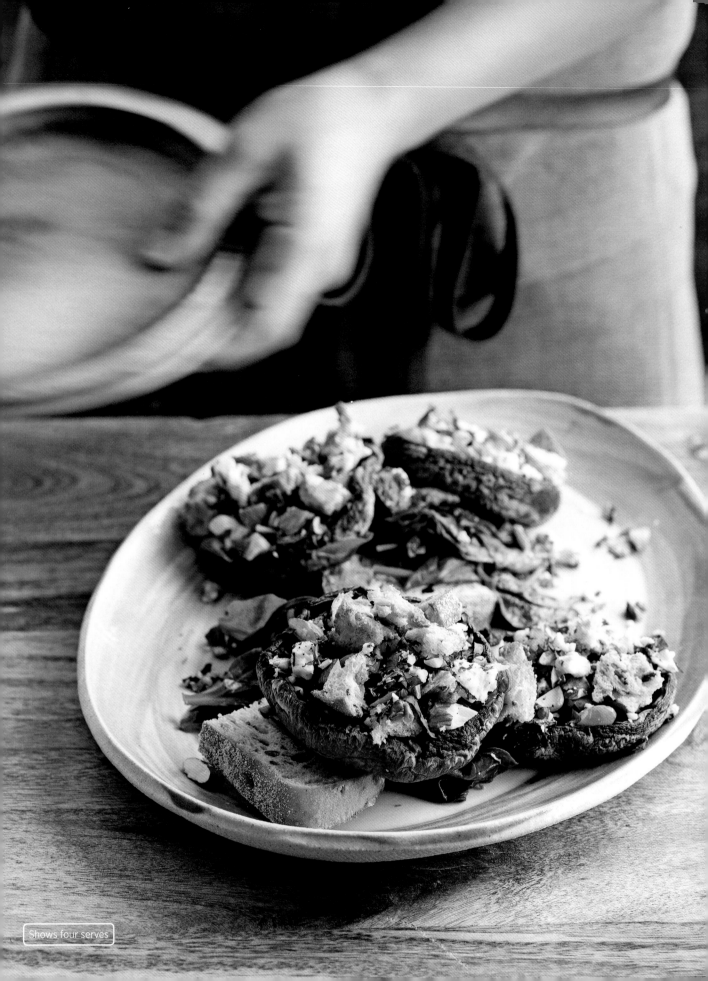

Shows four serves

Breads, cereals, legumes,
starchy vegetables **1**
Dairy **1**
Low-carb vegetables **1**
Healthy fats **1.5**

Mushrooms with feta croutons

15 G
CARB
PER
SERVE

🍴 Serves 4   🕐 Preparation: 15 minutes   ♨ Cooking: 25 minutes

4 large portobello or 8 medium
   mushrooms (about 400 g),
   stems trimmed
3 cloves garlic, 2 very thinly sliced,
   1 halved lengthways
4 sprigs lemon thyme, plus extra
   to serve
olive oil spray, for cooking
4 x 35 g slices mixed grain bread
   (preferably sourdough)
80 g salt-reduced low-fat feta,
   crumbled
60 g raw almonds,
   roughly chopped
small handful flat-leaf parsley,
   roughly chopped
160 g baby spinach leaves

Preheat the oven to 200°C (180°C fan-forced) and line a baking tray with baking paper.

Put the mushrooms, cup side up, in a large baking dish. Scatter over the sliced garlic and the thyme and spray lightly with olive oil. Season with freshly ground black pepper. Roast on the bottom shelf of the oven for 15–20 minutes or until tender.

Meanwhile, rub two of the bread slices on both sides with the halved garlic clove. Roughly tear up the bread, including the crusts, into chunky croutons. Spray lightly with olive oil and spread over the prepared tray in a single layer. Place on the top shelf of the oven and bake for 10–12 minutes, stirring after 8 minutes, until lightly browned and crisp. Remove from the oven and transfer to a large bowl. Add the feta, almonds and parsley, and toss to combine.

Remove the mushrooms from the oven and discard the thyme sprigs. Scatter the crouton mixture over the mushrooms, then return to the oven and roast for 5 minutes or until the feta just starts to melt.

While the mushroom mixture is roasting, add the spinach to a large saucepan with 1 tablespoon water and cook over medium heat for 1–2 minutes or until wilted, turning the spinach occasionally.

Toast the remaining 2 bread slices and cut them in half. Place the mushrooms, feta croutons, wilted spinach and toast halves on a large platter, scatter with extra thyme and serve.

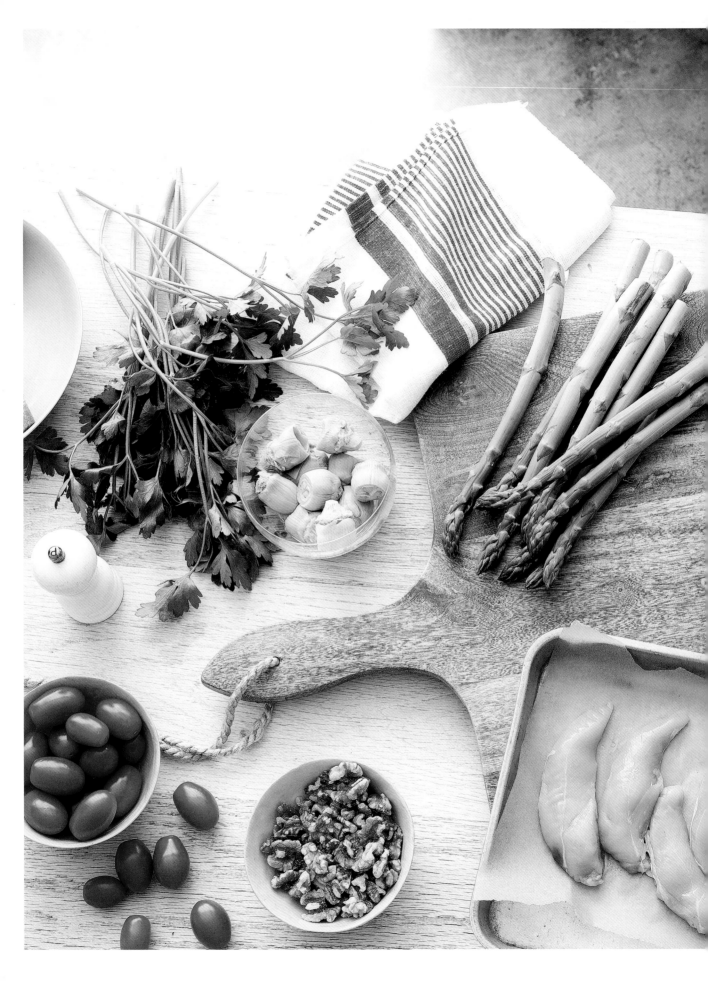

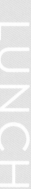

Chicken and asparagus salad, see page 154

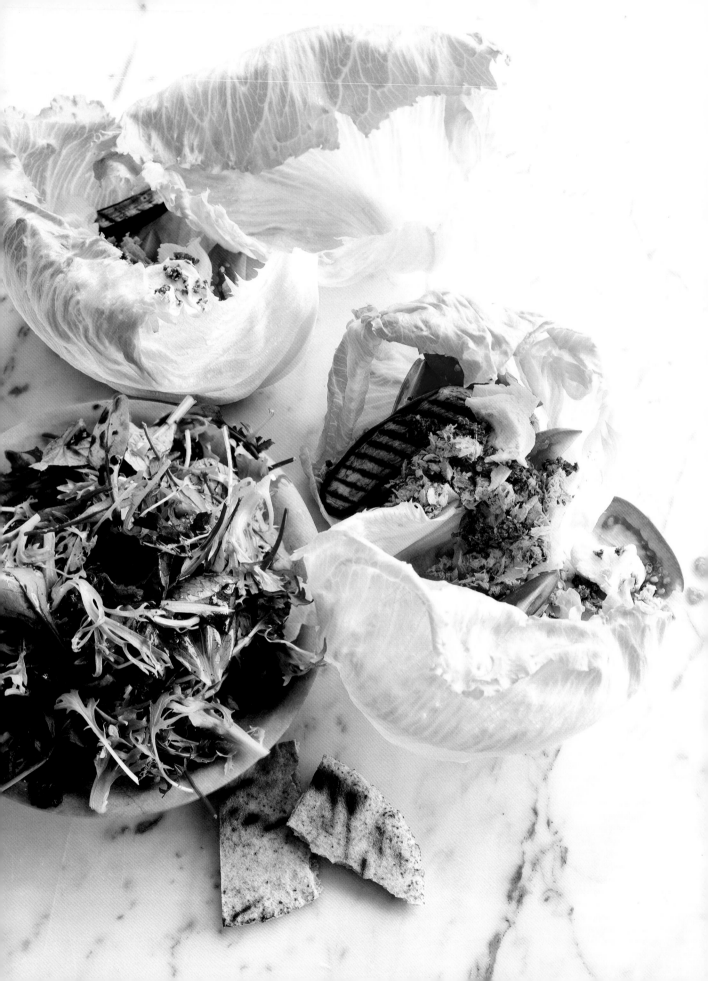

UNITS PER SERVE

Lean meat, fish, poultry, eggs, tofu **1**
Breads, cereals, legumes,
starchy vegetables **0.5**
Dairy **1**
Low-carb vegetables **2**
Mod-carb vegetables **1**
Healthy fats **4**

olive oil spray, for cooking
2 slender eggplants, halved
  lengthways and then halved
  again to give 8 pieces
1 wholemeal pita bread,
  cut into wedges
400 g tinned tuna in springwater,
  drained
2 tablespoons roughly chopped
  flat-leaf parsley
1 tablespoon tahini
40 g blanched almonds,
  finely chopped
16 inner iceberg lettuce leaves,
  trimmed to form cups
6 tomatoes, sliced
1 quantity Pesto (see page 114)
60 g bocconcini, sliced
400 g mixed salad leaves
1 teaspoon extra virgin olive oil
1 teaspoon white balsamic vinegar

Tuna and bocconcini lettuce cups

18 G
CARB
PER
SERVE

🍽 **Serves 4**   🕐 **Preparation: 20 minutes**   ◉ **Cooking: 15 minutes**

Heat a chargrill pan over medium heat and spray with olive oil. Spray the eggplant with oil, then add to the pan and chargrill for 2–3 minutes on each side or until tender and grill marks appear. Set aside. Spray the pita wedges with oil and grill for 2–3 minutes on each side or until golden and crisp. Set aside.

Place the tuna, parsley, tahini and blanched almonds in a bowl and mix to combine.

Place eight of the iceberg leaves on a chopping board and spoon one-eighth of the tuna mixture into each leaf. Top evenly with the grilled eggplant, tomato, pesto and bocconcini, then finish with the remaining iceberg leaves to form 8 'sandwiches'.

Place the mixed salad leaves in a bowl, then drizzle in the olive oil and balsamic vinegar and toss gently to combine. Divide the 'sandwiches', salad and pita triangles evenly among four plates and serve.

> **WEEKS 7–12 CARB EXTRAS**
>
> For an extra 10 g carbs per serve, add 200 g (50 g per person) drained and rinsed tinned salt-reduced cannellini beans to the salad before dressing.

Note: 1 x 400 g tin salt-reduced cannellini beans drained and rinsed will yield 240 g beans.

UNITS PER SERVE

Lean meat, fish, poultry, eggs, tofu **1**
Breads, cereals, legumes,
starchy vegetables **0.5**
Dairy **1**
Low-carb vegetables **2**
Healthy fats **3**

---

220 g low-fat cottage cheese
400 g tinned salmon, drained, skin
   and bones removed, flesh flaked
40 g pecans or walnuts, finely chopped
2 tablespoons finely chopped basil
finely grated zest of ½ lemon
4 large Lebanese cucumbers
   (170 g each) or 2 telegraph
   cucumbers, ends trimmed, if desired
2 x 35 g slices mixed grain bread
300 g mixed salad leaves
300 g cherry or grape tomatoes, halved
1 tablespoon extra virgin olive oil
2 teaspoons lemon juice
80 g avocado, sliced or diced

Cucumber and salmon 'sandwiches'

15 G CARB PER SERVE

🍴 **Serves 4**   🕐 **Preparation: 25 minutes**   ⊛ **Cooking: nil**

Place the cottage cheese, salmon, pecans, basil and lemon zest in a bowl, season with freshly ground black pepper and stir to combine.

If desired, peel strips of skin from the cucumbers, leaving some skin intact, then cut a thin slice lengthways from one side to form a stable base, if necessary. Cut the cucumbers in half lengthways, then, using a teaspoon, scrape out the seeds, leaving at least a 5 mm thick layer of the flesh intact, to form a hollow. (If using telegraph cucumbers, cut them in half widthways first.)

Toast the bread and cut into quarters, then into small cubes.

Divide the salmon mixture evenly among half of the hollowed cucumber lengths, then top with the remaining cucumber lengths to form 'sandwiches'. (Alternatively, divide the filling among the hollowed cucumber pieces and serve as open 'sandwiches'.)

Place the salad leaves and tomato in a bowl, then drizzle with the olive oil and lemon juice and toss to coat.

Arrange the cucumber 'sandwiches', salad, toasted bread cubes and avocado on a large serving platter. Season with freshly ground black pepper and serve.

WEEKS 7–12 CARB EXTRAS

For an extra 10 g carbs per serve, add 320 g (80 g per person) drained tinned lentils or 120 g (40 g per person) cooked corn kernels to the salad before dressing.

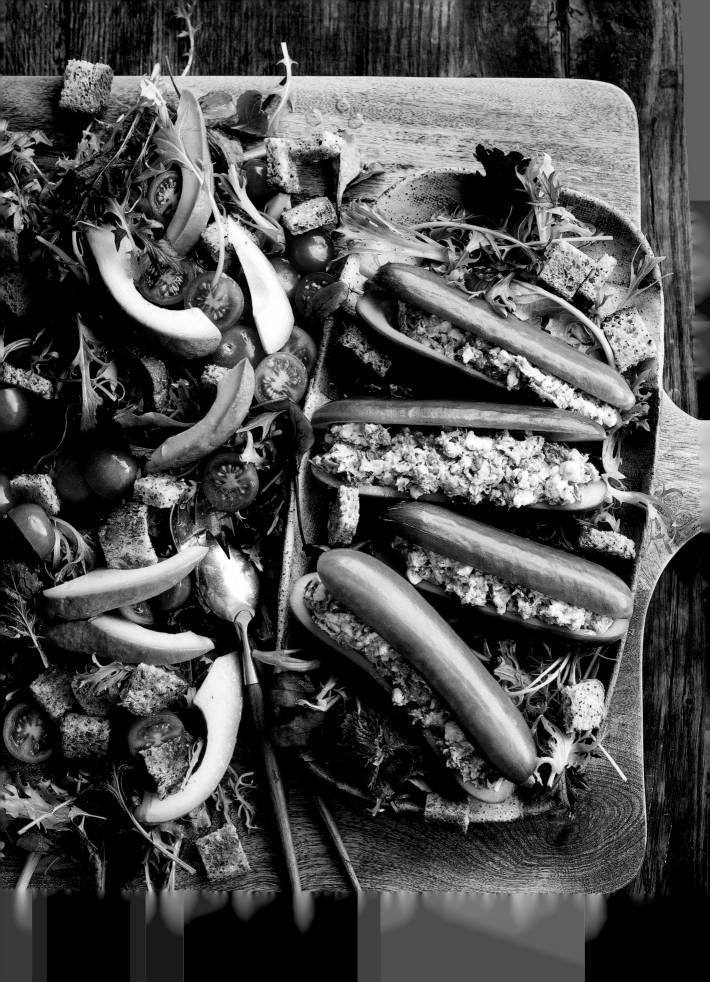

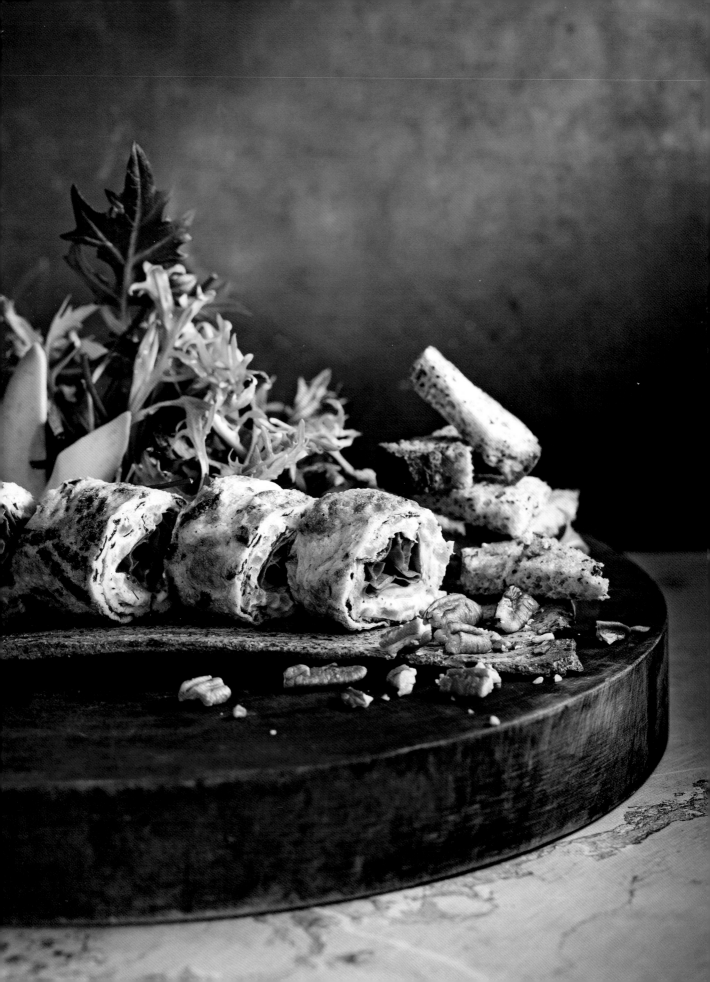

UNITS PER SERVE

Lean meat, fish, poultry, eggs, tofu **1**
Breads, cereals, legumes,
starchy vegetables **0.5**
Dairy **1**
Low-carb vegetables **2**
Healthy fats **4**

---

100 g smoked salmon,
   roughly chopped
100 g low-fat cream cheese
1 tablespoon chopped dill
finely grated zest of ½ lemon
6 eggs
2 tablespoons buttermilk
2 sheets nori, quartered lengthways
   then cut widthways into thin strips
2 teaspoons salt-reduced soy sauce
1 tablespoon olive oil
200 g rocket leaves
2 Lebanese cucumbers,
   shaved into ribbons
350 g mixed salad leaves
1 tablespoon extra virgin olive oil
2 teaspoons lemon juice
40 g pecans or walnuts
80 g avocado, diced
2 x 35 g slices mixed grain bread

Nori omelette rolls with smoked salmon

🍴 Serves 4   🕐 Preparation: 20 minutes   ♨ Cooking: 10 minutes

Place the smoked salmon, cream cheese, dill and lemon zest in a small food processor and pulse until the salmon is finely chopped and the mixture has combined to form a spread; take care not to over-process as you want the salmon to still have some texture. Set aside.

Break the eggs into a measuring jug and whisk to break the yolks, then whisk in the buttermilk. Add the nori and soy sauce and gently whisk to combine.

Heat a 24 cm, heavy-based non-stick frying pan over medium–high heat and add 1 teaspoon of the olive oil. Pour in one-quarter of the egg mixture and cook, gently tilting the pan to cover the base with an even layer. As the omelette sets, use a spatula to gently lift and stir, allowing any uncooked egg to run underneath. Cook for 1–2 minutes or until the egg is set. Carefully turn and cook the other side for 30 seconds or until light golden. Transfer to a serving plate and repeat with the remaining oil and egg mixture to cook 4 omelettes in all.

Gently spread one-quarter of the salmon mixture over each omelette. Top with the rocket and cucumber and roll the omelette over to enclose the filling (it should look like sushi). Cut into rounds and transfer to a plate or board.

Place the salad leaves in a bowl and drizzle with the olive oil and lemon juice, then toss gently to coat. Divide the salad evenly among the plates and scatter evenly with the pecans and avocado. Toast the bread and serve ½ a slice per person, cut into pieces.

> ### WEEKS 7–12 CARB EXTRAS
>
> For an extra 10 g carbs per serve, add 160 g (40 g per person) drained and rinsed tinned salt-reduced chickpeas to the salad before dressing.

 12 G CARB PER SERVE

Lean meat, fish, poultry, eggs, tofu **1**
Dairy **1**
Low-carb vegetables **3**
Healthy fats **2**

Mushroom and spiced chicken 'burgers'

4 G
CARB
PER
SERVE

🍴 **Serves 4**   🕐 **Preparation: 15 minutes**   🍲 **Cooking: 25 minutes**

8 large portobello mushrooms
   (about 800 g), stems trimmed
olive oil spray, for cooking
2 × 200 g chicken breast fillets
1 teaspoon sweet smoked paprika
2 teaspoons olive oil
1 small onion, thinly sliced
2 cloves garlic, thinly sliced
75 g baby rocket leaves
40 g pecans or walnuts,
   roughly chopped
2 tomatoes, thickly sliced
80 g thinly sliced Swiss cheese
20 g flaked almonds, toasted

Preheat a barbecue grill, chargrill pan or heavy-based frying pan over medium heat. Spray the mushrooms lightly with olive oil and cook, cup-side down, for 5 minutes. Turn and cook for a further 3–5 minutes or until tender. Transfer to a plate and cover with foil to keep warm.

Halve the chicken breast fillets horizontally to give 4 × 100 g thin pieces and sprinkle with the paprika.

Spray the chicken with olive oil, add to the pan and cook for 3–4 minutes each side or until just cooked through. (You can cook the mushrooms and chicken at the same time if you have a pan large enough.)

Meanwhile, heat the 2 teaspoons olive oil in a heavy-based frying pan or on a barbecue flat plate over medium heat. Add the onion and garlic and cook, stirring occasionally, for 5–6 minutes or until softened.

To assemble the burgers, place four mushroom 'buns', cup side up, on serving plates. Top evenly with the rocket, pecans and sliced tomato, then add the grilled chicken, cheese and the onion mixture. Sandwich together with the remaining mushrooms. Insert a skewer through the burgers to keep them standing tall if you like, then scatter over the flaked almonds and serve immediately.

> **WEEKS 7–12 CARB EXTRAS**
>
> For an extra 10 g carbs per serve, accompany the burgers with 200 g salt-reduced baked beans (50 g per person).

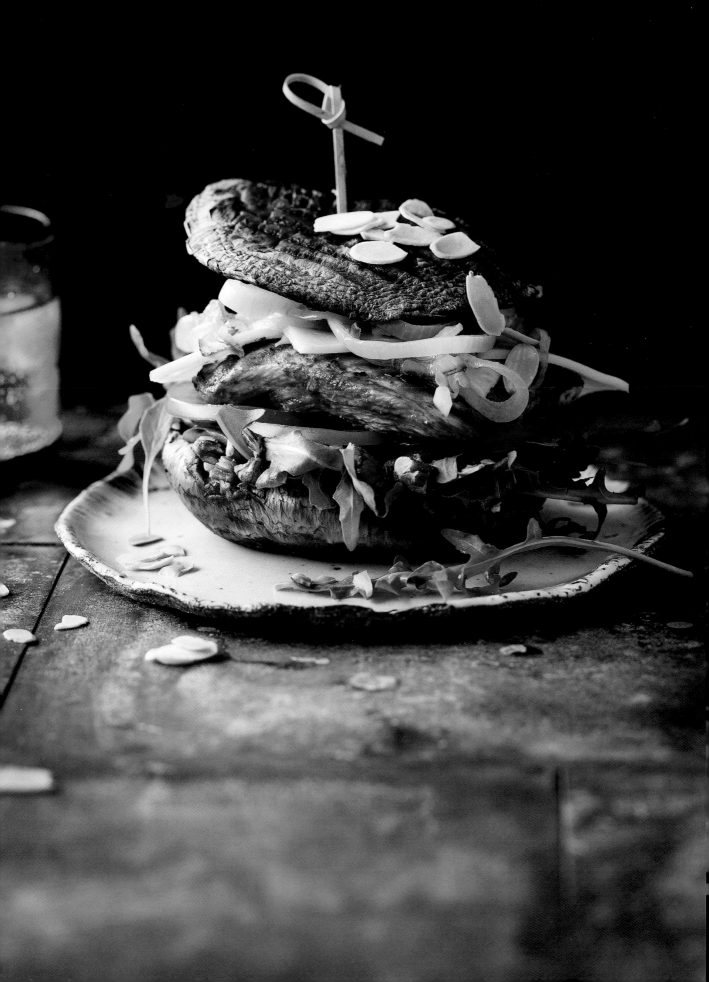

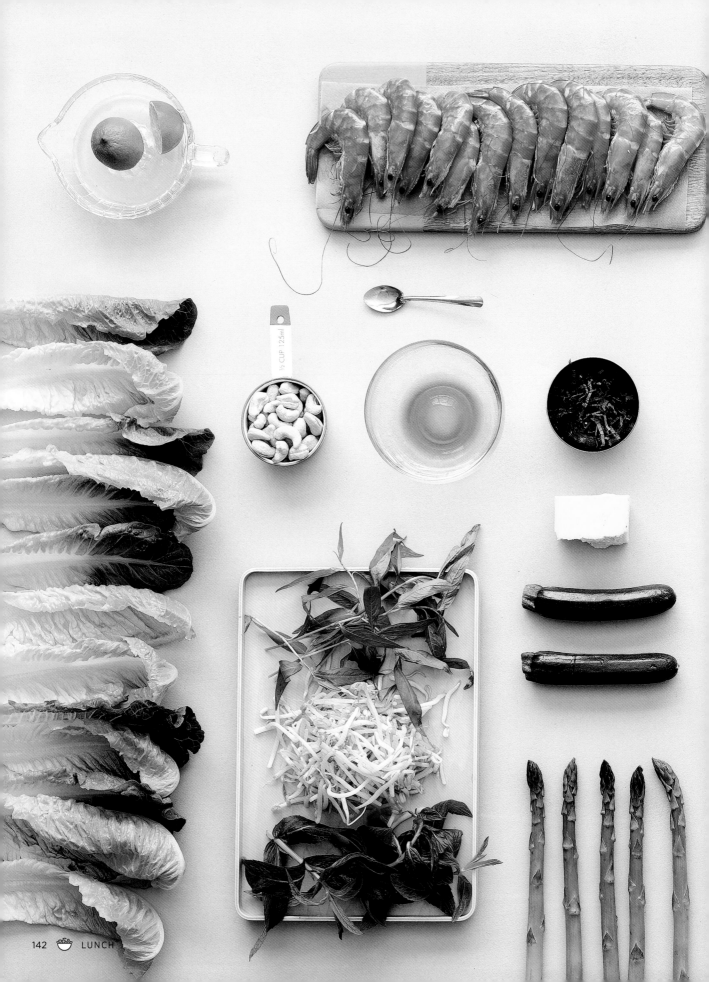

UNITS PER SERVE
Lean meat, fish, poultry, eggs, tofu **1**
Dairy **1**
Low-carb vegetables **2**
Healthy fats **2**

Prawn no-rice paper rolls

9 G CARB PER SERVE

🍴 Serves 4   ⏱ Preparation: 20 minutes   🍳 Cooking: nil

2 tablespoons lime or lemon juice
1 tablespoon fish sauce
½ teaspoon sesame oil
1 tablespoon finely shredded mint
   leaves, plus 1 handful extra leaves
300 g (12–16) cos lettuce leaves
400 g cooked, peeled and
   cleaned medium king prawns
   (weight after peeling)
80 g cheddar, grated
80 g raw unsalted cashews
   or raw almonds, roughly chopped
2 bunches asparagus, trimmed and
   thinly sliced or shaved lengthways
3 zucchini, spiralised
2 cups (160 g) bean sprouts
small handful Vietnamese mint leaves

Combine the lime or lemon juice, fish sauce, sesame oil, 1 tablespoon water and the shredded mint in a small serving dish.

Arrange the lettuce leaves on a platter or divide evenly among four serving plates, along with the prawns, cheese, nuts, asparagus, zucchini, bean sprouts and both types of mint. Serve the sauce alongside. Pile the fillings onto the lettuce leaves, drizzle with a little sauce and roll up to enclose the filling.

WEEKS 7–12 CARB EXTRAS

For an extra 10 g carbs per serve, add 160 g (40 g per person) drained and rinsed tinned salt-reduced chickpeas to the filling ingredients.

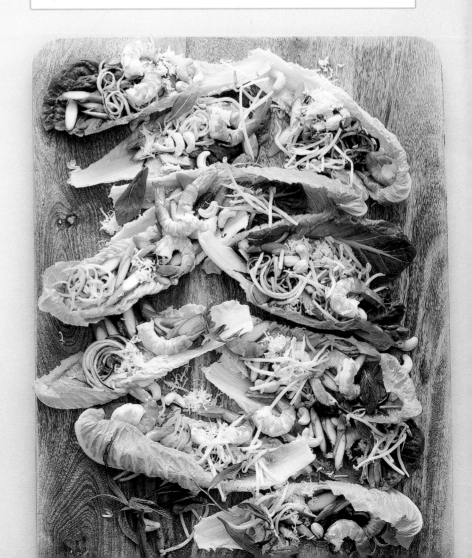

Shows four serves

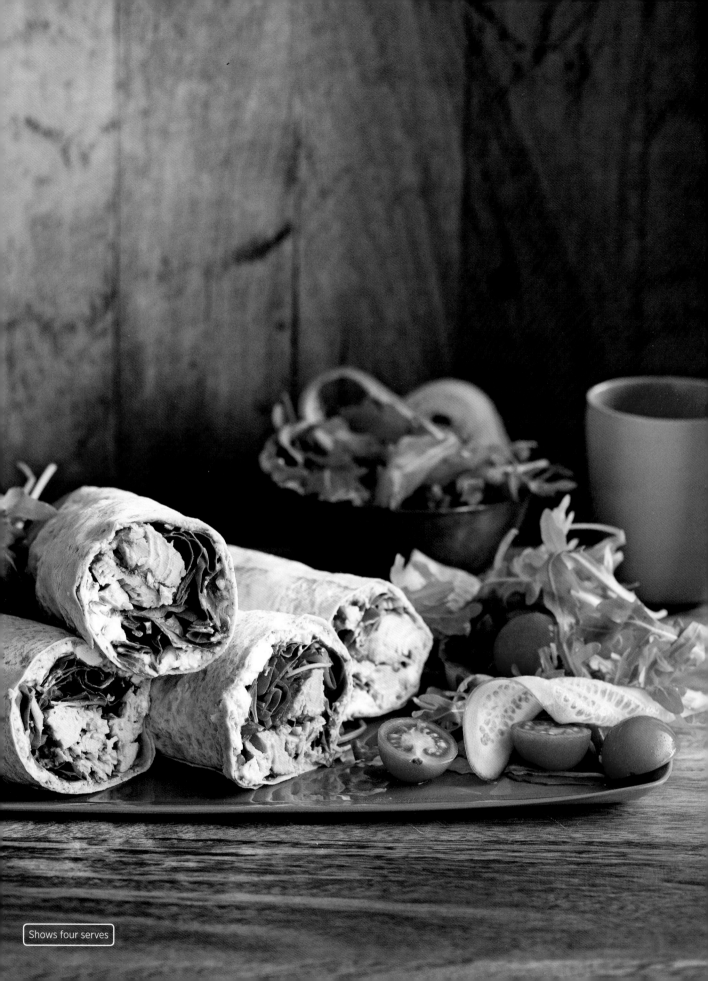

Shows four serves

UNITS PER SERVE

Lean meat, fish, poultry, eggs, tofu **1**
Breads, cereals, legumes,
starchy vegetables **0.5**
Dairy **1**
Low-carb vegetables **2**
Healthy fats **2**

---

2 pieces mountain bread
   (or 2 slices Herman Brot bread)
220 g low-fat cottage cheese or
   low-fat fresh ricotta
400 g tinned salmon, drained, skin
   and bones removed, flesh flaked
200 g baby rocket leaves
2 Lebanese cucumbers, thinly sliced
   lengthways into ribbons or chopped
300 g cherry tomatoes, halved

BROCCOLI PESTO

150 g broccoli florets
40 g pecans or walnuts
80 g avocado
2 teaspoons lemon juice

Salmon and broccoli pesto wraps

13 G CARB PER SERVE

🍴 **Serves 4**　🕐 **Preparation: 15 minutes**　🍳 **Cooking: 5 minutes**

To make the broccoli pesto, steam the broccoli in a steamer basket over a saucepan of simmering water for 3 minutes or until tender but still crisp. Set aside to cool. Place the pecans in a food processor and pulse until the nuts are roughly chopped. Add the cooled broccoli and pulse until finely chopped and combined. Add the avocado and lemon juice and blend until just combined. Season with freshly ground white pepper.

Spread the pesto evenly down the centre of the wraps. Top with the cottage cheese or ricotta, the salmon and half of the rocket. Roll up to enclose the filling. Serve with the cucumber, tomatoes and remaining rocket alongside.

> **WEEKS 7-12 CARB EXTRAS**
>
> For an extra 10 g carbs per serve, add 160 g (40 g per person) drained and rinsed tinned salt-reduced chickpeas or kidney beans to the salad.

UNITS PER SERVE

Lean meat, fish, poultry, eggs, tofu **1**
Breads, cereals, legumes,
starchy vegetables **0.5**
Dairy **1**
Low-carb vegetables **3**
Healthy fats **3**

400 g chicken breast tenderloins
½ teaspoon dried oregano
juice of 1 lemon
2 teaspoons extra virgin olive oil
olive oil spray, for cooking
4 cups mixed salad greens
2 baby cos lettuces, bases trimmed
    and leaves halved lengthways or
    torn into bite-sized pieces
1 Lebanese cucumber,
    quartered lengthways
1 × 340 g jar marinated artichoke
    hearts, drained
60 g salt-reduced low-fat feta,
    cut into small dice
⅓ cup (80 g) hummus
1 wholemeal pita bread, cut into
    eight wedges
1 quantity (80 g) Spiced Nut Sprinkle
    (see page 120)

TZATZIKI

1 Lebanese cucumber, coarsely
    grated, then squeezed to
    remove excess liquid
⅓ cup (95 g) low-fat
    Greek-style yoghurt
1 small clove garlic, finely chopped
2 teaspoons lemon juice, or to taste
1 teaspoon finely grated lemon zest
1 tablespoon thinly sliced mint
2 teaspoons finely chopped dill

Chicken salad
with tzatziki

19 G CARB PER SERVE

🍴 Serves 4
🕐 Preparation: 20 minutes, plus marinating and cooling time
♨ Cooking: 15 minutes

Place the chicken in a shallow bowl, then mix the oregano, lemon juice and extra virgin olive oil and pour over the chicken. Season with freshly ground black pepper, then turn to coat. Cover with plastic film and marinate for 10 minutes at room temperature or in the refrigerator for up to 30 minutes.

Meanwhile, to make the tzatziki dressing, place all the ingredients in a small bowl and whisk to combine, then season to taste with pepper. Cover with plastic film and refrigerate until required.

Heat a chargrill pan over medium heat and spray with olive oil. Chargrill the chicken tenderloins for 6 minutes on each side or until cooked through. Transfer to a chopping board and, when cool enough to handle, thinly slice on the diagonal (or leave them whole if you prefer).

Meanwhile, place the salad leaves, cucumber, artichokes and feta in a bowl and toss gently to combine. Spread the hummus evenly over the pita bread, then scatter with the nut sprinkle.

Divide the salad and chicken evenly among four plates or shallow bowls. Spoon one-quarter of the tzatziki dressing over each plate and serve with the pita bread.

WEEKS 7–12 CARB EXTRAS

For an extra 10 g carbs per serve, add 160 g (40 g per person) drained and rinsed tinned salt-reduced chickpeas to the salad.

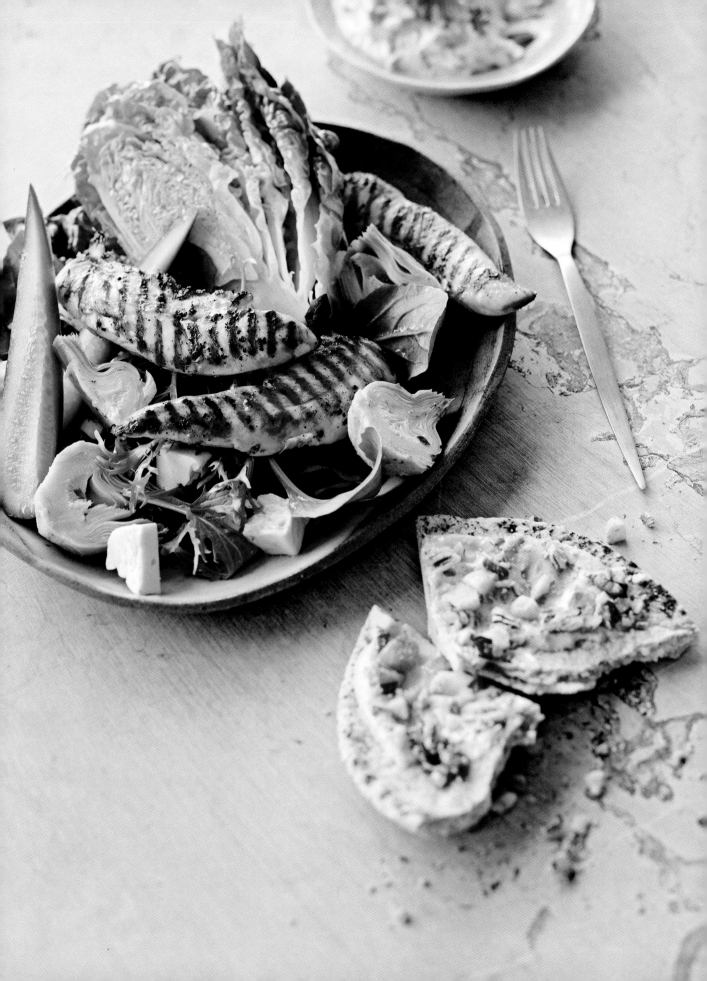

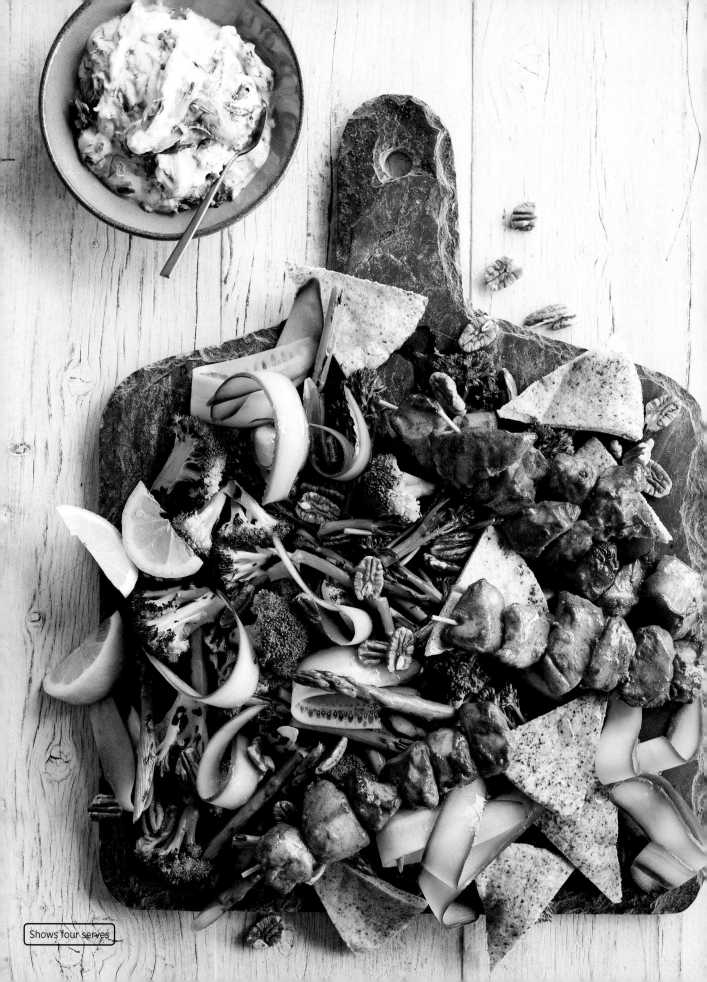

Shows four serves

Lean meat, fish, poultry, eggs, tofu **1**
Breads, cereals, legumes,
starchy vegetables **0.5**
Dairy **1**
Low-carb vegetables **2.5**
Healthy fats **2.5**

olive oil spray, for cooking
300 g broccoli, cut into small florets
1 bunch broccolini, trimmed and halved
1 bunch asparagus, trimmed and halved
2 cups spinach leaves, trimmed
2 Lebanese cucumbers, peeled
 into ribbons
40 g pecans or walnuts,
 roughly chopped
1 tablespoon extra virgin olive oil
2 teaspoons lemon juice
1 small wholemeal pita bread,
 cut into 8 wedges
lemon wedges, to serve

TANDOORI CHICKEN

220 g low-fat Greek-style yoghurt
1 clove garlic, finely chopped
1 × 2 cm piece ginger, peeled and
 finely grated
1 tablespoon lemon juice
1 × 50 g sachet salt-reduced
 tomato paste
1½ teaspoons garam masala
1½ teaspoons ground coriander
1 teaspoon sweet paprika
1 teaspoon hot paprika or chilli powder
½ teaspoon ground turmeric
400 g chicken breast fillets, cut into
 2 cm cubes
olive oil spray, for cooking

SPICED RAITA

180 g low-fat Greek-style yoghurt
1 clove garlic, finely chopped
1 Lebanese cucumber, coarsely
 grated, then squeezed to
 remove excess liquid
3 tablespoons thinly sliced mint
2 tablespoons finely chopped
 coriander leaves
½ teaspoon garam masala

Tandoori chicken with grilled vegetable salad

20 G CARB PER SERVE

🍴 **Serves 4**   🕐 **Preparation: 30 minutes, plus marinating time**
🍲 **Cooking: 25 minutes**

To make the tandoori chicken, place the yoghurt, garlic, ginger, lemon juice, tomato paste, garam masala, coriander, sweet paprika, hot paprika or chilli powder and turmeric in a small bowl and whisk to combine, then season to taste with freshly ground black pepper. Thread the chicken evenly onto the soaked skewers (see note), then place in a baking dish and add the tandoori paste, rubbing it in well to coat evenly. Cover with plastic film and marinate in the refrigerator for at least 30 minutes (or up to 3 hours).

Preheat the oven to 200°C (180°C fan-forced). Line a roasting tin with baking paper.

Place the chicken on a wire rack over the lined tin, spoon over any marinade remaining in the dish and roast, turning halfway through cooking, for 25 minutes or until cooked through and starting to crisp around the edges.

Meanwhile, to make the raita, place all the ingredients in a bowl and season to taste with pepper. Whisk to combine, cover with plastic film and refrigerate until required.

Heat a chargrill pan over medium heat and spray with olive oil. Working in batches, chargrill the broccoli and broccolini, turning occasionally, for 3–4 minutes or until tender and grill marks have appeared. Repeat with the asparagus, grilling for 2–3 minutes. Transfer to a large bowl and set aside until cool.

Add the spinach, cucumber and pecans to the broccoli mixture, drizzle with extra virgin olive oil and lemon juice and toss gently to coat.

Divide the salad and chicken evenly among four plates or pile onto a large serving platter, then serve with the raita, pita and lemon wedges to the side.

Note: You will need to soak eight long bamboo skewers in cold water for 30 minutes for this recipe.

UNITS PER SERVE

Lean meat, fish, poultry, eggs, tofu **1**
Breads, cereals, legumes,
starchy vegetables **0.5**
Dairy **1**
Low-carb vegetables **2**
Healthy fats **3**

---

4 cups mixed salad leaves
1 cup watercress sprigs
½ cup coriander leaves, torn
250 g grape or cherry tomatoes, halved
2 Lebanese cucumbers, cut into
    rounds or 1.5 cm dice
1 small red capsicum, seeded and
    thinly sliced
1½ teaspoons sweet paprika
1 teaspoon dried oregano
½ teaspoon ground allspice
30 g polenta
40 g raw almonds, coarsely crushed
400 g chicken breast fillets, cut
    into halves or thirds horizontally
    to form thin slices
olive oil spray, for cooking
1 tablespoon extra virgin olive oil
2 teaspoons lime juice
80 g avocado, sliced or cut into
    1.5 cm dice
80 g salt-reduced low-fat feta,
    crumbled or cut into 1.5 cm dice
lime wedges, to serve

Polenta-crusted chicken and avocado salad

16 G CARB PER SERVE

🍴 **Serves 4**   🕐 **Preparation: 25 minutes**   🍲 **Cooking: 15 minutes**

Place the salad leaves, watercress, coriander, tomatoes, cucumber and capsicum in a large bowl and toss to combine. Set aside.

Combine the paprika, oregano, allspice, polenta and almonds in a shallow bowl and season with freshly ground black pepper. Press the chicken pieces onto the spice mix to coat evenly.

Heat a heavy-based non-stick frying pan over medium heat and spray with olive oil. Pan-fry the chicken for 5–6 minutes on each side or until golden brown and cooked through.

Drizzle the salad with extra virgin olive oil and lime juice and gently toss to coat. Divide the salad and chicken evenly among four plates or pile onto a large platter and top with the avocado and feta. Serve with lime wedges to the side.

> **WEEKS 7–12 CARB EXTRAS**
>
> For an extra 10 g carbs per serve, add 160 g (40 g per person) cooked frozen or drained tinned salt-reduced corn kernels to the salad before dressing.

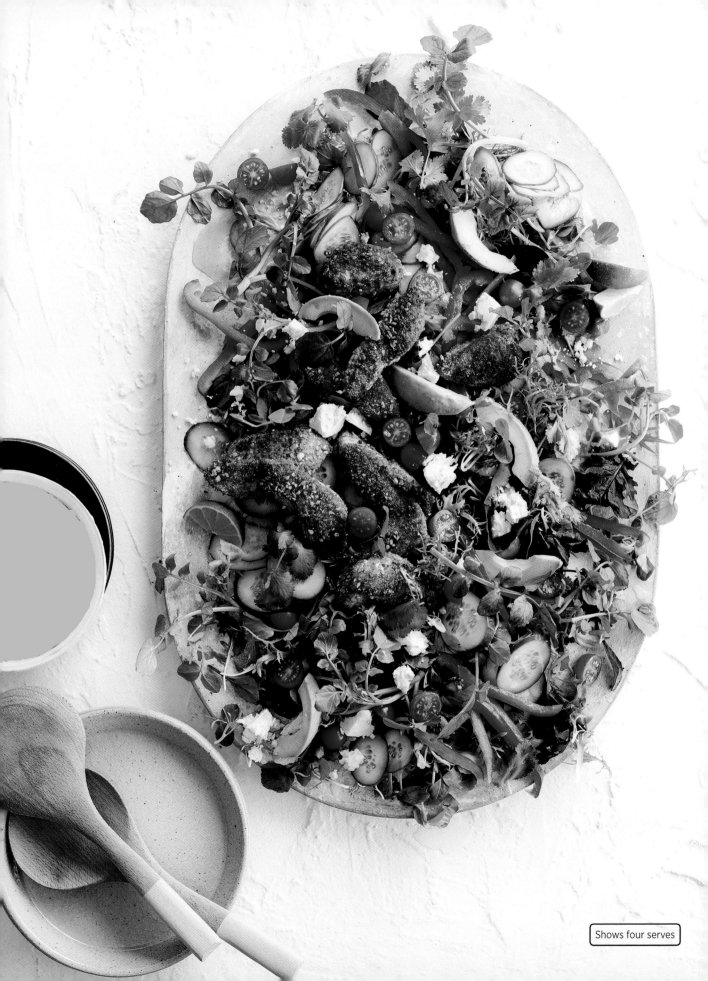

Shows four serves

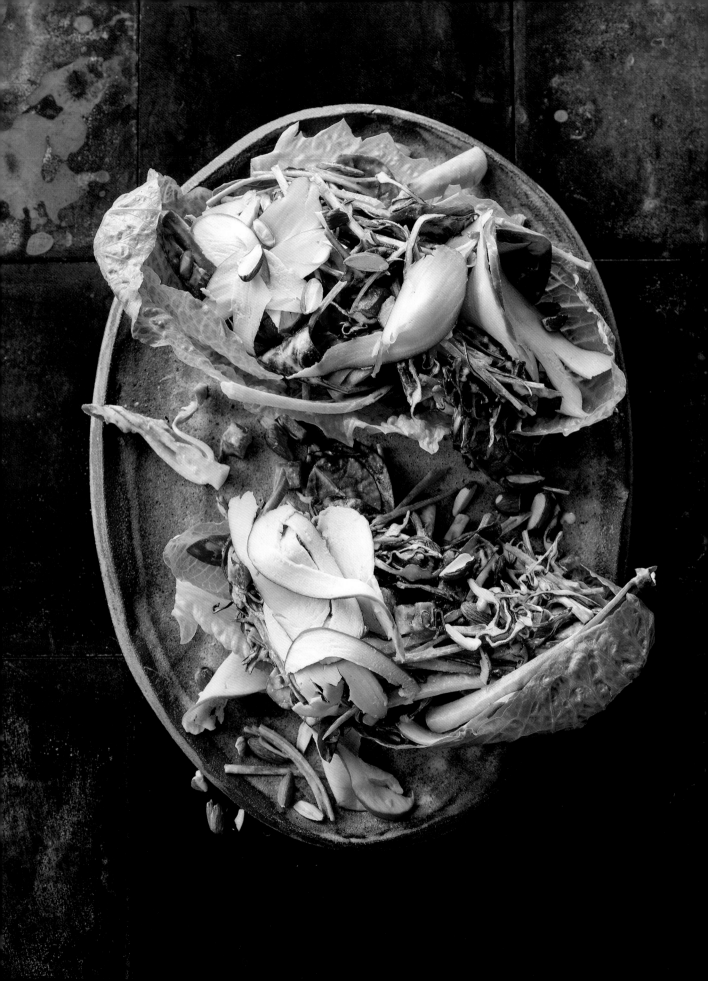

UNITS PER SERVE

Lean meat, fish, poultry, eggs, tofu **1**
Dairy **1**
Low-carb vegetables **1.5**
Mod-carb vegetables **0.5**
Healthy fats **2**

150 g finely shredded red cabbage
2 baby bok choy, shredded
1 large carrot, shredded
1 tomato, chopped
75 g baby spinach leaves, trimmed
300 g cos lettuce
400 g smoked chicken breast fillet,
    thinly sliced or shredded
40 g toasted or raw almonds,
    roughly chopped

CREAMY AVOCADO DRESSING

80 g avocado
110 g low-fat fresh ricotta
200 g low-fat Greek-style yoghurt
2 teaspoons lemon juice

Smoked chicken slaw with creamy avocado dressing

11 G CARB PER SERVE

🍽 Serves 4   🕐 Preparation: 20 minutes   🍚 Cooking: nil

To make the creamy avocado dressing, place all the ingredients in a food processor and pulse until combined and smooth. Season with freshly ground white pepper.

Combine the cabbage, bok choy, carrot, tomato and spinach in a large bowl. Add the avocado dressing and toss well to coat.

Divide the lettuce evenly among four bowls or place on a platter. Spoon the slaw and chicken on top and scatter over the almonds.

> **WEEKS 7–12 CARB EXTRAS**
>
> For an extra 10 g carbs per serve, add 200 g (50 g per person) drained and rinsed tinned salt-reduced cannellini beans to the salad.

Note: This dressing would make a great mayonnaise substitute.

QUICK TUNA SALAD FOR ONE

5 G CARB PER SERVE

Flake 1 small (95 g) drained tin of tuna in springwater into a salad bowl, then add 20 g salt-reduced low-fat feta and 300 g low-carb vegetables (such as leafy greens, rocket, cherry tomato, cucumber or steamed asparagus). Dress with 2 teaspoons of olive oil and 1 teaspoon of balsamic vinegar, lemon juice or apple cider vinegar and toss together gently.

UNITS PER SERVE

Lean meat, fish, poultry, eggs, tofu **1**
Dairy **1**
Low-carb vegetables **2**
Healthy fats **2**

EASY CHICKEN SALAD FOR ONE

5 G CARB PER SERVE

Shred 100 g poached chicken into a salad bowl, then add 25 g bocconcini and 300 g low-carb vegetables (such as leafy greens, rocket, cherry tomato, cucumber or steamed asparagus). Mix together 2 teaspoons of olive oil, 2 teaspoons of white wine vinegar and ½ teaspoon grain mustard, then use this to dress the salad.

UNITS PER SERVE

Lean meat, fish, poultry, eggs, tofu **1**
Dairy **1**
Low-carb vegetables **2**
Healthy fats **2**

Chicken and asparagus salad

4 G CARB PER SERVE

🍴 Serves 4

🕐 Preparation: 15 minutes, plus marinating and resting time

🍳 Cooking: 10 minutes

400 g chicken tenderloins

2 teaspoons lemon juice

1 clove garlic, crushed

2 bunches asparagus, trimmed

olive oil spray, for cooking

250 g marinated artichoke hearts from a jar, halved lengthways

300 g cherry or grape tomatoes, halved

200 g baby rocket leaves

40 g parmesan, shaved

WALNUT, HERB AND LEMON DRESSING

⅓ cup (40 g) finely chopped walnuts

2 tablespoons finely chopped flat-leaf parsley

1½ tablespoons olive oil

finely grated zest of 1 lemon

2 tablespoons lemon juice

Combine the chicken, lemon juice and garlic in a bowl and set aside to marinate for 10 minutes.

To make the walnut, herb and lemon dressing, place all the ingredients in a screw-top jar. Seal the jar and shake until combined. Season with freshly ground black pepper.

Thinly slice half a bunch of the asparagus on the diagonal and set aside in a large bowl.

Heat a chargrill pan or barbecue over medium–high heat. Drain the chicken, shaking off any excess marinade, and spray lightly all over with olive oil. Chargrill the chicken for 3 minutes, then turn and cook for a further 2–3 minutes or until cooked through. Transfer to a plate and set aside to rest.

Spray the artichoke hearts and remaining asparagus lightly with olive oil and chargrill for 3–4 minutes, turning occasionally until nicely charred. Cut the asparagus in half widthways. Add to the bowl with the raw asparagus, along with the artichokes and cherry or grape tomatoes. Pour over the dressing and toss to combine, then set aside for 5 minutes to allow the flavours to develop.

Add the rocket and toss until combined. Pile onto a serving platter or divide evenly among four bowls and top with the chicken and parmesan.

WEEKS 7–12 CARB EXTRAS

For an extra 10 g carbs per serve, add 160 g (40 g per person) drained and rinsed tinned salt-reduced chickpeas to the salad when you add the tomatoes and artichokes.

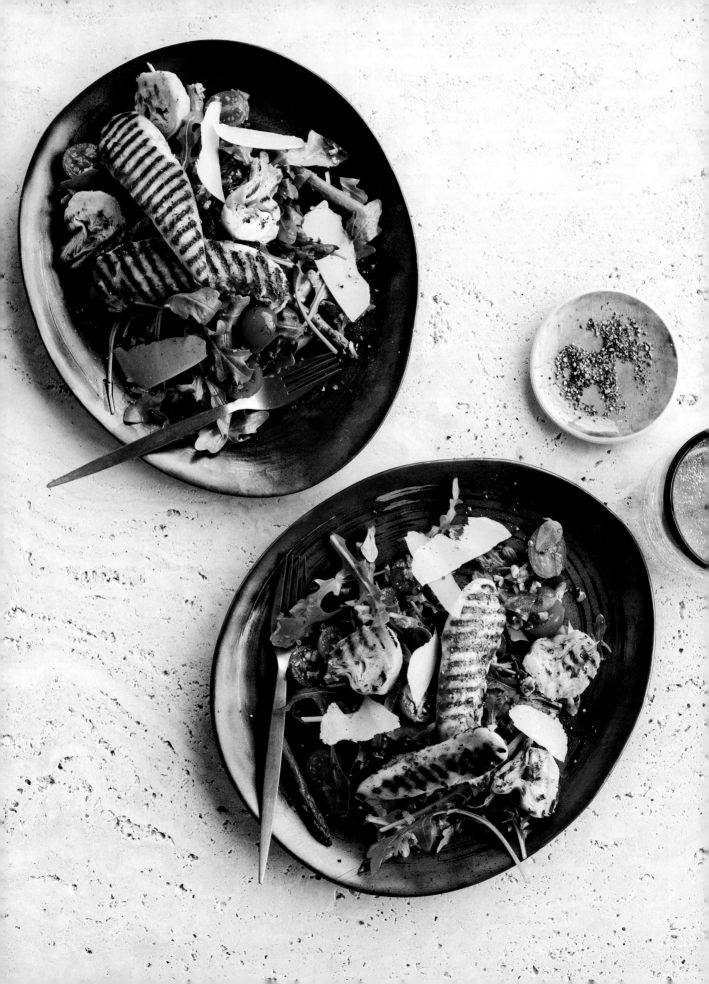

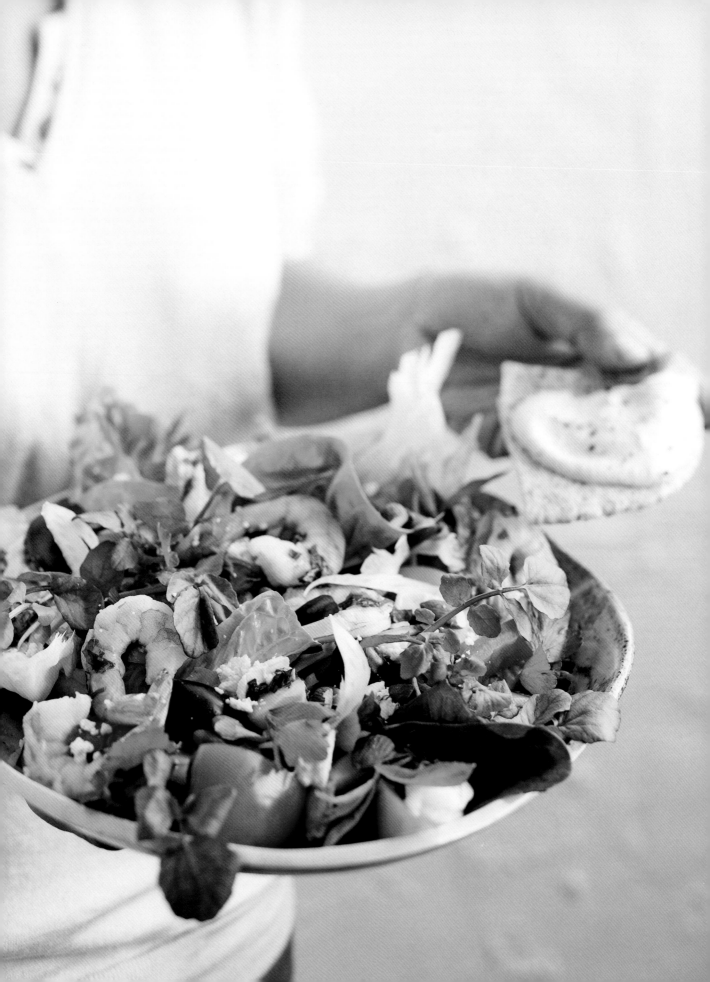

UNITS PER SERVE

Lean meat, fish, poultry, eggs, tofu **1**
Breads, cereals, legumes,
starchy vegetables **0.5**
Dairy **1**
Low-carb vegetables **3**
Mod-carb vegetables **0.5**
Healthy fats **4**

4 cups rocket leaves or watercress
   sprigs (or a mixture of both)
2 baby cos lettuces, trimmed and
   leaves separated
1 cup spinach leaves, trimmed
1 telegraph cucumber, halved
   lengthways and thickly sliced
   on the diagonal
5 tomatoes, halved widthways and
   cut into thin wedges
1 bulb baby fennel, trimmed, halved
   lengthways and thinly sliced
2 tablespoons small mint leaves
2 tablespoons flat-leaf parsley leaves
400 g cooked, peeled and cleaned
   king prawns, with tails intact
   (weight after peeling)
80 salt-reduced low-fat feta, sliced
12 kalamata olives
40 g raw almonds, roughly chopped
1 wholemeal pita bread
⅓ cup (80 g) hummus

SOFT-HERB DRESSING

1½ tablespoons extra virgin olive oil
2 teaspoons red wine vinegar
1 tablespoon finely chopped oregano
1 tablespoon finely chopped mint
1 tablespoon finely chopped basil

Greek salad with fennel and prawns

🍽 **Serves 4**   🕐 **Preparation: 25 minutes**   ♨ **Cooking: nil**

Place the rocket or watercress leaves, cos, spinach, cucumber,
tomato, fennel, mint and parsley in a bowl and toss gently to combine.

To make the dressing, place all the ingredients in a small bowl, season
to taste with freshly ground black pepper and whisk to combine.

Drizzle the dressing over the salad, then divide evenly among four
plates. Top with one-quarter each of the prawns, feta, olives and
almonds. Spread the pita bread with hummus, then cut into eight
wedges and place two wedges on each plate. Serve immediately.

WEEKS 7–12 CARB EXTRAS

For an extra 10 g carbs per serve, add 160 g (40 g per person)
drained and rinsed tinned salt-reduced chickpeas to the salad.

UNITS PER SERVE

Lean meat, fish, poultry, eggs, tofu **1**
Breads, cereals, legumes,
starchy vegetables **0.5**
Dairy **1**
Low-carb vegetables **2**
Healthy fats **2**

1 bunch asparagus, trimmed and
   thinly sliced on the diagonal
4 cups finely shredded inner
   iceberg lettuce leaves
1 cup rocket leaves
1 cup watercress sprigs
2 Lebanese cucumbers, peeled
   and shaved into ribbons with
   a vegetable peeler
400 g cooked, peeled and cleaned
   king or tiger prawns, with tails intact
   (weight after peeling)
160 g avocado, thinly sliced or diced
2 x 35 g slices mixed grain bread
110 g low-fat cottage cheese
2 teaspoons finely chopped
   flat-leaf parsley

**BUTTERMILK AND
YOGHURT DRESSING**

½ cup (125 ml) buttermilk
100 g low-fat Greek-style yoghurt
2½ tablespoons salt-reduced
   tomato passata
1½ teaspoons Worcestershire sauce
1–2 teaspoons lemon juice, to taste
Tabasco sauce, to taste

Prawn cocktail salad with buttermilk and yoghurt dressing

🍴 **Serves 4**   🕐 **Preparation: 20 minutes**   ♨ **Cooking: 3 minutes**

To make the dressing, place the buttermilk and yoghurt in a bowl and whisk to combine. Whisk in the passata, Worcestershire sauce, lemon juice and Tabasco to taste, then season to taste with freshly ground black pepper.

Steam the asparagus in a steamer basket over a saucepan of simmering water for 3 minutes or until just tender and still firm to the bite.

Place one-quarter of the iceberg lettuce in each of four bowls, then layer with the rocket, watercress, asparagus and cucumber. (Alternatively, place the iceberg, rocket, watercress, asparagus and cucumber in a bowl and toss gently to combine, then divide evenly among four bowls.) Spoon over a little of the dressing, then top each bowl with one-quarter of the prawns and avocado and spoon over the remaining dressing.

Toast the bread and mix the cottage cheese with the parsley. Spread the cottage cheese evenly over the toast, then cut in half and divide among the bowls. Serve immediately.

WEEKS 7–12 CARB EXTRAS

For an extra 10 g carbs per serve, cook 480 g (120 g per person) frozen peas in a saucepan of simmering water for 3 minutes or until tender, then drain, cool and add to the salad with the asparagus.

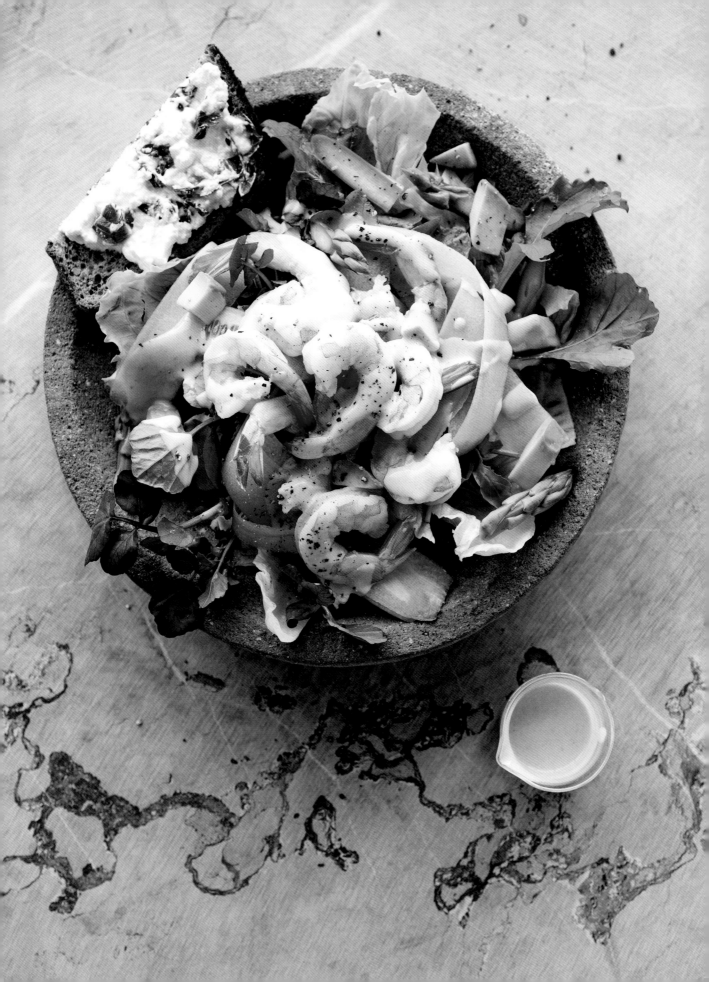

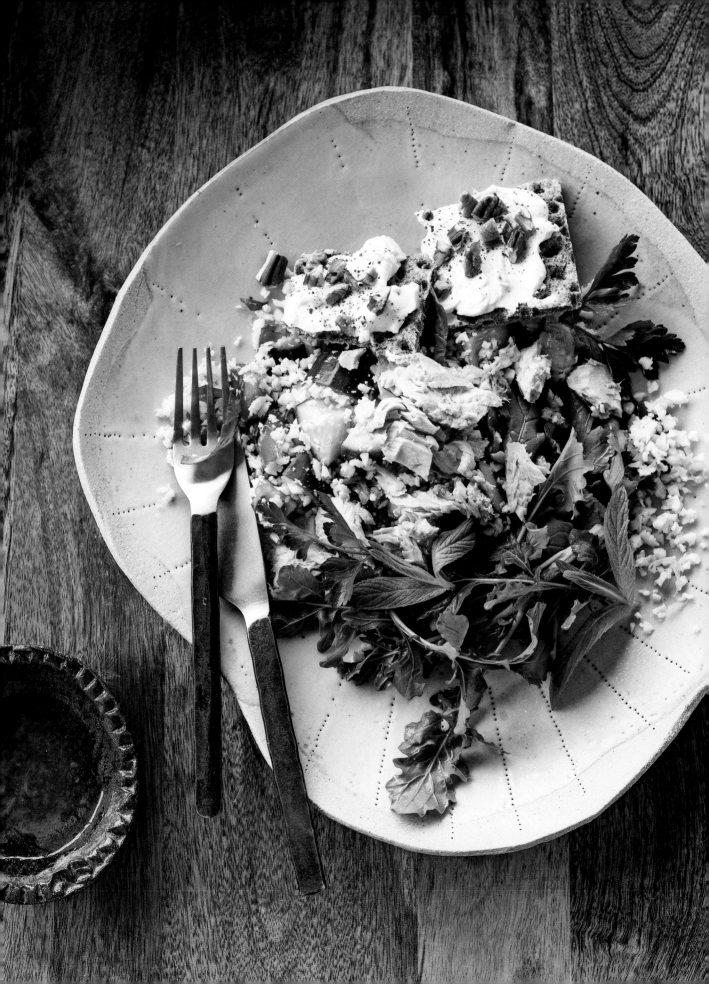

UNITS PER SERVE

Lean meat, fish, poultry, eggs, tofu **1**
Breads, cereals, legumes,
starchy vegetables **0.5**
Dairy **0.5**
Low-carb vegetables **1.5**
Mod-carb vegetables **0.5**
Healthy fats **2.5**

150 g cauliflower florets
150 g rocket leaves
3 tomatoes, chopped
2 Lebanese cucumbers (unpeeled),
   chopped
finely grated zest of 1 lemon
2 tablespoons lemon juice
1½ tablespoons extra virgin olive oil
100 g labne (see note) or plain yoghurt
4 wholegrain crispbreads (Ryvita)
½ teaspoon sumac
40 g pecans or walnuts,
   toasted and roughly chopped
400 g tinned salmon, drained, skin
   and bones removed, flesh flaked
few sprigs mint and flat-leaf parsley,
   to garnish

Salmon and cauliflower 'tabbouleh' with crispbreads

🍴 **Serves 4**   🕐 **Preparation: 15 minutes, plus cooling time**
〰 **Cooking: 5 minutes**

Steam the cauliflower in a steamer basket over a large saucepan of simmering water for 4 minutes or until barely tender. Set aside to cool.

Place the cooled cauliflower in a food processor and pulse until finely chopped. Do not over-process as you want the cauliflower to retain a coarse grain-like texture. Transfer to a large bowl.

Roughly chop 100 g of the rocket and add to the cauliflower with the remaining whole rocket and the tomato and cucumber. Toss to combine, then stir in the lemon zest, lemon juice and olive oil. Season with freshly ground black pepper.

Spread the labne or yoghurt evenly over the crispbreads, sprinkle with the sumac and gently press the pecans on top. Roughly chop the crispbreads into chunky 'croutons'. Pile the salad onto four plates or a serving platter, top with the salmon and scatter with the 'croutons'. Garnish with the herb sprigs and serve.

> **WEEKS 7–12 CARB EXTRAS**
>
> For an extra 10 g carbs per serve, add 160 g (40 g per person) drained and rinsed tinned salt-reduced lentils to the salad.

Note: Labne is a Middle Eastern yoghurt-based cheese that's easy to make at home: just strain plain pot-set yoghurt overnight in a sieve placed over a bowl in the fridge.

Lean meat, fish, poultry, eggs, tofu **1**
Breads, cereals, legumes,
starchy vegetables **0.5**
Dairy **1**
Low-carb vegetables **2**
Mod-carb vegetables **1**
Healthy fats **3**

2 teaspoons olive oil
1 leek, white part only, thinly sliced
600 g mixed mushrooms
   (button, portobello and oyster)
2 cloves garlic, crushed
2½ tablespoons white wine vinegar
1 bunch broccolini, halved widthways,
   steamed
8 eggs
150 g mesclun or baby spinach leaves
1 wholemeal pita bread, quartered
   and toasted

FETA AND PECAN SALSA

40 g pecans or walnuts, chopped
80 g salt-reduced low-fat feta,
   crumbled
1 tomato, finely chopped
1½ tablespoons extra virgin olive oil
1 tablespoon white wine vinegar

Warm mushroom salad with poached eggs

15 G CARB PER SERVE

🍽 **Serves 4**　🕐 **Preparation: 20 minutes**　♨ **Cooking: 30 minutes**

For the feta and pecan salsa, combine the pecans, feta and tomato in a bowl. Add the olive oil and vinegar and mix gently to combine. Season with freshly ground black pepper. Set aside for the flavours to develop.

Heat the olive oil in a large heavy-based frying pan or saucepan over medium heat. Add the leek and cook, covered, stirring occasionally, for 5 minutes or until softened. Slice the mushrooms into varying thicknesses and leave some of the oyster mushrooms whole, so that the textures will vary when cooked. Add the mushrooms, garlic and 1½ tablespoons of the vinegar to the pan and cook, covered for 5 minutes until softened, stirring occasionally. Remove the lid and cook for 1 minute or until there is only a small amount of moisture remaining.

Steam the broccolini in a steamer basket over a saucepan of simmering water for 3 minutes or until tender but still crisp. Add to the mushroom mixture and toss to combine.

Meanwhile, bring a large saucepan of water to the boil, then reduce the heat so the water is just simmering. Add the remaining vinegar to the water. Working quickly, crack an egg into a small cup. Use a spoon to stir the water to make a whirlpool, then carefully tip the egg into the centre of the whirlpool. Crack in the remaining eggs one by one, then cook for 4 minutes for a soft yolk or until cooked to your liking. Transfer to a plate with a slotted spoon.

Divide the mesclun or baby spinach, mushrooms, poached eggs and salsa among four plates or between two platters. Serve the toasted pita on the side.

WEEKS 7–12 CARB EXTRAS

For an extra 10 g carbs per serve, add 160 g (40 g per person) drained and rinsed tinned salt-reduced red kidney beans to the salsa.

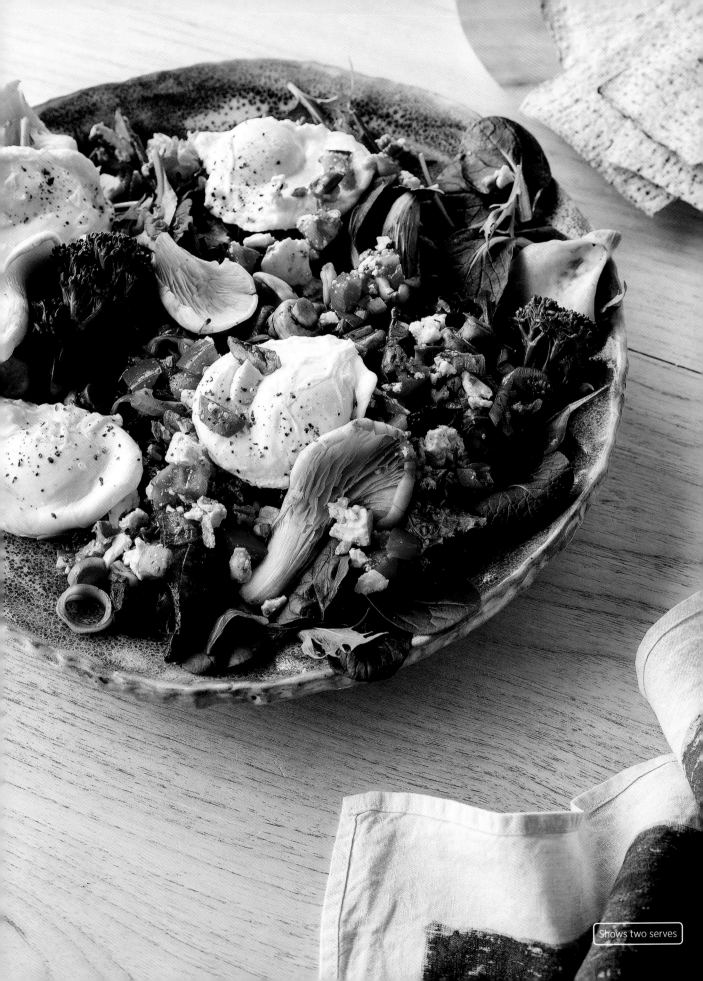

Shows two serves

Lean meat, fish, poultry, eggs, tofu **1**
Breads, cereals, legumes,
starchy vegetables **0.5**
Dairy **1**
Low-carb vegetables **3**
Healthy fats **4**

2 x 35 g slices mixed grain bread,
    torn into large crumbs
olive oil spray, for cooking
4 zucchini
3 cups rocket leaves
1 cup watercress sprigs
400 g tinned tuna in springwater,
    drained
4 tomatoes, finely chopped
    or cut into thin wedges
2 tablespoons torn basil or small
    basil leaves
40 g parmesan, shaved, flaked or
    finely grated

ALMOND AND TOMATO PESTO

40 g raw almonds
160 g semi-dried tomatoes, drained
3 tomatoes, seeds removed,
    roughly chopped
1 small clove garlic, finely chopped
3 tablespoons roughly chopped basil
¼ cup (60 ml) extra virgin olive oil
40 g finely grated parmesan

Tuna 'pasta' salad with almond and tomato pesto

25 G CARB PER SERVE

🍴 **Serves 4**   🕐 **Preparation: 25 minutes**   ⓦ **Cooking: 5 minutes**

To make the pesto, place the almonds, semi-dried tomatoes, chopped tomato, garlic and basil in a small food processor and process until finely chopped. With the motor running, pour in the olive oil in a thin, steady stream until the mixture comes together to form a paste. Stir in the parmesan and season to taste with freshly ground black pepper, then set aside. Just before using, stir in 1–2 tablespoons boiling water if a thinner consistency is preferred for coating the zucchini.

Preheat the oven to 180°C (160°C fan-forced) and line a baking tray with baking paper.

Place the bread on the prepared tray and spray with olive oil. Toast in the oven for 3–5 minutes or until golden, then leave to cool.

Thinly slice the zucchini lengthways, then cut into long, thin strands (alternatively, use a spiral cutter or julienne peeler, if you have one, or grate on the large side of a box grater). Squeeze well to remove any excess liquid. Transfer to a bowl, add the pesto and stir gently to coat the zucchini. Add the rocket, watercress, tuna, tomato and basil and stir gently to mix, then season with pepper.

Divide the zucchini salad evenly among four bowls or plates and top with the parmesan and toasted breadcrumbs. Serve immediately.

UNITS PER SERVE

Lean meat, fish, poultry, eggs, tofu **1**
Dairy **0.5**
Low-carb vegetables **1.5**
Mod-carb vegetables **0.5**
Healthy fats **2**

1 tablespoon olive oil
1 onion, thinly sliced
2 cloves garlic, crushed
2 teaspoons Madras-style Spice Mix
   (page 264)
1 teaspoon ground turmeric
150 g button mushrooms, sliced
1.5 litres salt-reduced chicken stock
400 g chicken breast fillets,
   cut into 1.5 cm pieces
3 baby bok choy, quartered lengthways
1 tablespoon lemon juice
2 small zucchini, spiralised
handful coriander leaves
80 g raw unsalted cashews, toasted
1 quantity Raita (see page 264)

Spiced chicken broth with bok choy

12 G
CARB
PER
SERVE

🍴 **Serves 4**   🕐 **Preparation: 15 minutes**   ⓦ **Cooking: 15 minutes**

Heat the olive oil in a large heavy-based saucepan over medium heat. Add the onion, garlic, spice blend and turmeric and cook, stirring, for 5–6 minutes or until the onion is starting to soften. Add the mushrooms and chicken stock and bring to the boil over medium heat. Reduce the heat to a simmer, add the chicken and cook for 5 minutes or until the chicken is just cooked through. Add the bok choy and simmer for 30 seconds, then remove from the heat and add the lemon juice.

Divide the zucchini 'noodles' among four large serving bowls and ladle in the soup, ensuring each bowl gets an even share of the chicken and vegetables. Scatter with the coriander and cashews and serve with the raita.

WEEKS 7–12 CARB EXTRAS

For an extra 10 g carbs per serve, add 160 g drained and rinsed tinned salt-reduced chickpeas to the broth when you add the chicken.

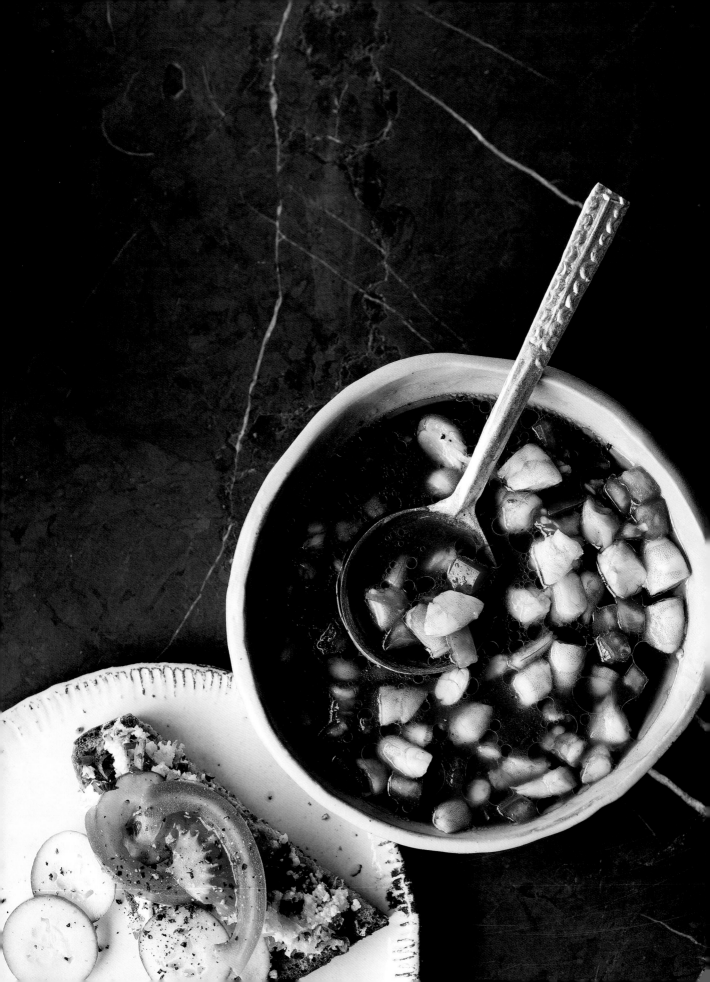

UNITS PER SERVE

Lean meat, fish, poultry, eggs, tofu **1**
Breads, cereals, legumes,
starchy vegetables **0.5**
Dairy **1**
Low-carb vegetables **2**
Mod-carb vegetables **0.5**
Healthy fats **4**

2 cloves garlic, crushed
3 spring onions, finely chopped
1 green capsicum, seeded and
    roughly chopped
1 telegraph cucumber, seeded and
    roughly chopped
4 cups roughly chopped iceberg lettuce
2 cups rocket leaves
1 cup flat-leaf parsley leaves
1 cup (250 ml) salt-reduced chicken
    stock, plus extra if needed
40 g ground almonds
¼ cup (60 ml) extra virgin olive oil
2 tablespoons white balsamic
    condiment or sherry vinegar,
    or to taste
400 g cooked, peeled and cleaned
    king prawns (weight after peeling),
    finely chopped
1 tomato, seasoned and finely chopped
lemon juice, to taste

HERBED RICOTTA TOAST

220 g low-fat fresh ricotta
2 tablespoons finely chopped chives
2 tablespoons finely chopped
    flat-leaf parsley
1 teaspoon finely grated lemon zest
2 x 35 g slices mixed grain bread
1 Lebanese cucumber, thinly sliced
1 tomato, sliced

Green gazpacho with prawns and herbed ricotta toast

🍽 **Serves 4** 🕐 **Preparation: 25 minutes, plus chilling time**
🍲 **Cooking: 2 minutes**

Working in batches, process the garlic, spring onion, capsicum, cucumber, lettuce, rocket, parsley and chicken stock in a blender or food processor until a smooth puree forms. Strain the puree through a fine-mesh sieve over a bowl, then stir in the almonds, olive oil and balsamic condiment or vinegar and season to taste with freshly ground black pepper. If you prefer a thinner soup, stir in a little extra stock until the desired consistency is achieved. Cover with plastic film and chill for 3 hours.

Meanwhile, to make the herbed ricotta toast, place the ricotta, chives, parsley and lemon zest in a small bowl and stir to combine, then season to taste with pepper. Just before serving, toast the bread and spread evenly with the herbed ricotta, then top with the cucumber and tomato and any remaining herbed ricotta.

Place the prawn meat and tomato in a bowl. Squeeze over some lemon juice and season with pepper.

Divide the soup evenly among four bowls, then top with one-quarter of the prawn and tomato mixture. Serve with ½ slice herbed ricotta toast per person.

WEEKS 7–12 CARB EXTRAS

For an extra 10 g carbs per serve, cook 480 g (120 g per person) frozen peas in a saucepan of simmering water for 3 minutes or until tender, drain and cool under cold running water, then add to the food processor with the vegetables.

Lean meat, fish, poultry, eggs, tofu **1**
Low-carb vegetables **3**
Mod-carb vegetables **0.5**
Healthy fats **3**

Roasted tomato, capsicum and fish soup

11 G
CARB
PER
SERVE

🍴 **Serves 4**   🕐 **Preparation: 20 minutes**
🍲 **Cooking: 2 hours 10 minutes**

1.5 kg tomatoes, quartered
4 cloves garlic, unpeeled
1 small carrot, roughly chopped
¼ bulb baby fennel, trimmed and
   finely chopped
½ small red capsicum, peeled with
   a vegetable peeler, seeded and
   finely chopped
¼ cup (60 ml) extra virgin olive oil
400 g flathead, whiting or monkfish
   fillets, skin removed, pin-boned
   and cut into bite-sized pieces
2 tablespoons roughly chopped basil

Preheat the oven to 200°C (180°C fan-forced) and line a roasting tin with baking paper.

Place the tomato, garlic, carrot, fennel and capsicum in the prepared tin and drizzle over the olive oil, then season to taste with freshly ground black pepper. Cover tightly with foil and roast for 1½ hours. Remove the foil and roast for a further 30 minutes or until the vegetables are very tender and slightly caramelised around the edges.

Remove and peel the garlic. Transfer the tomato mixture and garlic to a high-speed blender and blend until a smooth puree forms. Transfer the soup to a heavy-based saucepan and bring to the boil, then add the fish. Reduce the heat to low, then cover and cook for 5 minutes or until the fish is just cooked through.

Divide the soup and fish evenly among four bowls, sprinkle with the basil and serve immediately with freshly ground black pepper.

WEEKS 7–12 CARB EXTRAS

For an extra 10 g carbs per serve, add 200 g (50 g per person) drained and rinsed tinned salt-reduced cannellini beans to the food processor with the vegetables (add a little boiling water if necessary to thin the soup).

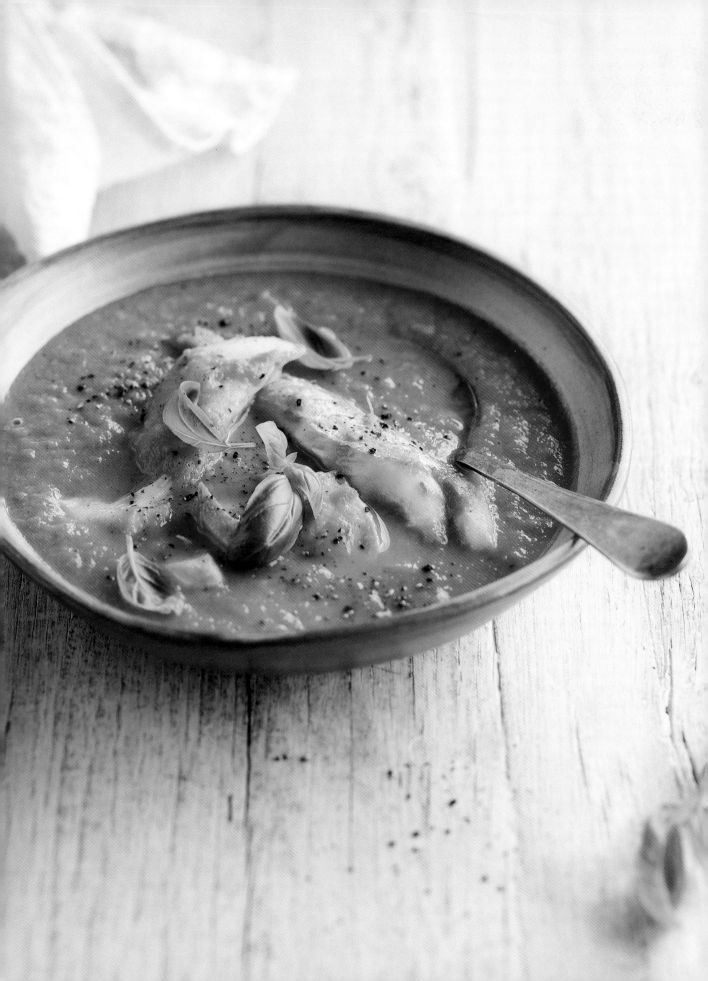

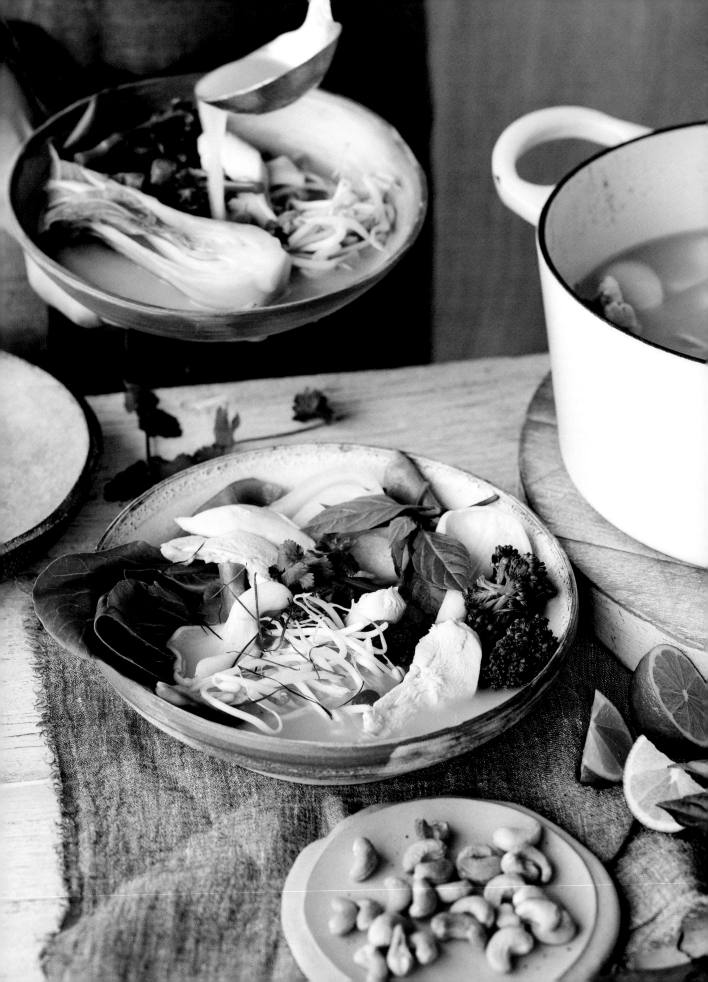

Thai chicken soup with greens

11 G CARB PER SERVE

🍴 Serves 4   🕐 Preparation: 15 minutes   ♨ Cooking: 15 minutes

1 large stalk lemongrass, cut into
   6 cm lengths
1 × 5 cm piece ginger, peeled and
   thinly sliced
1 small fresh red chilli, thinly sliced
   (optional)
1.5 litres salt-reduced chicken stock
400 g chicken breast fillets, thinly
   sliced on the diagonal
150 g oyster mushrooms, torn in
   half if large
2 bunches broccolini, trimmed and
   stalks cut into 2 cm lengths
2 baby bok choy, halved lengthways
100 g snow peas, halved on
   the diagonal
100 ml light coconut-flavoured
   evaporated milk
1 tablespoon lime juice
3 teaspoons fish sauce
5 kaffir lime leaves, finely shredded
150 g bean sprouts, trimmed
small handful Thai basil leaves
small handful coriander leaves
40 g raw unsalted cashews, toasted
lime wedges, to serve (optional)

Combine the lemongrass, ginger, chilli (if using) and stock in a large saucepan and bring to the boil over medium heat. Add the chicken, mushrooms and broccolini stalks and bring back to a simmer. Add the broccolini florets, bok choy, snow peas and evaporated milk and bring to the boil. Remove the pan from the heat and stir in the lime juice, fish sauce and kaffir lime leaves.

Place the bean sprouts in four large serving bowls. Ladle the soup evenly into the bowls and scatter over the Thai basil, coriander and cashews. Serve with lime wedges, if you like.

Note: A good alternative to light coconut-flavoured evaporated milk is to use 100 ml light evaporated milk with ½ teaspoon natural coconut essence added.

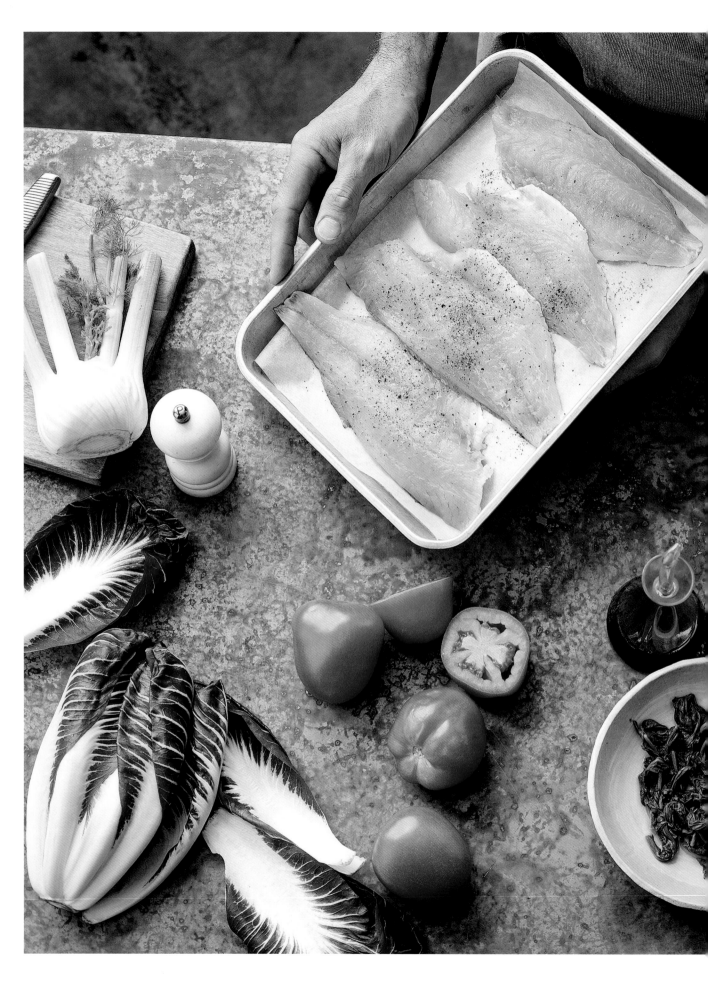

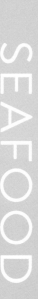

SEAFOOD

Baked snapper with gremolata and roasted vegetables, see page 180

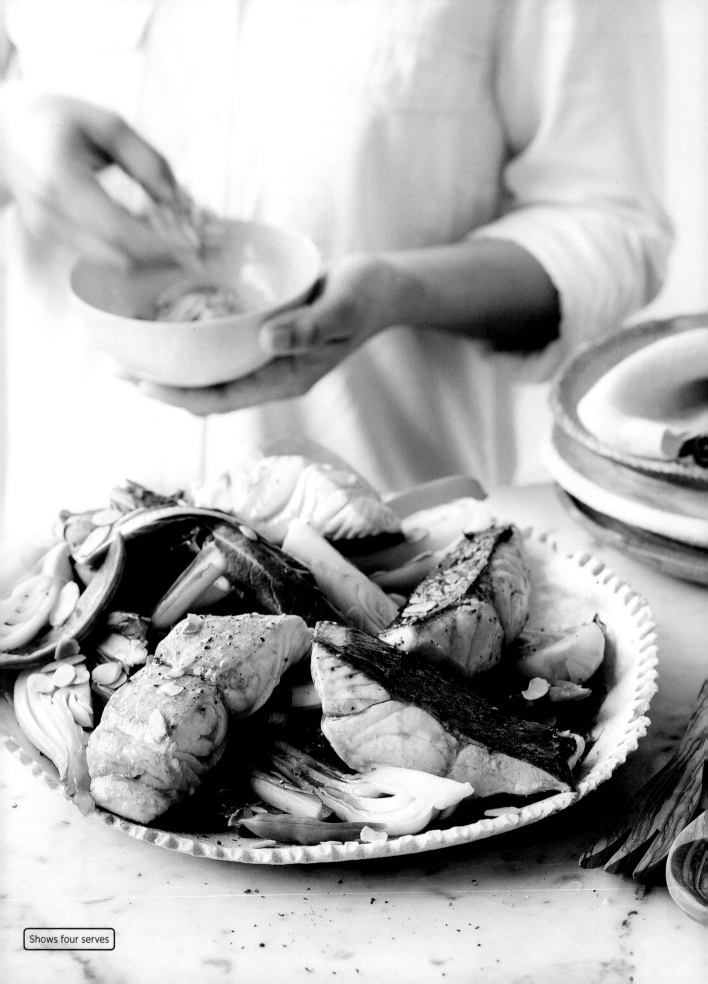

Shows four serves

UNITS PER SERVE

Lean meat, fish, poultry, eggs, tofu **1.5**
Low-carb vegetables **3**
Mod-carb vegetables **0.5**
Healthy fats **3**

Crisp-skin blue-eye trevalla with steamed Asian greens

🍴 **Serves 4**   🕐 **Preparation: 20 minutes**   ◎ **Cooking: 15 minutes**

3 baby bok choy, trimmed and halved
    or quartered lengthways
1 bunch choy sum, trimmed and cut
    into 5 cm lengths
150 g snow peas, halved on
    the diagonal
1 tablespoon olive oil
4 × 150 g blue-eye trevalla fillets,
    skin on and pin-boned
1 teaspoon salt-reduced soy sauce
40 g flaked almonds

DRESSING

3 teaspoons extra virgin olive oil
2 teaspoons rice vinegar
2 teaspoons lime juice
1½ teaspoons salt-reduced soy sauce

Working in batches, steam the bok choy, choy sum and snow peas in a steamer basket over a saucepan of simmering water for 2–3 minutes or until tender but still crisp, setting each batch aside in a heatproof bowl, while you cook the remainder.

Meanwhile, heat 2 teaspoons of the olive oil in a heavy-based frying pan over medium–high heat. Pat the fish dry with paper towel, then season with freshly ground black pepper. Add to the pan, skin-side down, and cook for 3–4 minutes or until the skin is golden and crisp, then carefully turn and cook for another 1 minute or until the fish is just cooked through.

Wipe the pan clean with paper towel, then add the remaining olive oil, soy sauce and almonds and heat over medium heat for 1 minute or until the nuts are glazed in the soy mixture.

To make the dressing, whisk together all the ingredients in a small bowl. Add the steamed vegetables and dressing to the pan and toss to coat.

Divide the steamed vegetables and fish among four plates or pile onto a platter and serve immediately.

> **WEEKS 7–12 CARB EXTRAS**
>
> For an extra 10 g carbs per serve, add 480 g (120 g per person) cooked and drained frozen peas to the steamed vegetables.

Lean meat, fish, poultry, eggs, tofu **1.5**
Low-carb vegetables **3**
Healthy fats **3.5**

Thai fish cakes with broccoli salad

9 G CARB PER SERVE

🍴 Serves 4 🕐 Preparation: 20 minutes, plus refrigerating time
🍲 Cooking: 10 minutes

300 g broccoli, cut into small florets
4 cups mixed salad leaves (Asian salad mix, if available)
2 cups watercress sprigs
2 cups (160 g) bean sprouts, trimmed
4 Lebanese cucumbers, cut lengthways into ribbons with a vegetable peeler
300 g cherry tomatoes, halved
1 tablespoon fish sauce
1 tablespoon extra virgin olive oil
juice of 1 lime
1 small fresh red chilli, seeded and finely chopped
80 g avocado, sliced
40 g macadamias, coarsely crushed

THAI FISH CAKES

600 g firm white fish fillets, skin removed and pin-boned
3 kaffir lime leaves, very thinly sliced
2 coriander roots, well washed and finely chopped
⅓ cup finely chopped coriander leaves and stems
1 small fresh red chilli, seeded and finely chopped
50 g green beans, trimmed and finely chopped
2 tablespoons finely chopped water chestnuts
1 tablespoon fish sauce
olive oil spray, for cooking

To make the fish cakes, place the fish in a food processor and process until a coarse paste forms. Transfer to a bowl, then add the kaffir lime leaves, coriander root, leaves and stems, chilli, beans, water chestnuts and fish sauce and stir to mix well. Season with freshly ground white pepper, then cover with plastic film and refrigerate for 15 minutes to chill and firm.

Divide the fish mixture into 12 even-sized portions, then shape into patties. Heat a large heavy-based non-stick frying pan over medium heat and spray with olive oil. Add the fish cakes and cook for 5 minutes on each side or until golden and cooked through.

Meanwhile, steam the broccoli in a steamer basket over a saucepan of simmering water for 3 minutes or until tender but still crisp. Set aside to cool. Place the salad leaves, watercress, bean sprouts, cucumber and tomatoes in a large bowl and toss gently to combine. Place the fish sauce, olive oil, lime juice and chilli in a small bowl and stir to mix well. Add to the salad and toss gently to coat. Just before serving, add the cooled broccoli and toss to mix through.

Divide the salad among four plates or large bowls and top with one-quarter of the avocado and fish cakes. Sprinkle over the crushed macadamias and serve immediately.

WEEKS 7–12 CARB EXTRAS

For an extra 10 g carbs per serve, roast 480 g (120 g per person) pumpkin cubes at 200°C (180°C fan-forced) for 30 minutes or until golden and tender, then add to the salad.

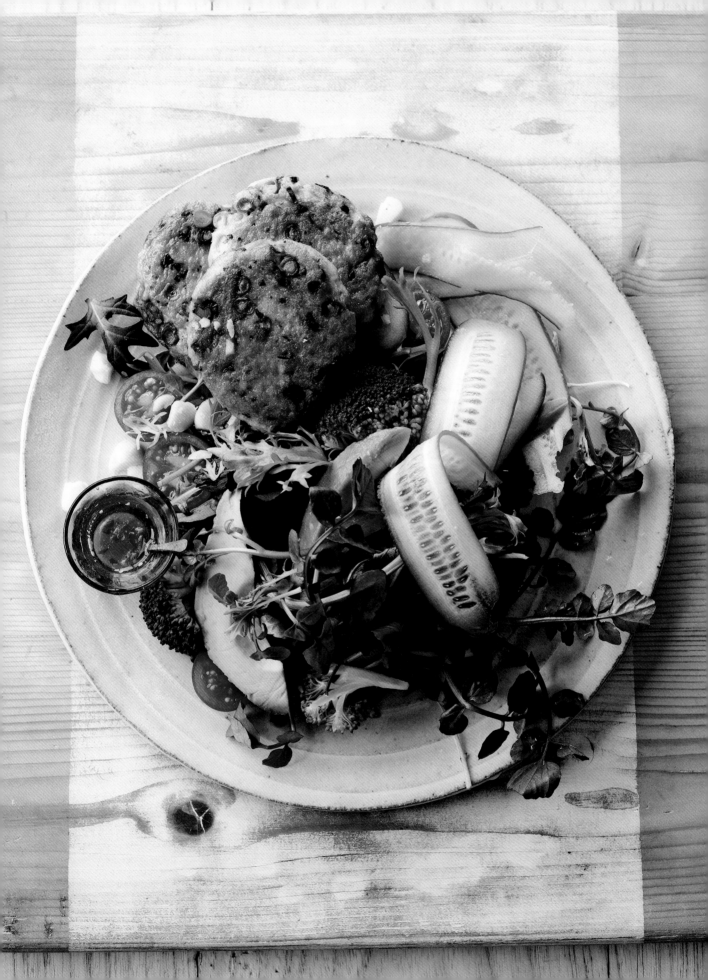

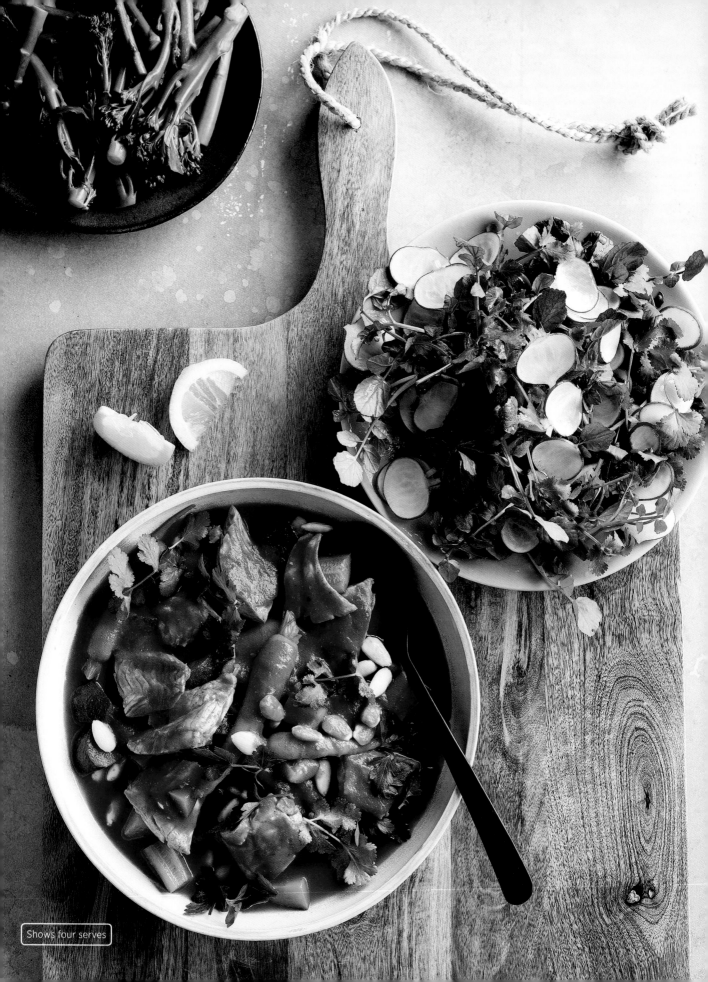

Shows four serves

UNITS PER SERVE

Lean meat, fish, poultry, eggs, tofu **1.5**
Low-carb vegetables **2**
Mod-carb vegetables **1**
Healthy fats **3**

Fish tagine with watercress, coriander and radish salad

🍴 Serves 4   🕐 Preparation: 25 minutes   ♨ Cooking: 25 minutes

1 tablespoon olive oil
½ small onion or 1 golden shallot,
    finely chopped
2 cloves garlic, finely chopped
3 coriander roots and stems, well
    washed and finely chopped
2 teaspoons sweet paprika
1 teaspoon ground cumin
1 teaspoon ground coriander
½ teaspoon ground turmeric
¼ teaspoon ground cinnamon
¼ teaspoon ground cardamom
1 bunch baby carrots, trimmed
    and scrubbed (8 carrots)
400 g salt-reduced tomato passata
600 g snapper, blue-eye trevalla or
    other firm white fish fillets, skin
    removed, pin-boned and cut into
    bite-sized pieces or strips
4 small zucchini, quartered and cut
    into batons
40 g blanched almonds
½ cup roughly chopped flat-leaf parsley
½ cup roughly chopped
    coriander leaves
1 bunch broccolini, trimmed and halved
1 bunch asparagus, trimmed and halved
lemon wedges, to serve

WATERCRESS, CORIANDER AND RADISH SALAD

3 cups watercress sprigs
½ cup coriander leaves, torn if desired
2 radishes, shaved
1 tablespoon extra virgin olive oil
2 teaspoons lemon juice

Heat the olive oil in a large heavy-based deep frying pan with a lid over medium heat. Add the onion or shallot, garlic and coriander root and stem and cook, stirring, for 5 minutes or until softened. Add the paprika, cumin, ground coriander, turmeric, cinnamon and cardamom and cook, stirring, for 30 seconds or until fragrant. Add the carrots, tomato passata and ¼ cup (60 ml) water and bring to a simmer over high heat. Cover, reduce the heat to low and cook for 15 minutes or until the carrots are tender. Add the fish, zucchini and 2 tablespoons water, if desired, return to the simmer and cook, covered, over medium heat for 5 minutes or until the fish is cooked through and the zucchini is tender. Stir in the almonds, parsley and coriander leaves and season to taste with freshly ground black pepper.

Meanwhile, blanch the broccolini in a saucepan of simmering water for 3 minutes or until tender but crisp. Transfer to a plate and set aside, then repeat with the asparagus.

To make the salad, place the watercress, coriander and radish in a large bowl and toss gently to mix. Drizzle over the olive oil and lemon juice and toss gently to coat.

Serve the tagine with the salad, broccolini and asparagus, with lemon wedges to the side.

> **WEEKS 7–12 CARB EXTRAS**
>
> For an extra 10 g carbs per serve, serve the tagine with 100 g (25 g per person) cooked couscous alongside (this is 50 g raw couscous; 12.5 g per person).

UNITS PER SERVE
Lean meat, fish, poultry, eggs, tofu **1.5**
Low-carb vegetables **3**
Mod-carb vegetables **1**
Healthy fats **4**

Baked snapper with gremolata and roasted vegetables

8 G CARB PER SERVE

🍴 Serves 4   🕐 Preparation: 25 minutes   〰 Cooking: 1 hour

2 cups rocket leaves, trimmed
40 g blanched almonds
1 large clove garlic, finely chopped
½ cup flat-leaf parsley leaves,
    finely chopped
finely grated zest of 1 lemon
4 × 150 g pink snapper or barramundi
    fillets, skin on and pin-boned
¼ cup (60 ml) dry white wine
1 tablespoon extra virgin olive oil
3 cups baby spinach leaves, trimmed
100 g green beans, trimmed
40 g flaked almonds, toasted

ROASTED RADICCHIO, TOMATO AND FENNEL

4 tomatoes, halved crossways
1 tablespoon extra virgin olive oil
1 bulb baby fennel, trimmed and
    quartered lengthways
1 head radicchio, quartered lengthways
1 tablespoon balsamic vinegar

To make the roasted vegetables for the salad, preheat the oven to 210°C (190°C fan-forced) and line a roasting tin with baking paper.

Place the tomatoes, cut-side up, in the prepared tin, drizzle with a little of the olive oil and roast for 30 minutes. Add the fennel and radicchio, drizzle with the balsamic vinegar and remaining olive oil and roast for another 25–30 minutes or until the tomatoes and fennel are tender and golden and the radicchio has wilted and caramelised.

Meanwhile, place the rocket in a heatproof bowl, cover with boiling water and leave to stand for 2 minutes. Drain, then cool under cold running water and drain well, squeezing out the excess liquid.

Place the blanched almonds in a mortar and coarsely crush with the pestle. Stir in the garlic, parsley and lemon zest, then set the gremolata aside.

Place the fish in a small roasting tin lined with baking paper or foil, skin-side down, and season to taste with freshly ground black pepper. Place one-quarter of the rocket leaves on top of each piece of fish, then spoon on the gremolata, gently pressing it down. Drizzle evenly with the wine and olive oil. Place in the oven when adding the radicchio and fennel to the tomatoes, and roast for 20–25 minutes or until the fish is cooked through and the topping is crisp and golden.

Wash the spinach leaves and place in a heavy-based saucepan over medium–high heat. Cook, stirring, for 1–2 minutes or until wilted. Blanch the beans in a saucepan of simmering water for 3 minutes or until tender but still crisp, then drain.

Divide the roasted vegetables among four plates and top each with one piece of fish. Serve immediately with one-quarter of the spinach and beans to the side, scattered with the flaked almonds.

WEEKS 7–12 CARB EXTRAS

For an extra 10 g carbs per serve, cut 200 g sweet potato (50 g per person) into 1.5 cm dice and add to the roasting tin along with the fennel and radicchio. Roast until golden and tender.

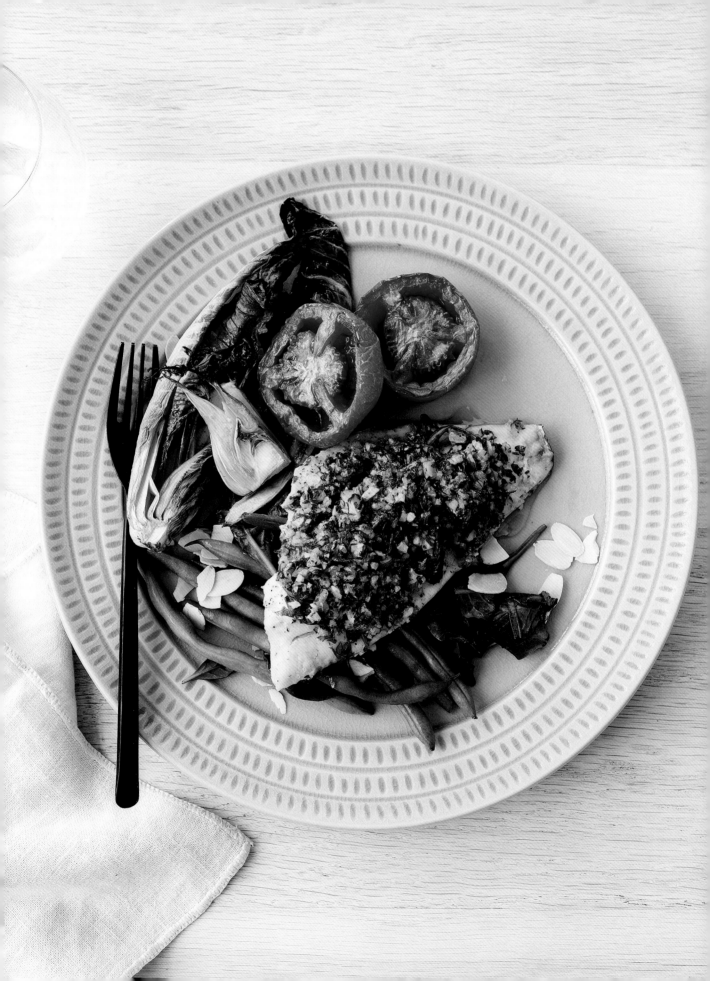

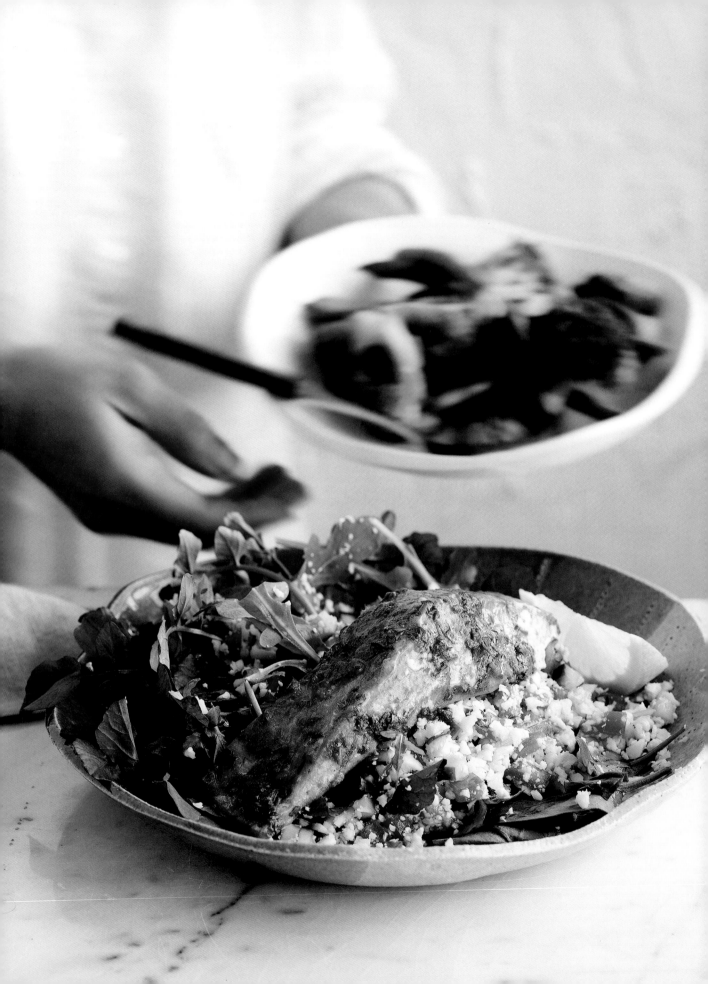

UNITS PER SERVE
Lean meat, fish, poultry, eggs, tofu **1.5**
Low-carb vegetables **2.5**
Mod-carb vegetables **2**
Healthy fats **3**

Spiced salmon fillets with cauliflower 'couscous'

11 G CARB PER SERVE

🍴 Serves 4   🕐 Preparation: 25 minutes, plus marinating time
🍲 Cooking: 25 minutes

2 teaspoons extra virgin olive oil
2 tablespoons lemon juice
2 tablespoons roughly chopped
   flat-leaf parsley
2 tablespoons roughly
   chopped coriander leaves
1 teaspoon ground cumin
1 teaspoon sweet paprika
1 teaspoon ground coriander
1 teaspoon ground turmeric
1 clove garlic, finely chopped
4 × 150 g salmon fillets, skin removed
   and pin-boned
300 g broccoli, trimmed and cut into
   small florets
100 g green beans, trimmed
40 g flaked almonds, lightly toasted
lemon wedges, to serve

CAULIFLOWER 'COUSCOUS'

550 g cauliflower, cut into small florets
1½ tablespoons extra virgin olive oil
2 cups watercress sprigs
2 cups baby rocket leaves
2 cups baby spinach leaves, trimmed
2 Lebanese cucumbers, cut into
   5 mm dice
2 tomatoes, seeded and cut into
   5 mm dice
1 tablespoon lemon juice
few sprigs mint and flat-leaf parsley,
   to garnish

Place the olive oil, lemon juice, parsley, coriander, cumin, paprika, ground coriander, turmeric and garlic in a bowl and stir to combine. Place the salmon in a baking dish, then spread evenly with the herb mixture. Cover with plastic film and marinate in the refrigerator for 30 minutes.

Meanwhile, to prepare the cauliflower for the 'couscous', working in batches if necessary, process the cauliflower in a food processer until finely chopped to resemble grains of rice or couscous. Heat 2 teaspoons of the olive oil in a heavy-based non-stick frying pan over medium heat. Add the cauliflower and cook, stirring occasionally, for 5–6 minutes or until tender. Transfer to a large bowl and set aside to cool.

Preheat the oven to 200°C (180°C fan-forced).

Cut out four squares of foil large enough to enclose the salmon, then place a piece of salmon and any marinade left in the dish in the centre of each square. Fold the edges over to enclose the salmon in a neat parcel. Transfer to a baking tray and bake for 15 minutes for medium or continue until cooked to your liking.

Meanwhile, steam the broccoli and beans in a steamer basket over a saucepan of simmering water for 3 minutes or until tender but still crisp.

Add the watercress, rocket, spinach, cucumber and tomato to the cauliflower 'couscous', then drizzle in the lemon juice and remaining olive oil and stir gently to mix. Garnish with the parsley and mint sprigs.

Divide the cauliflower 'couscous' evenly among four plates and add a salmon fillet. Scatter the almonds evenly over the greens and divide among the plates. Serve immediately, with lemon wedges to the side.

WEEKS 7–12 CARB EXTRAS

For an extra 10 g carbs per serve, add 100 g (25 g per person) cooked couscous to the cauliflower 'couscous' (this is 50 g raw couscous; 12.5 g per person).

UNITS PER SERVE

Lean meat, fish, poultry, eggs, tofu **1.5**
Low-carb vegetables **3**
Healthy fats **3**

Crisp-skin salmon with herb and cashew 'butter'

🍴 Serves 4   🕐 Preparation: 25 minutes   ▨ Cooking: 10 minutes

olive oil spray, for cooking
4 × 150 g salmon fillets, skin on
    and pin-boned
2 bunches asparagus, trimmed
2 bunches broccolini, trimmed

HERB AND CASHEW 'BUTTER'

80 g raw unsalted cashew butter
1 small clove garlic, finely chopped
juice of ½ lemon
¼ cup basil leaves, roughly chopped
¼ cup flat-leaf parsley leaves,
    roughly chopped
¼ cup coriander leaves,
    roughly chopped
2 tablespoons boiling water

TOMATO, CUCUMBER AND SUMAC SALAD

4 tomatoes, cut into thin wedges
2 Lebanese cucumbers, halved
    lengthways and thinly sliced on
    the diagonal
2 cups baby rocket leaves
2 teaspoons extra virgin olive oil
2 teaspoons lemon juice
pinch of sumac

To make the herb and cashew 'butter', place the cashew butter, garlic, lemon juice, basil, parsley and coriander in a small food processor and process until a paste forms. Add the boiling water and pulse until well combined and emulsified. Transfer to a bowl, season to taste with freshly ground black pepper and cover with plastic film. Set aside until required.

To make the salad, place the tomato, cucumber and rocket in a bowl and gently mix to combine. Just before serving, drizzle over the olive oil and lemon juice and sprinkle with sumac.

Heat a heavy-based non-stick frying pan over medium heat and spray with olive oil. Season the salmon with pepper, then cook, skin-side down, for 3–4 minutes or until golden. Turn and cook for another 2 minutes for medium or continue until cooked to your liking.

Meanwhile, working in batches, steam the asparagus and broccolini in a steamer basket over a saucepan of simmering water for 3 minutes or until tender but still crisp.

Place one salmon fillet and one-quarter of the steamed greens and salad on each of four plates. Serve the herb and cashew 'butter' in a small dish on the side for spooning over.

WEEKS 7-12 CARB EXTRAS

For an extra 10 g carbs per serve, add 200 g cooked quinoa (50 g per person) to the salad to make 'tabbouleh'. (This is 60 g raw quinoa; 15 g per person.) Cut the tomato and cucumber into fine dice and add ¼ cup each roughly chopped flat-leaf parsley and mint.

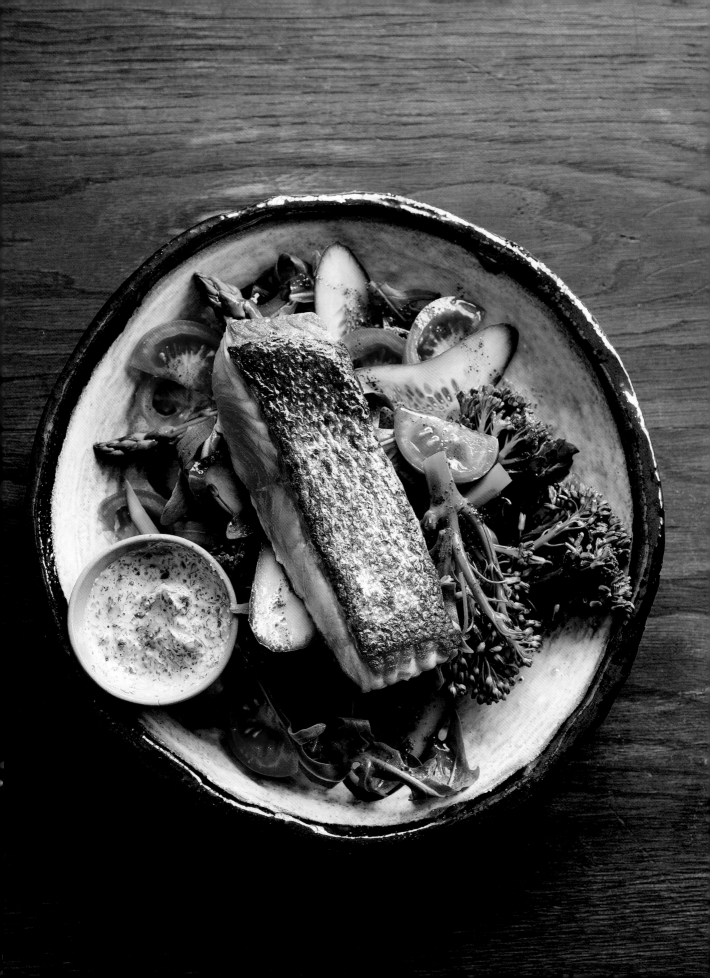

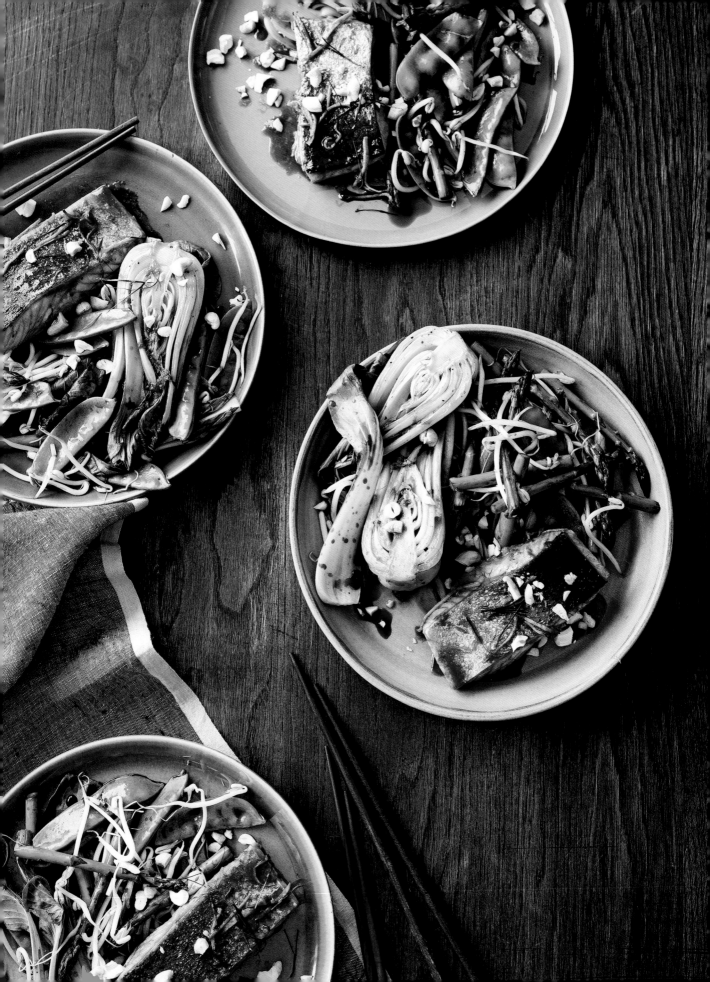

Lean meat, fish, poultry, eggs, tofu **1.5**
Low-carb vegetables **3**
Mod-carb vegetables **0.5**
Healthy fats **3**

Asian-glazed salmon with stir-fried greens

12 G CARB PER SERVE

🍴 Serves 4   🕐 Preparation: 25 minutes   ⧉ Cooking: 15 minutes

olive oil spray, for cooking
2 teaspoons kecap manis
2 teaspoons finely grated lime zest
1½ tablespoons lime juice
2 teaspoons extra virgin olive oil
1 tablespoon julienned ginger
4 × 150 g salmon fillets, skin on
    and pin-boned
40 g raw unsalted cashews,
    roughly chopped
2 kaffir lime leaves,
    very finely shredded

STIR-FRIED GREENS

1½ tablespoons extra virgin olive oil
4 baby bok choy, halved or quartered
    if large
1 bunch choy sum, trimmed and
    cut into 5 cm lengths, stems
    and leaves separated
2 bunches asparagus, trimmed and
    cut into 5 cm lengths
200 g snow peas, halved on
    the diagonal
100 g bean sprouts, trimmed
1 clove garlic, finely chopped
1 × 2 cm piece ginger, peeled and
    finely grated
1 tablespoon mirin
1½ tablespoons rice wine vinegar
1 tablespoon salt-reduced soy sauce

Preheat the oven grill to high. Line a roasting tin with foil or baking paper and place an ovenproof wire rack on top for grilling the salmon. Spray the rack with olive oil.

Place the kecap manis, lime zest, lime juice, olive oil and ginger in a small bowl and stir to combine. Place the salmon on the wire rack, skin-side down, then spoon half of the kecap manis mixture over and rub to coat the salmon. Turn and spoon the remaining kecap manis mixture over the skin-side, rubbing it in evenly. Set aside while you start stir-frying the vegetables.

Heat 2 teaspoons of the olive oil in a wok over high heat. Add the bok choy and choy sum stems and stir-fry for 2–3 minutes or until softened, then add the choy sum leaves and stir-fry until wilted. Transfer to a large bowl. Add another teaspoon of oil to the wok and stir-fry the asparagus and snow peas for 2 minutes or until tender but still crisp, then add to the bowl with the bok choy and choy sum. Add another 2 teaspoons of the oil to the wok and stir-fry the bean sprouts for 1–2 minutes or until warmed through. Transfer to the bowl with the other vegetables. Add the remaining oil to the wok, then add the garlic and ginger and cook for 30 seconds or until fragrant. Pour in the mirin, rice wine vinegar and soy sauce and bring to the boil, then boil for 1 minute. Return the vegetables to the wok, then turn off the heat and toss to coat in the sauce.

Meanwhile, place the salmon under the hot oven grill and grill for 4–5 minutes or until the skin has become crisp and golden. Carefully turn each fillet over, taking care not to tear the flesh, and grill for another 2 minutes for medium or continue until cooked to your liking.

Place one-quarter of the stir-fried vegetables on each of four plates. Top with a salmon fillet, scatter evenly with the cashews and sprinkle with shredded kaffir lime leaves, then serve immediately.

> ### WEEKS 7-12 CARB EXTRAS
>
> For an extra 10 g carbs per serve, add 160 g (40 g per person) baby corn, halved lengthways, to the vegetable stir-fry when adding the bean sprouts.

UNITS PER SERVE

Lean meat, fish, poultry, eggs, tofu **1.5**
Low-carb vegetables **2**
Mod-carb vegetables **1**
Healthy fats **3**

Herb fish skewers with cauliflower and almond puree

9 G CARB PER SERVE

🍴 Serves 4   🕐 Preparation: 30 minutes, plus marinating time
🍲 Cooking: 20 minutes

600 g blue-eye trevalla or other firm
   white fish fillets, skin removed,
   pin-boned and cut into 2 cm cubes
2 cloves garlic, crushed
1 tablespoon chopped flat-leaf parsley
1 teaspoon chopped lemon thyme
½ teaspoon finely chopped rosemary
2 teaspoons olive oil
2 teaspoons lemon juice
2 bunches broccolini, trimmed

CAULIFLOWER AND ALMOND PUREE

1 teaspoon olive oil
1 onion, chopped
2 cloves garlic, crushed
300 g cauliflower, cut into
   3–4 cm pieces
40 g blanched almonds, chopped
1½ cups (375 ml) salt-reduced
   vegetable stock or water

GREEN SALAD WITH DIJON DRESSING

200 g mixed salad leaves
1 bunch watercress, leaves picked
1 Lebanese cucumber, halved
   lengthways and sliced on
   the diagonal
1 tomato, sliced
1 tablespoon olive oil
2 tablespoons white wine vinegar
   or lemon juice
3 teaspoons Dijon mustard

To make the cauliflower and almond puree, heat the olive oil in a large heavy-based saucepan over medium heat. Add the onion and garlic and cook, covered, for 5 minutes, then stir in the cauliflower. Add the almonds and stock or water and bring to the boil, then reduce the heat to low and simmer, partially covered, stirring occasionally, for 13–15 minutes or until very tender. Drain, reserving 2 tablespoons of the cooking liquid.

Return the cauliflower mixture to the pan and blend with a stick blender until smooth. (Or allow to cool slightly, then puree in a food processor or blender.) Add a little of the reserved cooking liquid to the mash to adjust the consistency if required. Season to taste with freshly ground black pepper and reheat over low–medium heat if necessary.

Meanwhile, combine the fish, garlic, herbs, olive oil and lemon juice in a large bowl. Set aside to marinate for 5 minutes. Thread the fish on to eight bamboo skewers (see note).

To make the salad, combine the salad leaves, watercress, cucumber and tomato in a large bowl. Place the olive oil, vinegar or lemon juice and mustard in a screw-top jar, secure the lid and shake until combined. Season to taste with freshly ground black pepper. Add the dressing to the salad just before serving and toss to combine.

Heat a chargrill pan, barbecue or heavy-based frying pan over medium–high heat. Reduce the heat to medium and cook the fish skewers, in batches if necessary, turning occasionally, for 4–5 minutes or until cooked to your liking.

Steam the broccolini in a steamer basket over a large saucepan of simmering water for 2–3 minutes or until just tender.

Divide the fish skewers, cauliflower puree, broccolini and salad evenly among four plates and serve.

WEEKS 7–12 CARB EXTRAS

For an extra 10 g carbs per serve, add 200 g (50 g per person) drained and rinsed tinned salt-reduced cannellini beans to the cauliflower puree and reheat over medium heat.

Note: You will need to soak eight long bamboo skewers in cold water for 30 minutes for this recipe.

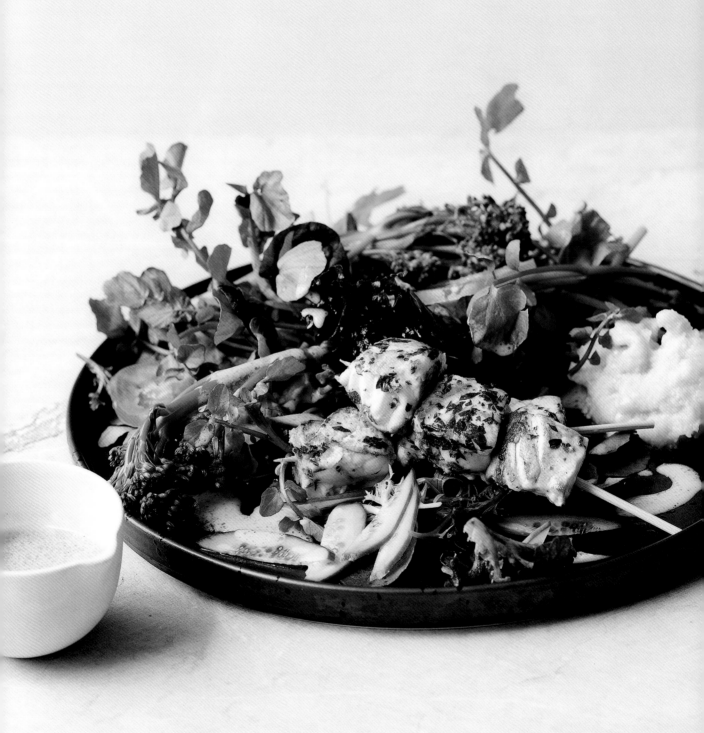

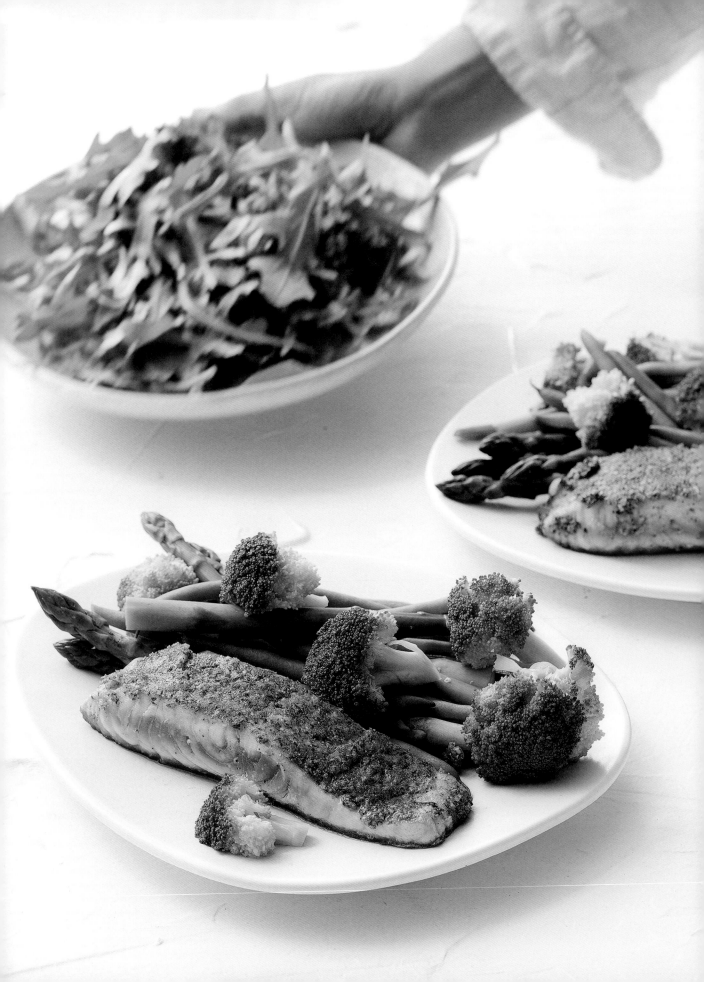

UNITS PER SERVE

Lean meat, fish, poultry, eggs, tofu **1.5**
Dairy **0.5**
Low-carb vegetables **2**
Mod-carb vegetables **1**
Healthy fats **2**

---

4 × 150 g salmon fillets, skin removed
    and pin-boned
olive oil spray, for cooking
2 bunches asparagus, trimmed
300 g broccoli florets
200 g green beans, trimmed
150 g cabbage, finely shredded
1 Lebanese cucumber, coarsely grated
100 g rocket leaves

MACADAMIA AND WATERCRESS PESTO

40 g macadamias
handful basil leaves
½ cup watercress sprigs
½ cup (40 g) finely grated parmesan
½ small clove garlic, crushed
1 tablespoon extra virgin olive oil
1 tablespoon lemon juice

Salmon with macadamia and watercress pesto

6 G CARB PER SERVE

🍴 Serves 4   🕐 Preparation: 20 minutes   ♨ Cooking: 10 minutes

To make the pesto, place all the ingredients in a food processor and process until finely chopped and combined. Season to taste with freshly ground black pepper. Transfer ¼ cup (65 g) of the mixture to a separate bowl to dress the salad. Coat the salmon fillets evenly with the remaining pesto.

Heat a heavy-based frying pan over medium heat. Spray the pan lightly with olive oil, then cook the salmon on one side for 3–4 minutes or until golden. Turn and cook for another 2 minutes for medium or continue until cooked to your liking.

Meanwhile, working in batches, steam the asparagus, broccoli and beans in a steamer basket over a saucepan of simmering water for 3 minutes or until tender but still crisp.

Toss the cabbage, cucumber and rocket together in a large bowl. Add the reserved pesto and toss to combine.

Divide the salmon and steamed vegetables evenly among four plates and serve with the salad on the side.

WEEKS 7–12 CARB EXTRAS

For an extra 10 g carbs per serve, add 160 g (40 g per person) baby corn to the steamer with the vegetables, or 480 g (120 g per person) cooked and cooled green peas to the salad.

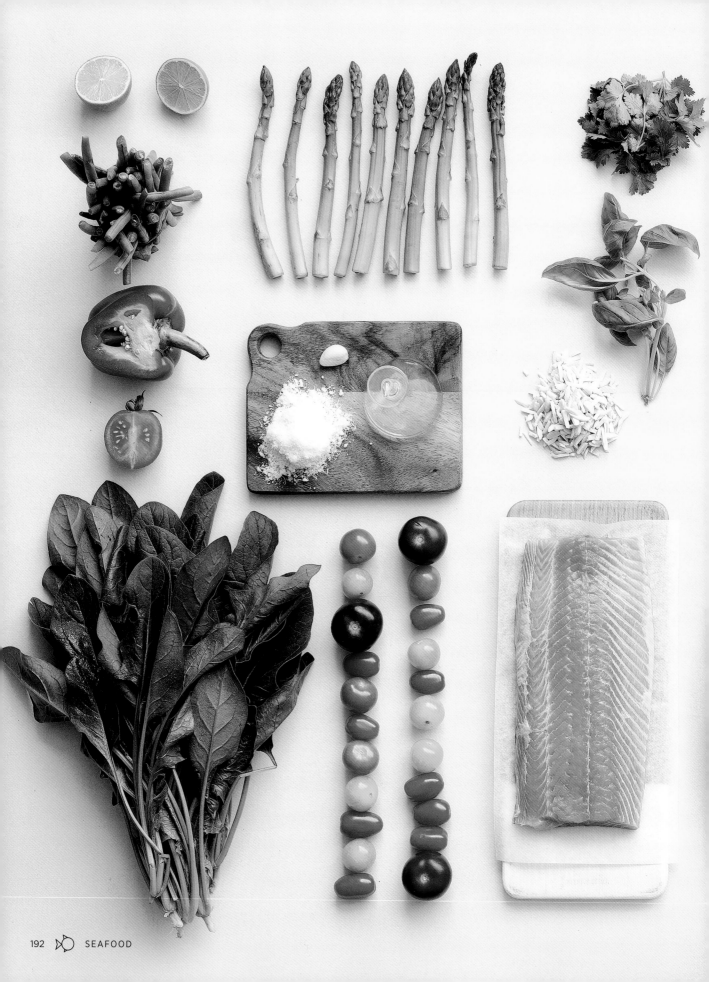

Roasted salmon with vegetable parcels and pistou

UNITS PER SERVE
Lean meat, fish, poultry, eggs, tofu **1.5**
Low-carb vegetables **1.5**
Mod-carb vegetables **1**
Healthy fats **2**

🍽 Serves 4   🕐 Preparation: 20 minutes   ♨ Cooking: 30 minutes

300 g green beans, trimmed
½ (100 g) red capsicum, seeded
  and cut into 3 cm pieces
2 bunches asparagus, trimmed
350 g mixed baby tomatoes, halved
finely grated zest of 1 lime
600 g piece salmon (centre-cut),
  skin on and pin-boned
40 g slivered almonds
1 bunch (600 g) spinach,
  leaves trimmed, washed
lime wedges, to serve

CORIANDER, BASIL AND LIME PISTOU
½ tomato
½ cup coriander leaves
handful basil leaves
¼ cup (20 g) finely grated parmesan
1 small clove garlic, crushed
1 tablespoon extra virgin olive oil
finely grated zest and juice of 1 lime

Preheat the oven to 190°C (170°C fan-forced). Cut four 30 cm squares of baking paper.

To make the pistou, squeeze the seeds from the tomato half and roughly chop the flesh. Place in a food processor with the remaining ingredients and process until finely chopped and combined. Season to taste with freshly ground black pepper.

Divide the beans, capsicum, asparagus and baby tomatoes among the baking paper squares, sprinkle with the lime zest and season with a little freshly ground black pepper. For each parcel, fold together two diagonally opposite sides of the baking paper to enclose the vegetables securely, then twist the ends to seal. Place the parcels on a large baking tray.

Line another baking tray with baking paper. Place the salmon on the tray, skin-side down, spread the pistou evenly over the top and scatter over the almonds. Place the vegetable parcels on the lower shelf of the oven and the salmon on the upper shelf and bake for 25–30 minutes or until the fish flakes easily and is cooked to your liking. The vegetable parcels should be ready at the same time.

Meanwhile, heat a large heavy-based saucepan over medium heat. Add the spinach and cook, covered, turning regularly, for 4–5 minutes or until wilted.

Flake the salmon into large chunks and serve with the vegetable parcels, spinach and lime wedges alongside.

> **WEEKS 7–12 CARB EXTRAS**
>
> For an extra 10 g carbs per serve, cut 200 g sweet potato (50 g per person) into chunks, place on a tray lined with baking paper and roast with the salmon and parcels.

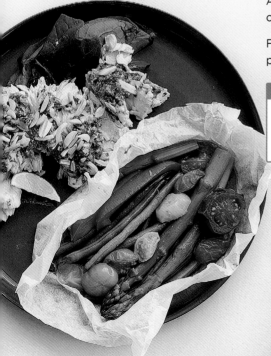

Lean meat, fish, poultry, eggs, tofu **1.5**
Dairy **0.5**
Low-carb vegetables **3**
Mod-carb vegetables **1**
Healthy fats **2**

Mediterranean vegetable and fish bake

8 G
CARB
PER
SERVE

3 zucchini, cut into 3 cm chunks
1 small (230 g) eggplant, cut into
    3 cm chunks
½ (100 g) red capsicum, seeded
    and cut into 3 cm chunks
200 g mushrooms, halved or
    quartered if large
½ teaspoon fennel seeds
olive oil spray, for cooking
3 tomatoes, quartered
600 g blue-eye trevalla fillets or other
    white fish fillets, skin removed,
    pin-boned and cut into 2 cm cubes
1 quantity Macadamia and Watercress
    Pesto (see page 191)
basil leaves or flat-leaf parsley, to serve

⊗ Serves 4   ⊘ Preparation: 15 minutes   ⊛ Cooking: 45 minutes

Preheat the oven to 200°C (180°C fan-forced).

Place the zucchini, eggplant, capsicum, mushrooms and fennel seeds in a large roasting tin. Spray with olive oil, season to taste with freshly ground black pepper and toss to combine. Roast for 20 minutes.

Remove from the oven, stir gently and scatter the tomato over the top. Return to the oven and roast for 15 minutes.

Meanwhile, place the fish in a large bowl and add the pesto. Toss gently to coat the fish.

Remove the vegetables from the oven and stir gently. Scatter the fish over the vegetables and return to the oven to roast for a further 10 minutes or until the vegetables are tender and lightly browned around the edges and the fish is cooked to your liking.

Divide the fish and vegetables evenly among four deep serving bowls and drizzle with the pan juices. Scatter with basil or parsley and serve.

> **WEEKS 7–12 CARB EXTRAS**
>
> For an extra 10 g carbs per serve, serve with 200 g (50 g per person) cooked quinoa (this is 60 g raw quinoa; 15 g per person).

Chermoula prawns with cauliflower mash

UNITS PER SERVE
Lean meat, fish, poultry, eggs, tofu **1.5**
Low-carb vegetables **2**
Mod-carb vegetables **1**
Healthy fats **2**

🍴 Serves 4   🕐 Preparation: 20 minutes   ♨ Cooking: 20 minutes

1 bunch kale (400 g trimmed),
    stalks removed and leaves
    coarsely shredded
2 bunches broccolini, trimmed
600 g raw medium king prawns,
    peeled and cleaned, with tails intact
    (weight after peeling)
1 teaspoon Moroccan seasoning
olive oil spray, for cooking
lemon wedges, to serve

CAULIFLOWER MASH

1 teaspoon olive oil
1 onion, chopped
2 cloves garlic, crushed
300 g cauliflower, chopped into
    3–4 cm pieces
1½ cups (375 ml) salt-reduced
    vegetable stock or water

CHERMOULA

40 g raw almonds, toasted
½ cup coriander leaves
½ cup flat-leaf parsley leaves
1 clove garlic
1 small fresh red chilli, seeds removed
1 teaspoon ground cumin
2 tablespoons lemon juice
2 teaspoons olive oil

To make the cauliflower mash, heat the olive oil in a large heavy-based saucepan over medium heat. Add the onion and garlic and cook, covered, for 5 minutes or until soft. Stir in the cauliflower. Add the stock and bring to the boil, then reduce the heat to low and simmer, partially covered, stirring occasionally, for 13–15 minutes or until very tender. Strain well, reserving 2 tablespoons of the cooking liquid.

Return the cauliflower mixture to the pan and mash well with a potato masher. Add a little of the reserved cooking liquid to the mash if a looser mash is desired. Season to taste with freshly ground black pepper and reheat over low–medium heat if necessary. (If you would like a smoother puree, blend with a stick blender or leave to cool slightly and puree in a food processor or blender.)

Meanwhile, to make the chermoula, place all the ingredients in a food processor and process until finely chopped and well combined. Season to taste with freshly ground black pepper. Cover and set aside.

Steam the kale in a steamer basket over a large saucepan of simmering water for 7–8 minutes or until tender. Remove. Steam the broccolini for 3 minutes or until just tender but still crisp.

Heat a chargrill pan, barbecue or heavy-based frying pan over medium–high heat. Toss the prawns with the Moroccan seasoning, then spray lightly with olive oil. Cook for 1–2 minutes on each side or until just cooked through. Transfer to a large bowl, add the chermoula and toss until well coated.

Serve one-quarter of the prawns with one-quarter of the cauliflower mash, kale and broccolini, on each of four plates, with lemon wedges to the side.

> **WEEKS 7–12 CARB EXTRAS**
>
> For an extra 10 g carbs per serve, serve with ½ piece of pita bread per person.

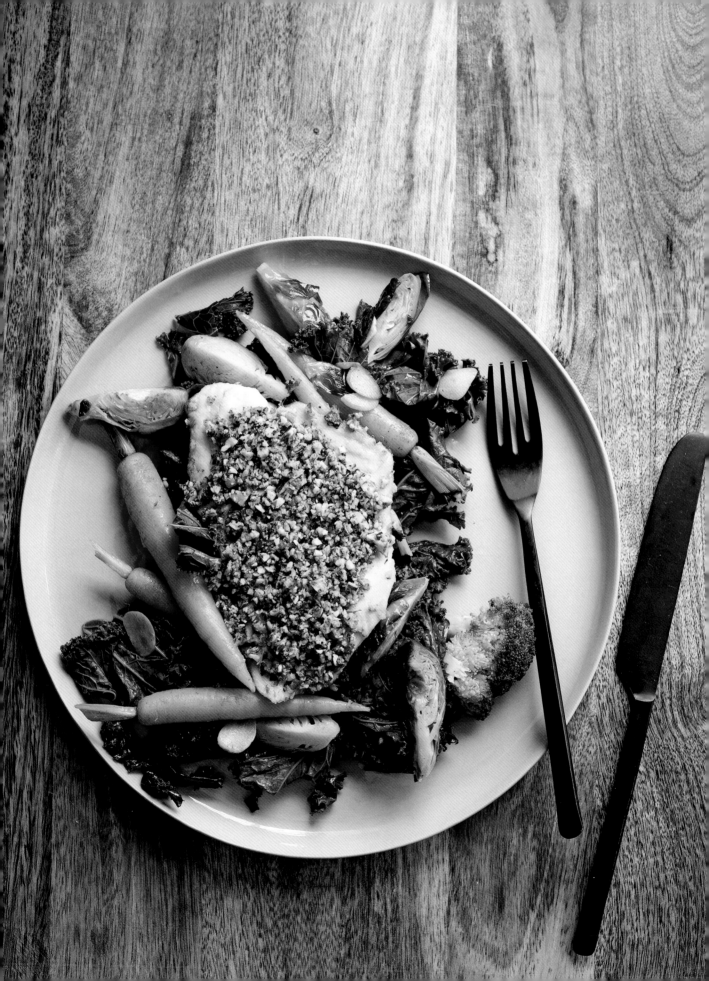

Baked fish with thyme and fennel-seed crust

UNITS PER SERVE
Lean meat, fish, poultry, eggs, tofu **1.5**
Low-carb vegetables **2**
Mod-carb vegetables **1**
Healthy fats **3**

🍴 Serves 4   🕐 Preparation: 20 minutes   ♨ Cooking: 20 minutes

4 × 150 g rockling or other firm
    white fish fillets, skin removed
    and pin-boned
1 bunch kale (400 g trimmed),
    stalks removed and leaves
    coarsely shredded
2 bunches baby carrots, trimmed
    and scrubbed
300 g broccoli florets
olive oil spray, for cooking
150 g brussels sprouts, trimmed
    and quartered
2 cloves garlic, thinly sliced
finely grated zest of 1 lemon
1 tablespoon lemon juice

THYME AND FENNEL-SEED CRUST
40 g raw almonds
40 g pecans or walnuts
1 tablespoon flat-leaf parsley
1 teaspoon thyme leaves
1 teaspoon finely grated lemon zest
½ teaspoon fennel seeds
2 teaspoons olive oil

Preheat the oven to 200°C (180°C fan-forced) and line a baking tray with baking paper.

To make the crust, place all the ingredients in a food processor and process until finely chopped and well combined. Season to taste with freshly ground black pepper.

Place the fish on the prepared tray and press one-quarter of the crust mixture over the top of each fillet. Bake for 12–15 minutes or until the fish is just cooked through and the topping is lightly browned; the cooking time will depend on the thickness of the fillets.

Meanwhile, steam the kale in a steamer basket over a large saucepan of simmering water for 7–8 minutes or until tender. Remove and set aside. Steam the carrots for 4–5 minutes or until just tender, then steam the broccoli for 3 minutes or until just tender.

Heat a heavy-based frying pan over medium–high heat. Spray lightly with olive oil and cook the sprouts and garlic, stirring occasionally, for 3–4 minutes or until just tender and caramelised. Add the steamed kale and broccoli, lemon zest and lemon juice and toss to combine.

Divide the fish, lemony kale mixture and carrots evenly among four plates and serve.

> **WEEKS 7–12 CARB EXTRAS**
>
> For an extra 10 g carbs per serve, cut 200 g (50 g per person) sweet potato or 480 g (120 g per person) pumpkin into wedges and pop it in the oven for 20 minutes before adding the fish (it should be tender when the fish is done).

UNITS PER SERVE

Lean meat, fish, poultry, eggs, tofu **1.5**
Low-carb vegetables **2**
Mod-carb vegetables **1**
Healthy fats **2.5**

Aromatic steamed fish with vegetable stir-fry

10 G CARB PER SERVE

 Serves 4   Preparation: 20 minutes   Cooking: 10 minutes

handful coriander leaves
1 × 3 cm piece ginger, peeled and
    cut into thin strips
2 cloves garlic, thinly sliced
1 long fresh red chilli, seeded and
    cut into thin strips
3 kaffir lime leaves, finely shredded
4 × 150 g blue-eye trevalla or
    other firm white fish fillets,
    skin on and pin-boned
4 baby bok choy, halved lengthways
olive oil spray, for cooking
500 g mixed mushrooms
    (button, shiitake, oyster, shimeji),
    sliced if large
1 large red or yellow capsicum,
    seeded and cut into thin strips
150 g snow peas, halved on
    the diagonal
40 g blanched or raw almonds
40 g raw unsalted cashews
2 teaspoons hoisin sauce
2 teaspoons salt-reduced soy sauce
few drops sesame oil

Line the base of a large steamer basket with baking paper. Add enough water to a saucepan or wok so the level is just under the steamer and bring to a gentle simmer.

Combine the coriander, ginger, garlic, chilli and kaffir lime leaves in a small bowl. Place the fish on the paper in the steamer, leaving space between them and sprinkle with the aromatic mixture. Cover and steam for 6–7 minutes or until the fish is just cooked through; the time will depend on the thickness of the fillets. Transfer the fish to a plate, cover with foil to keep warm and set aside briefly. Add the bok choy to the steamer basket and steam for 2 minutes or until just tender.

Meanwhile, spray a large heavy-based frying pan or wok with olive oil and place over high heat. Add the mushrooms, capsicum, snow peas and nuts and stir-fry for 5 minutes or until just tender.

Combine the hoisin sauce, soy sauce, sesame oil and 1 tablespoon water in a small bowl. Add to the pan or wok and stir-fry until heated through.

Divide the steamed fish, bok choy and stir-fried vegetables evenly among four plates and serve immediately.

WEEKS 7–12 CARB EXTRAS

For an extra 10 g carbs per serve, add 160 g (40 g per person) baby sweet corn to the stir-fry with the vegetables.

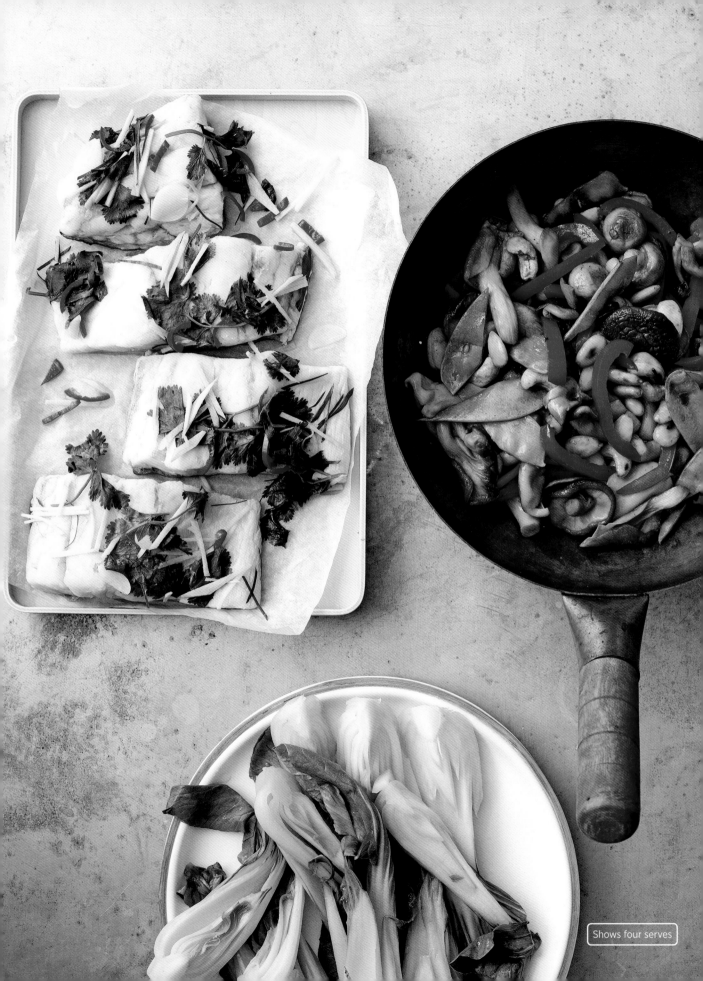

Shows four serves

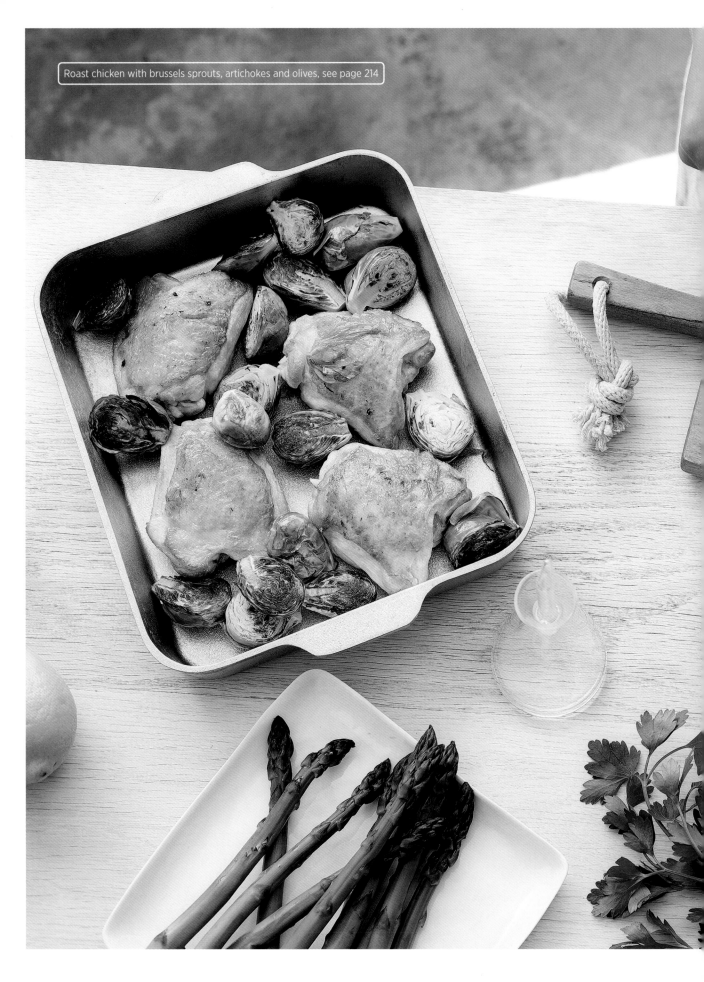

Roast chicken with brussels sprouts, artichokes and olives, see page 214

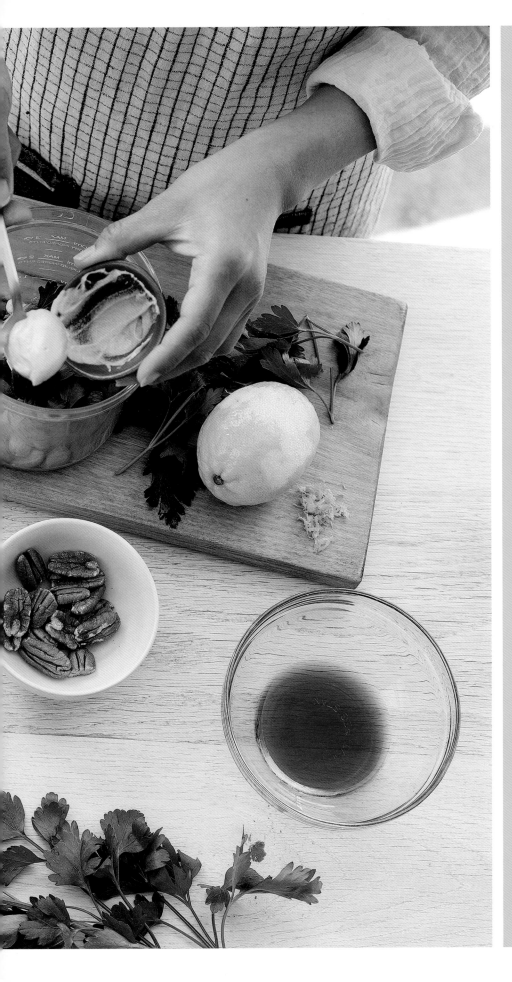

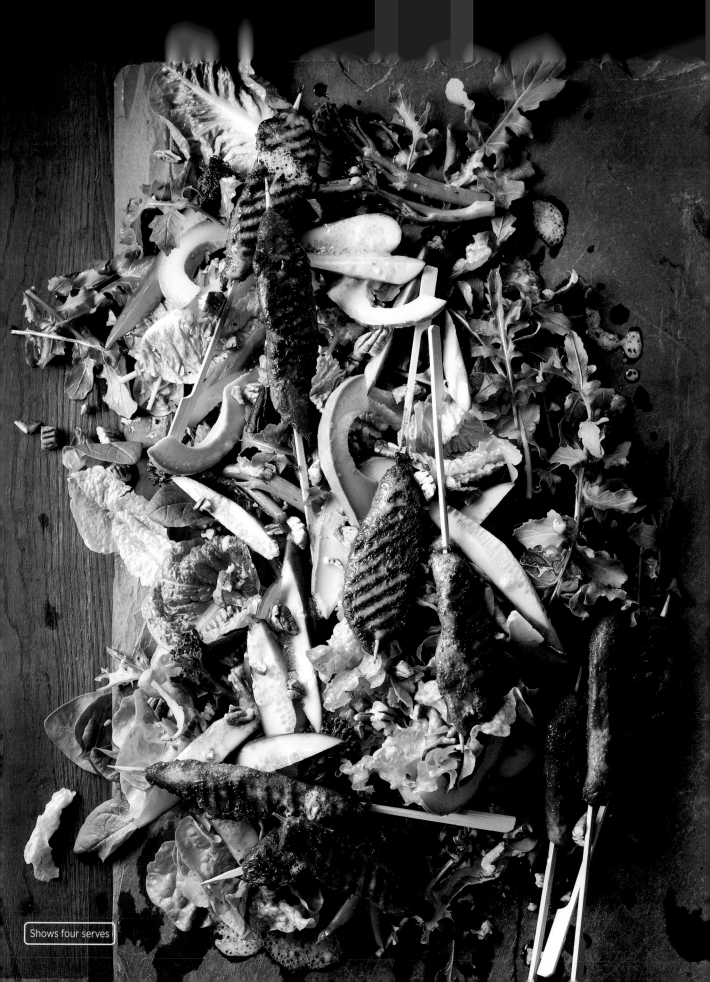

Shows four serves

Lean meat, fish, poultry, eggs, tofu **1.5**
Low-carb vegetables **3**
Healthy fats **4**

Chargrilled Cajun chicken and broccolini with salad

10 G CARB PER SERVE

🍴 Serves 4   🕐 Preparation: 25 minutes   ♨ Cooking: 15 minutes

1 tablespoon sweet paprika
2 teaspoons garlic powder
2 teaspoons onion powder
1 teaspoon dried oregano
½ teaspoon dried thyme
¼ teaspoon cayenne pepper
600 g chicken breast tenderloins
olive oil spray, for cooking
2 bunches broccolini, trimmed

MIXED LEAF AND AVOCADO SALAD

2 baby cos lettuce hearts, trimmed,
   leaves separated
1 green oak lettuce heart, trimmed,
   leaves separated
2 cups baby rocket leaves
2 cups mixed baby salad leaves
2 cups baby spinach leaves, trimmed
2 Lebanese cucumbers, halved
   lengthways and thinly sliced
   on the diagonal
1 small clove garlic, crushed
2 teaspoons Dijon mustard
2 teaspoons white wine vinegar
2 teaspoons extra virgin olive oil
160 g avocado, diced
40 g pecans or walnuts,
   roughly chopped

To make the salad, place the lettuce, rocket, salad leaves, spinach and cucumber in a large bowl and toss gently to mix. Place the garlic and mustard in a small bowl, season with freshly ground black pepper and stir to mix, then stir in the vinegar until combined. Whisk in the olive oil until emulsified. Add the dressing to the salad just before serving and toss to lightly coat, then add the avocado and pecans.

Place the paprika, garlic powder, onion powder, oregano and thyme in a shallow bowl large enough to fit the chicken, season with pepper and stir to mix well. Insert a skewer (see note) into each chicken tenderloin lengthways, then place in the Cajun spice mix, pressing to coat each chicken tenderloin evenly.

Heat a chargrill pan over medium heat and spray with olive oil. Spray the chicken tenderloins with oil, then add the chicken to the hot chargrill pan and cook for 4–5 minutes on each side or until golden and cooked through. Transfer to a plate, cover with foil and keep warm. Spray the broccolini with oil, then cook in the chargrill pan for 3 minutes on each side or until tender but still crisp and chargrilled on the edges.

Pile the salad, chicken and broccolini onto a large platter and serve.

> **WEEKS 7–12 CARB EXTRAS**
>
> For an extra 10 g carbs per serve, add 200 g (50 g per person) drained and rinsed tinned salt-reduced black-eye beans or 160 g (40 g per person) cooked corn kernels to the salad.

Note: You will need to soak twelve long bamboo skewers in cold water for 30 minutes for this recipe.

UNITS PER SERVE

Lean meat, fish, poultry, eggs, tofu **1.5**
Low-carb vegetables **3.5**
Mod-carb vegetables **0.5**
Healthy fats **1**

Turkey larb with 'noodle' salad

🍽 **Serves 4**   🕐 **Preparation: 20 minutes**   ⓦ **Cooking: 20 minutes**

olive oil spray, for cooking
1 small onion, chopped
1 long fresh red chilli, seeded
    and thinly sliced
2 cloves garlic, crushed
1 stalk lemongrass, white part only,
    finely chopped or grated
4 kaffir lime leaves, finely shredded
600 g lean minced turkey
1 bunch broccolini, trimmed and
    thinly sliced
300 g green cabbage, finely shredded
2 tablespoons lime juice
1½ tablespoons fish sauce
1½ cups (120 g) bean sprouts, trimmed
2 zucchini, spiralised
2 Lebanese cucumbers, spiralised
small handful Thai basil leaves
small handful mint leaves
40 g raw almonds or peanuts, toasted,
    roughly chopped
lime wedges, to serve

Heat a large heavy-based frying pan over medium heat and spray lightly with olive oil. Add the onion, chilli and garlic and cook, stirring, for 1–2 minutes or until fragrant. Increase the heat to high, add the lemongrass, kaffir lime leaves and half the turkey and cook, stirring occasionally for 5–6 minutes or until browned. Remove to a plate. Spray the pan with a little more oil if necessary and cook the remaining turkey for 5–6 minutes. Return the first batch of mince and flavourings to the pan, then add the broccolini and half the cabbage and cook for 1–2 minutes or until they are just tender.

Add the lime juice and fish sauce and stir-fry to combine. Toss through the bean sprouts.

Place the zucchini and cucumber 'noodles' in a large bowl and toss with the remaining cabbage.

Divide the larb and 'noodle' salad evenly among four plates. Scatter with the herbs and nuts and serve with lime wedges on the side.

> **WEEKS 7–12 CARB EXTRAS**
>
> For an extra 10 g carbs per serve, add 480 g (120 g per person) green peas or 160 g (40 g per person) corn kernels to the larb mixture when you add the broccolini and cabbage.

UNITS PER SERVE

Lean meat, fish, poultry, eggs, tofu **1.5**
Low-carb vegetables **3**
Mod-carb vegetables **0.5**
Healthy fats **4**

Lemon oregano roast chicken with rocket and tahini salad

🍽 **Serves 4**   🕐 **Preparation: 25 minutes, plus marinating time**
🍲 **Cooking: 45 minutes**

4 × 150 g chicken breast fillets, flattened
   with a meat mallet
finely grated zest and juice of 1 lemon
2 tablespoons extra virgin olive oil
3 teaspoons dried oregano
3 teaspoons finely chopped rosemary
9 cloves garlic, 8 unpeeled, 1 crushed
olive oil spray, for cooking
3 small zucchini, trimmed and
   halved lengthways
200 g broccoli, trimmed and cut
   into small florets
2 bunches broccolini, bases trimmed
150 g small brussels sprouts, trimmed
6 fresh bay leaves
¼ cup (60 ml) salt-reduced
   chicken stock
2 cups kale leaves, torn

ROCKET AND TAHINI SALAD

1 cup rocket leaves
250 g cherry tomatoes, halved
2 tablespoons tahini
2 teaspoons seasoned rice vinegar
1 small clove garlic, finely crushed
1 tablespoon boiling water, plus extra
   if needed

Place the chicken in a shallow bowl, then place the lemon zest and juice and 1 tablespoon of the olive oil in a small bowl and stir to combine. Stir in the oregano, rosemary and crushed garlic and mix to combine. Spoon over the chicken and rub to coat evenly. Season to taste with freshly ground black pepper, then cover with plastic film and marinate in the refrigerator for 30 minutes or up to 2 hours.

Preheat the oven to 200°C (180°C fan-forced).

Heat a large flameproof roasting tin over medium–high heat and spray with olive oil. Add the chicken and cook for 4 minutes on each side or until golden, then remove from the heat. Add the zucchini, broccoli, broccolini, brussels sprouts, whole garlic cloves and bay leaves to the tin, drizzle the remaining olive oil over the vegetables and pour in the chicken stock. Roast for 30–35 minutes or until the chicken is golden and cooked through and the vegetables are golden and tender. In the last 10 minutes, place the kale on a baking tray, spray with olive oil and add to the oven to roast until crisp; check after 8 minutes.

Meanwhile, to make the salad, place the rocket and tomato in a bowl. Place the tahini, vinegar, garlic and boiling water in a small bowl and stir to combine and emulsify; add a little more boiling water if a thinner consistency is preferred. Add to the salad and toss gently to coat.

Place a chicken breast on each of four plates, then add one-quarter of the roasted vegetables and salad to each plate and serve immediately.

WEEKS 7–12 CARB EXTRAS

For an extra 10 g carbs per serve, cut 200 g (50 g per person) sweet potato into 1.5 cm dice and add to the roasting tin with the chicken and other vegetables.

UNITS PER SERVE

Lean meat, fish, poultry, eggs, tofu **1.5**
Dairy **1**
Low-carb vegetables **3**
Mod-carb vegetables **1**
Healthy fats **4**

Hummus-crusted chicken with roasted cauliflower and haloumi salad

9 G
CARB
PER
SERVE

🍴 **Serves 4**   🕐 **Preparation: 25 minutes**   ♨ **Cooking: 30 minutes**

⅓ cup (80 g) hummus
1 clove garlic, finely chopped
1 teaspoon sweet paprika
1 teaspoon ground cumin
600 g chicken breast tenderloins
sumac, for sprinkling
extra virgin olive oil, for drizzling
lemon wedges, to serve (optional)

ROASTED CAULIFLOWER AND HALOUMI SALAD

1 small head cauliflower, cut into
    small florets
olive oil spray, for cooking
½ teaspoon sumac
40 g macadamias, roughly crushed
2 cups watercress sprigs
2 cups baby rocket leaves
2 cups frisee, torn
2 cups baby spinach leaves, trimmed
2 tomatoes, sliced
1 Lebanese cucumber, halved
    lengthways and thinly sliced
    on the diagonal
1 tablespoon extra virgin olive oil
2 teaspoons lemon juice
80 g haloumi, cut into 1 cm thick slices

Preheat the oven to 210°C (190°C fan-forced). Line two roasting tins with baking paper.

Place the hummus, garlic, paprika and cumin in a small bowl, season to taste with freshly ground black pepper and stir to combine.

Place the chicken tenderloins in one of the lined roasting tins and spread evenly with the hummus mixture. Sprinkle with sumac, then drizzle lightly with olive oil.

Roast for 20–25 minutes or until the hummus is golden and the chicken is cooked through.

Meanwhile, to start making the salad, place the cauliflower in the second lined roasting tin, spray with olive oil and sprinkle with sumac. Roast for 15–20 minutes or until tender and golden around the edges; add the macadamias to the tin to roast 5 minutes before the cauliflower is ready.

Place the watercress, rocket, frisee, spinach, tomato and cucumber in a large bowl and toss gently to mix. Just before serving, add the olive oil and lemon juice and toss to coat.

Heat a heavy-based non-stick frying pan over medium heat and spray with olive oil. Add the haloumi and cook for 2 minutes on each side or until golden.

Divide the salad, chicken, cauliflower and haloumi among four plates. Serve immediately with lemon wedges to the side, if using.

> **WEEKS 7-12 CARB EXTRAS**
>
> For an extra 10 g carbs per serve, cut 480 g (120 g per person) pumpkin into thin wedges. Add to the roasting tin with the cauliflower, spray with olive oil and sprinkle with sumac.

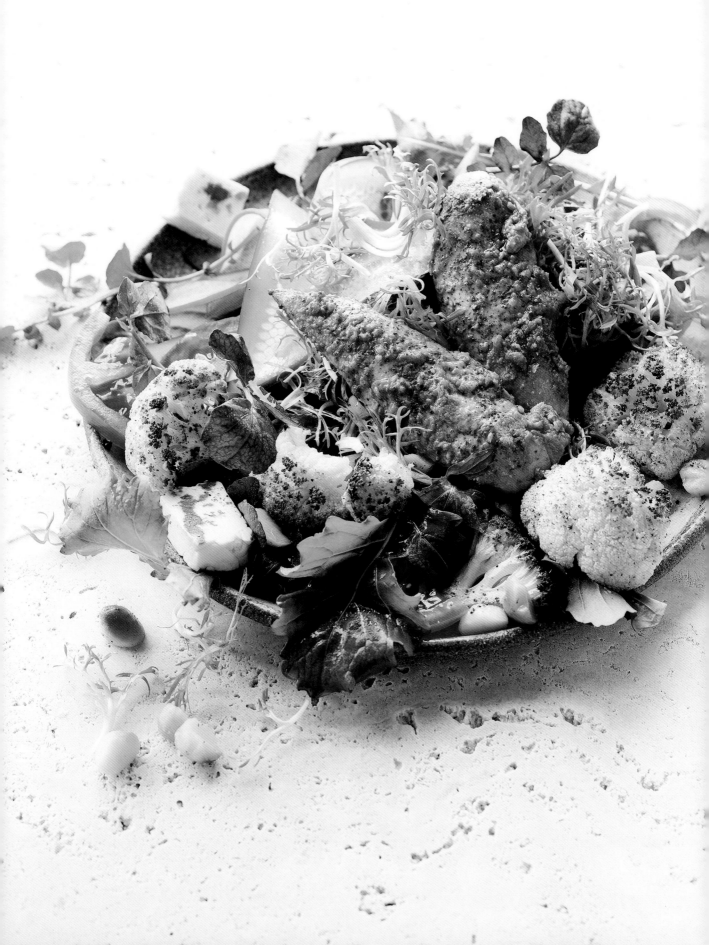

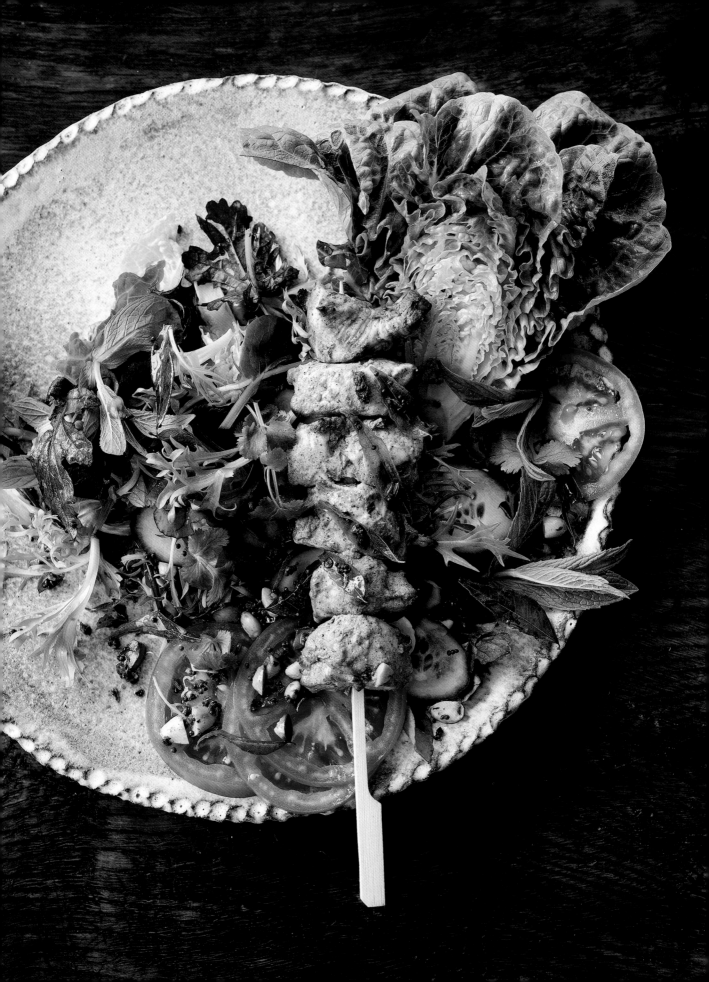

UNITS PER SERVE

Lean meat, fish, poultry, eggs, tofu **1.5**
Low-carb vegetables **3**
Mod-carb vegetables **0.5**
Healthy fats **2**

Chicken tikka skewers with Indian summer salad

14 G CARB PER SERVE

🍽 Serves 4   🕐 Preparation: 25 minutes, plus marinating time
🍳 Cooking: 30 minutes

2 teaspoons garam masala
1 teaspoon ground turmeric
½ teaspoon ground cumin
½ teaspoon ground coriander
¼ teaspoon chilli powder
¼ cup (70 g) low-fat
   Greek-style yoghurt
2 tablespoons roughly chopped mint
2 tablespoons roughly
   chopped coriander leaves
1 tablespoon lemon juice
600 g chicken breast fillets, cut
   into 2 cm cubes
olive oil spray, for cooking
lemon wedges, to serve (optional)

INDIAN DUKKAH

2 teaspoons extra virgin olive oil
40 g raw almonds, roughly chopped
1 teaspoon finely grated ginger
2 tablespoons fresh or dried
   curry leaves
2 teaspoons mustard seeds
¼ teaspoon fennel seeds
¼ teaspoon chilli flakes (optional)

INDIAN SUMMER SALAD

4 cups mixed salad leaves
2 baby cos lettuces, shredded
1 cup finely shredded red cabbage
1 cup finely shredded green cabbage
4 tomatoes, sliced
1 telegraph cucumber, sliced
1 zucchini, shaved lengthways
   with a vegetable peeler
½ cup mint leaves, torn
½ cup coriander leaves, torn
2 teaspoons extra virgin olive oil
lemon juice, to taste

Place the garam masala, turmeric, cumin, ground coriander, chilli powder, yoghurt, mint, chopped coriander and lemon juice in a small bowl and mix well to combine. Thread the chicken onto the skewers (see note) and place in a baking dish that fits them in a single layer, then add the tikka marinade and rub to coat the chicken all over. Cover with plastic film and marinate in the refrigerator for at least 30 minutes or up to 2 hours.

Meanwhile, to make the dukkah, heat the olive oil in a small heavy-based non-stick frying pan over medium heat. Add the almonds and cook, stirring frequently, for 2 minutes or until light golden. Add the ginger, curry leaves, mustard seeds, fennel seeds and chilli flakes (if using) and stir for 30 seconds or until fragrant. Set aside to cool.

Preheat the oven to 210°C (190°C). Line a roasting tin with foil or baking paper and place an ovenproof wire rack on top.

Place the chicken skewers on the wire rack, spoon over any remaining marinade and spray with olive oil, then bake for 20 minutes or until the chicken is almost cooked. Preheat the oven grill to high and grill the chicken for 5 minutes or until golden and cooked through.

Meanwhile, to make the salad, place the salad leaves, lettuce, cabbage, tomato, cucumber, zucchini, mint and coriander in a large bowl. Drizzle over the olive oil and lemon juice and toss gently to mix.

Place one-quarter of the salad on each of four plates or small platters, then top with the chicken tikka skewers. Scatter over the dukkah and serve immediately with lemon wedges, if using.

WEEKS 7–12 CARB EXTRAS

For an extra 10 g carbs per serve, add 160 g (40 g per person) drained and rinsed tinned salt-reduced chickpeas to the salad.

Note: You will need to soak twelve long bamboo skewers in cold water for 30 minutes for this recipe.

UNITS PER SERVE

Lean meat, fish, poultry, eggs, tofu **1.5**
Dairy **0.5**
Low-carb vegetables **3**
Mod-carb vegetables **0.5**
Healthy fats **2.5**

olive oil spray, for cooking
1 small onion, chopped
2 cloves garlic, crushed
4 tomatoes, chopped
1 teaspoon red wine vinegar
boiling water, to thin the sauce
  (optional)
3 zucchini, spiralised
100 g radicchio
100 g rocket leaves
1 bulb baby fennel, trimmed
  and thinly sliced
40 g parmesan, to serve (optional)

TURKEY AND LEMON MEATBALLS

600 g lean minced turkey
40 g flaked almonds
2 tablespoons ground almonds
2 tablespoons finely chopped
  flat-leaf parsley
finely grated zest of 1 lemon

DRESSING

1 tablespoon olive oil
2 tablespoons red wine vinegar
  or lemon juice
3 teaspoons wholegrain mustard

Turkey and lemon meatballs with 'spaghetti' Napolitana

🍴 Serves 4   🕐 Preparation: 20 minutes   ♨ Cooking: 35 minutes

To make the meatballs, combine all the ingredients in a bowl and season with freshly ground black pepper. Divide the mixture into 20 portions and roll into balls.

Heat a large heavy-based non-stick frying pan over medium heat. Spray the meatballs lightly with olive oil and, working in two batches if necessary, pan-fry the meatballs for 12–15 minutes, turning regularly until browned and cooked through.

Meanwhile, heat another heavy-based frying pan over low–medium heat. Spray the pan lightly with olive oil, add the onion and cook, stirring regularly, for 5 minutes or until softened. Add the garlic and cook for 1 minute or until fragrant. Add the tomato and cook, stirring occasionally, for 8–10 minutes or until the tomato has broken down to form a thick sauce. Stir in the vinegar; add a little boiling water to thin out the sauce slightly if necessary.

Add the meatballs to the sauce and turn to coat. Add the zucchini 'spaghetti' and toss to combine. Cook for 1–2 minutes or until just heated through.

To make the dressing, place all the ingredients in a screw-top jar, secure the lid and shake until combined. Season to taste with freshly ground black pepper.

Combine the radicchio, rocket and fennel in a large bowl. Add the dressing just before serving and toss to combine.

Divide the zucchini 'spaghetti' and meatballs evenly among four bowls and grate or shave the parmesan over the top, if using. Serve the salad on the side.

WEEKS 7–12 CARB EXTRAS

For an extra 10 g carbs per serve, add 200 g (50 g per person) drained and rinsed tinned salt-reduced cannellini beans, or 480 g (120 g per person) cooked green peas to the 'spaghetti'.

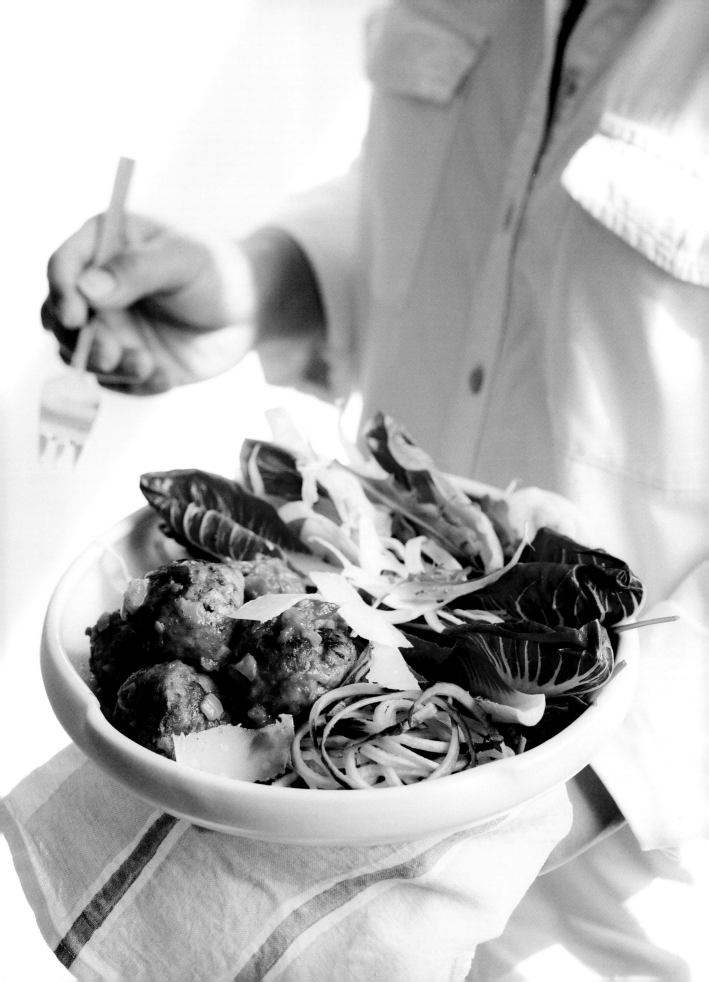

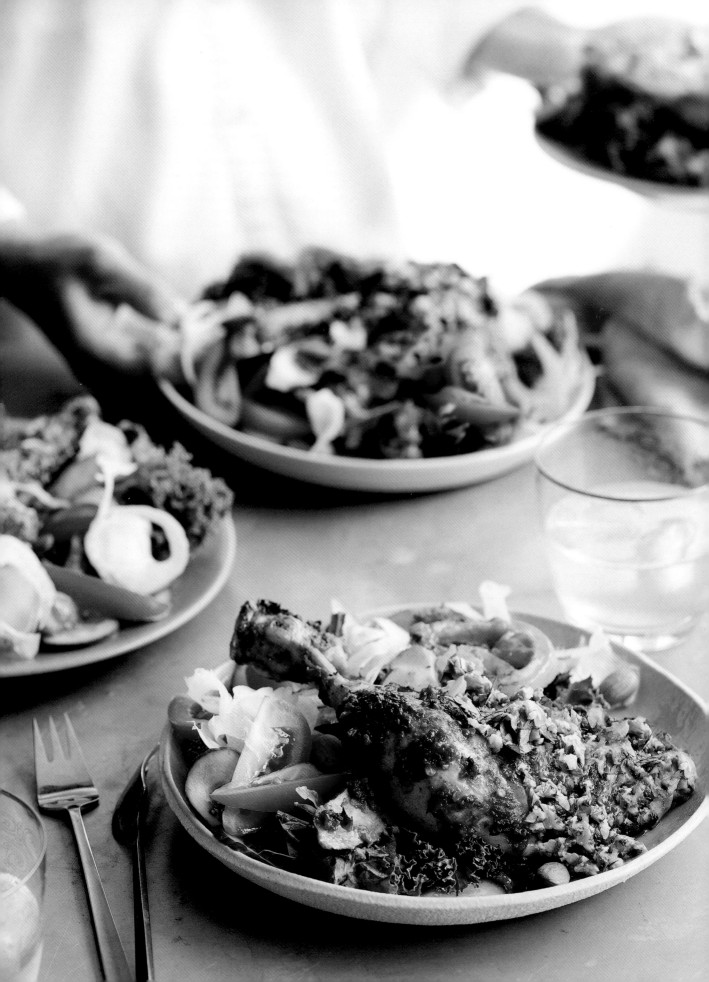

Portuguese chicken with cucumber and fennel salad

12 G CARB PER SERVE

🍴 Serves 4   🕐 Preparation: 20 minutes, plus refrigerating time
🍲 Cooking: 35 minutes

2 tablespoons finely grated lemon zest

2 long fresh red chillies,
   roughly chopped

1 tablespoon sweet paprika

4 cloves garlic

2 teaspoons olive oil

600 g chicken pieces,
   fat removed

4 small zucchini, halved lengthways

1 lemon, thickly sliced

olive oil spray, for cooking

2 tablespoons finely chopped
   flat-leaf parsley

40 g pecans or walnuts,
   finely chopped

2 tablespoons lemon juice

2 tomatoes, halved lengthways

2 Lebanese cucumbers, sliced

1 bulb baby fennel, trimmed and
   thinly sliced

200 g baby kale leaves

40 g raw almonds, toasted

Place the lemon zest, chilli, paprika and 3 of the garlic cloves in a mortar and pound with a pestle until a paste forms. Season to taste with freshly ground black pepper, then add the olive oil and stir to combine. (Alternatively, blend in a small food processor until combined.) Place in a large bowl or zip-lock bag with the chicken and rub over the chicken to coat well. Cover and refrigerate for 3 hours or overnight.

Preheat the oven to 180°C (160°C fan-forced).

Heat a chargrill pan or barbecue to medium heat. Cook the chicken for 2–3 minutes or until well marked on one side. Turn and cook for a further 3 minutes or until well marked on the other side.

Place the zucchini and sliced lemon in a large roasting tin and spray lightly with olive oil. Place the chicken on top of the zucchini and roast for 20–25 minutes or until the chicken is cooked through.

Meanwhile, crush the remaining garlic clove and place in a small bowl with the parsley, pecans and lemon juice. Stir to combine. Spread the mixture over the chicken as soon as it is removed from the oven.

Toss the tomato, cucumber, fennel, kale and almonds together. Divide among four plates and serve with the chicken, zucchini and lemon.

> **WEEKS 7–12 CARB EXTRAS**
>
> For an extra 10 g carbs per serve, cut 160 g (40 g per person) sweet corn into sections or 200 g (50 g per person) sweet potato into wedges and roast with the chicken and zucchini.

Roast chicken with brussels sprouts, artichokes and olives

8 G CARB PER SERVE

UNITS PER SERVE

Lean meat, fish, poultry, eggs, tofu **1.5**
Low-carb vegetables **2**
Mod-carb vegetables **1**
Healthy fats **4**

🍴 **Serves 4**   🕐 **Preparation: 20 minutes**   🍳 **Cooking: 40 minutes**

4 × 180 g chicken thigh cutlets
(thigh with bone in)
300 g brussels sprouts, trimmed
and halved lengthways
olive oil spray, for cooking
¾ cup (180 ml) salt-reduced
chicken stock
4 tomatoes, quartered lengthways
300 g marinated artichoke hearts
from a jar, halved lengthways
½ cup (70 g) pitted kalamata olives
2 bunches asparagus, trimmed

ALMOND AND MUSTARD CRUST

40 g raw almonds
1 tablespoon chopped flat-leaf parsley
1 teaspoon finely grated lemon zest
2 teaspoons Dijon mustard

DRESSING

40 g pecans or walnuts,
finely chopped
1 tablespoon chopped flat-leaf parsley
2 tablespoons red wine vinegar
1 tablespoon olive oil

Preheat the oven to 200°C (180°C fan-forced).

Heat a large flameproof baking dish over medium heat. Add the chicken and brussels sprouts and spray lightly with olive oil. Cook, turning occasionally, for 5–6 minutes or until browned all over. Transfer to a plate.

Meanwhile, to make the almond and mustard crust, place all the ingredients in a food processor and process until finely chopped and well combined. Season to taste with freshly ground black pepper. Press the mixture over the top of each piece of chicken.

Pour the chicken stock into the baking dish and stir to scrape any residue off the bottom. Cook for 1–2 minutes or until the liquid has reduced slightly. Remove from the heat and return the sprouts and chicken, crust-side up, to the dish, along with the tomato, artichoke hearts and olives. Spray the tomatoes and artichokes with oil, cover with foil and bake for 15 minutes. Remove the foil and cook for a further 15 minutes or until the chicken and vegetables are tender.

Meanwhile, to make the dressing, combine all the ingredients in a small bowl. Season to taste with freshly ground black pepper.

Steam the asparagus in a steamer basket over a large saucepan of simmering water for 3–4 minutes or until just tender.

Divide the chicken and vegetables evenly among four plates and pour over the pan juices. Serve with the asparagus, drizzled with the pecan dressing.

WEEKS 7–12 CARB EXTRAS

For an extra 10 g carbs per serve, accompany with 200 g (50 g per person) cooked quinoa (this is 60 g raw quinoa; 15 g per person).

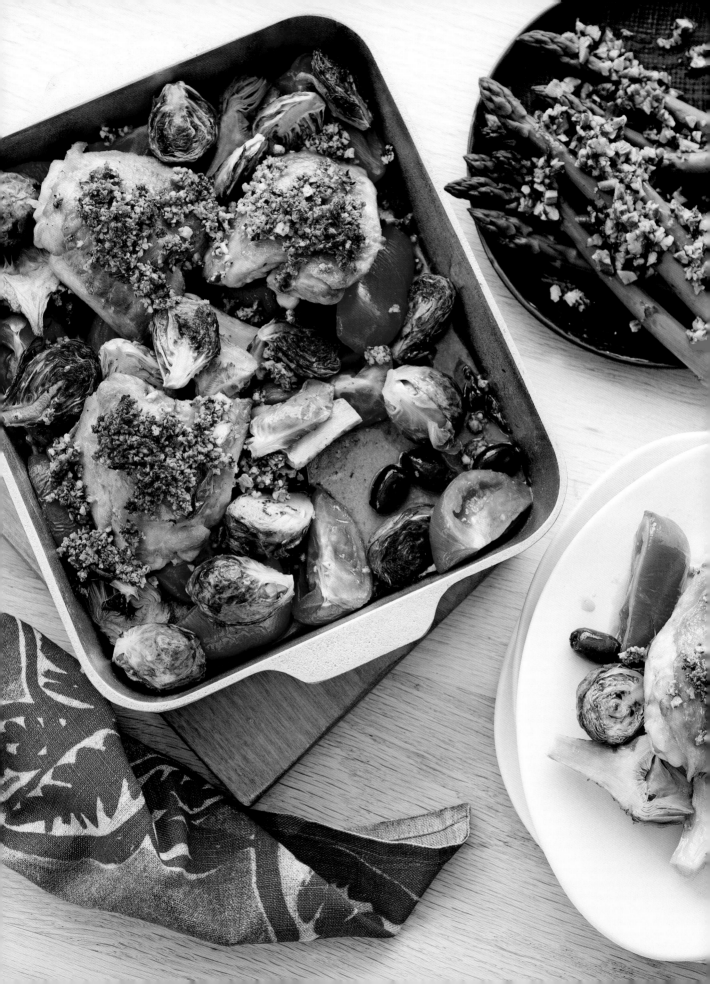

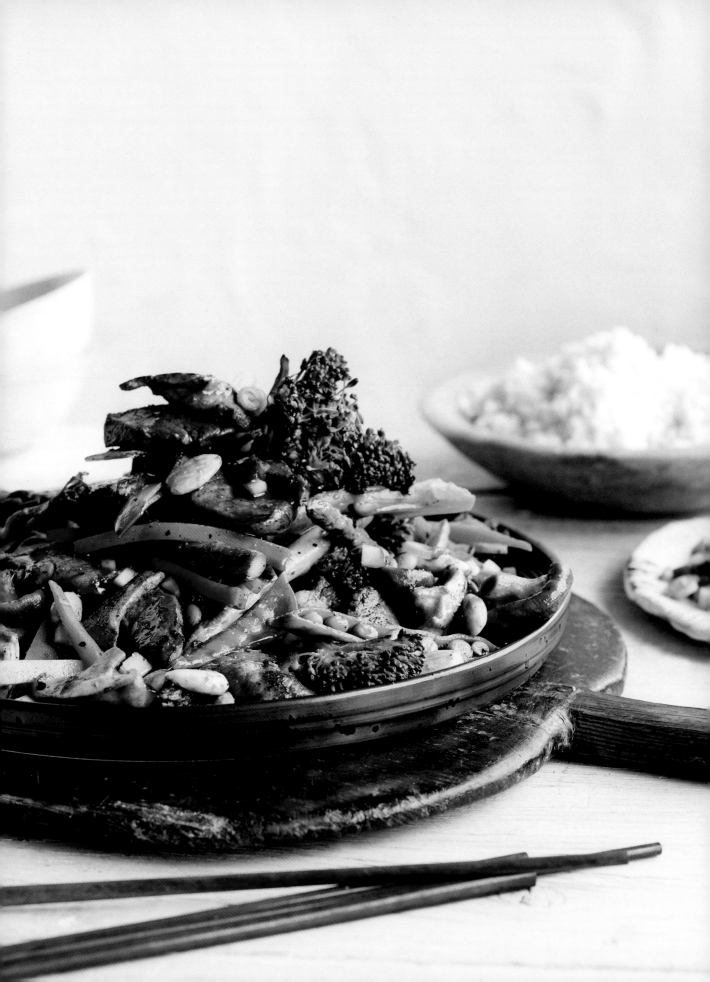

UNITS PER SERVE
Lean meat, fish, poultry, eggs, tofu **1.5**
Low-carb vegetables **2.5**
Mod-carb vegetables **2**
Healthy fats **3**

Mu shu pork stir-fry with cauliflower 'rice'

12 G CARB PER SERVE

🍽 **Serves 4**   🕐 **Preparation: 25 minutes, plus marinating time**
🍲 **Cooking: 30 minutes**

2 tablespoons salt-reduced soy sauce

2 tablespoons Shaoxing rice wine
 or dry sherry

1 tablespoon hoisin sauce

2 tablespoons extra virgin olive oil

1 × 600 g pork fillet, thinly sliced
 against the grain

40 g blanched almonds

pinch of five-spice powder

2 bunches broccolini, trimmed and
 halved lengthways

2 bunches thin asparagus

200 g snow peas, trimmed and
 halved lengthways

1 carrot, cut into thick julienne

300 g fresh shiitake or oyster
 mushrooms, trimmed and thinly sliced

¼ cup (60 ml) salt-reduced
 chicken stock

2 Lebanese cucumbers, finely diced

1 spring onion, sliced

CAULIFLOWER 'RICE'

1 small head cauliflower, cut into
 small florets

olive oil spray, for cooking

Place the soy sauce, rice wine or sherry, hoisin sauce and 2 teaspoons of the olive oil in a small bowl and mix to combine. Place the pork in a glass bowl, add the soy marinade and stir to coat. Cover with plastic film and marinate in the refrigerator for 30 minutes or up to 2 hours.

To make the cauliflower 'rice', working in batches, place the cauliflower in a food processor and process until finely chopped to resemble grains of rice. Heat a heavy-based non-stick frying pan over medium heat and spray with olive oil. Add the cauliflower and cook, stirring, for 5–6 minutes or until warmed through. Cover with a lid or foil to keep warm and set aside.

Heat 1 teaspoon of the oil in a wok over high heat, then add the almonds and five-spice powder and stir-fry for 1 minute or until golden and fragrant. Set aside. Add half the pork to the wok and stir-fry for 3–4 minutes or until cooked through. Set aside in a large heatproof bowl. Repeat with the remaining pork, adding a little more of the oil to the wok if necessary. Transfer to the bowl, cover with foil to keep warm and set aside. Reserve any remaining marinade.

Heat another teaspoon of the oil in the wok, then add the broccolini and asparagus and stir-fry for 2–3 minutes or until tender but still crisp. Add to the bowl with the pork. Heat another teaspoon of oil in the wok, then add the snow peas and carrot and stir-fry for 2–3 minutes or until tender but still crisp. Transfer to the bowl. Heat the remaining oil in the wok, then add the mushrooms and stir-fry for 3–4 minutes or until tender. Add the stock and any reserved marinade and bring to the boil. Return the pork and vegetables to the wok, reduce the heat to low and toss to combine. Remove from the heat.

Combine the cucumber and spring onion and stir through the pork mixture. Divide the pork and vegetable mixture among four plates or bowls and scatter with the five-spice almonds. Serve the cauliflower 'rice' to the side.

> **WEEKS 7–12 CARB EXTRAS**
>
> For an extra 10 g carbs per serve, add 200 g (50 g per person) cooked quinoa to the cauliflower 'rice' (this is 60 g raw quinoa; 15 g per person).

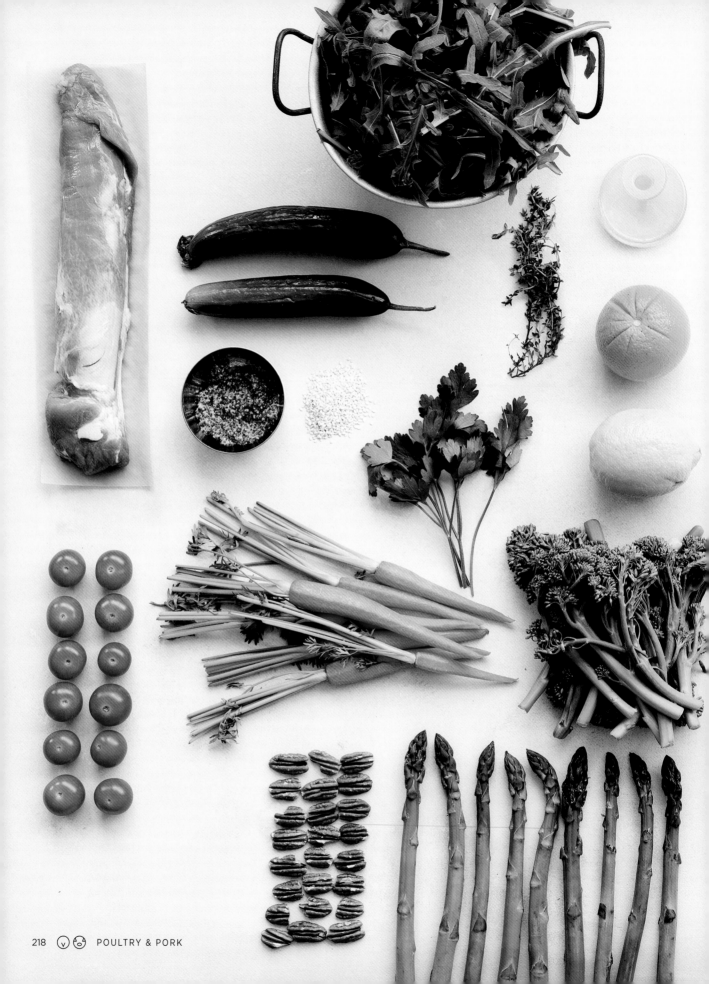

UNITS PER SERVE
Lean meat, fish, poultry, eggs, tofu **1.5**
Low-carb vegetables **2.5**
Mod-carb vegetables **0.5**
Healthy fats **2.5**

Orange and mustard roasted pork fillet

10 G CARB PER SERVE

🍴 **Serves 4**
🕐 **Preparation: 15 minutes, plus marinating and resting time**
🍳 **Cooking: 30 minutes**

1 tablespoon wholegrain mustard
1 tablespoon sesame seeds
1 teaspoon chopped thyme
1 teaspoon olive oil
1 teaspoon finely grated orange zest
1 × 600 g pork fillet
olive oil spray, for cooking
1 bunch baby carrots, trimmed
   and scrubbed
2 bunches broccolini, trimmed
2 bunches asparagus, trimmed and
   sliced into thirds on the diagonal
200 g baby rocket leaves
2 Lebanese cucumbers,
   thinly sliced on the diagonal
300 g cherry tomatoes, halved
1 lemon, cut into wedges

ORANGE AND PECAN VINAIGRETTE
40 g pecans or walnuts,
   roughly chopped
1 tablespoon chopped flat-leaf parsley
2 tablespoons orange juice
1 tablespoon olive oil

Preheat the oven to 180°C (160°C fan-forced).

Combine the mustard, sesame seeds, thyme, olive oil and orange zest in a bowl. Add the pork and turn to coat. Set aside to marinate for 5 minutes.

Heat a heavy-based frying pan over medium heat. Spray the pork lightly with olive oil and pan-fry, turning, for 4–5 minutes or until caramelised all over. Transfer to a roasting tin, then add the carrots and spray lightly with olive oil. Roast for 20–25 minutes or until the pork is just cooked through. Remove from the oven and cover loosely with foil, then set aside to rest for 10 minutes.

Meanwhile, to make the vinaigrette, combine all the ingredients in a small bowl and season to taste with freshly ground black pepper.

Steam the broccolini and asparagus in a steamer basket over a large saucepan of simmering water for 2–3 minutes or until just tender.

Combine the rocket, cucumber and tomatoes in a bowl.

Slice the pork thickly and divide evenly among four plates, along with the steamed vegetables, roast carrots and salad. Drizzle the vinaigrette over the vegetables, and serve the lemon wedges on the side.

WEEKS 7–12 CARB EXTRAS

For an extra 10 g carbs per serve, cut 480 g (120 g per person) pumpkin or 200 g (50 g per person) sweet potato into wedges and roast with the pork and carrots.

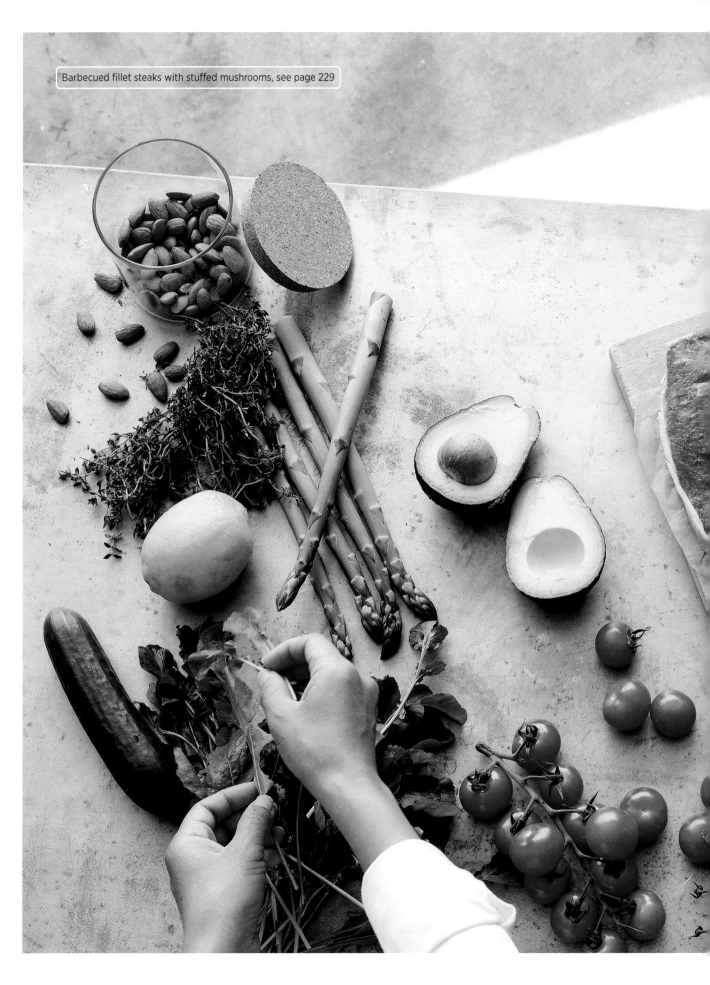

Barbecued fillet steaks with stuffed mushrooms, see page 229

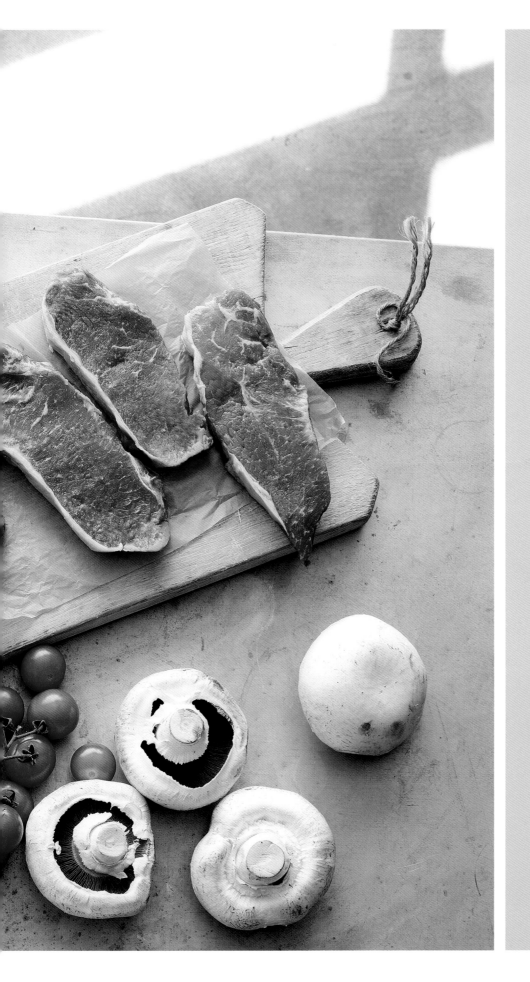

UNITS PER SERVE

Lean meat, fish, poultry, eggs, tofu **1.5**
Low-carb vegetables **3**
Mod-carb vegetables **0.5**
Healthy fats **3.5**

Lemongrass and chilli beef with zucchini 'noodles'

11 G CARB PER SERVE

🍴 **Serves 4**   🕐 **Preparation: 25 minutes, plus marinating time**
🍲 **Cooking: 20 minutes**

1 stalk lemongrass, white part only, finely chopped

1 tablespoon oyster sauce

2 teaspoons salt-reduced soy sauce

2 teaspoons fish sauce

1 small fresh red chilli, seeded and finely chopped

2 cloves garlic, finely chopped

600 g beef rump steak, all visible fat removed, thinly sliced on the diagonal

3 zucchini, spiralised

2 tablespoons extra virgin olive oil

3 baby bok choy, halved or quartered lengthways, depending on size

150 g broccoli, trimmed and cut into small florets

1 bunch asparagus, halved on the diagonal

150 g small snow peas

60 g raw unsalted cashews, coarsely crushed

¼ cup Thai basil leaves, torn

¼ cup small mint leaves

Place the lemongrass, oyster sauce, soy sauce, fish sauce, chilli and 1 clove of the garlic in a glass bowl and stir to combine. Add the beef and stir to coat, then cover with plastic film and marinate in the refrigerator for 30 minutes or up to 2 hours.

Just before cooking the stir-fry, steam the zucchini 'noodles' in a steamer basket over a large saucepan of simmering water for 2 minutes or until just tender. Place in a colander over a large bowl and set aside.

Heat 1 tablespoon of the olive oil in a wok over high heat. Working in two batches, stir-fry the beef for 3–4 minutes or until just cooked through. Transfer to a large heatproof bowl and set aside.

Heat 2 teaspoons of the oil in the wok, then add the bok choy and stir-fry for 2–3 minutes or until the stems are just tender. Transfer to the bowl with the beef. Add the remaining oil and garlic to the wok and stir-fry the broccoli, asparagus and snow peas for 2–3 minutes or until tender but still crisp. Add to the bowl of beef and bok choy, then add the basil and mint, season to taste with freshly ground white pepper and toss gently to mix well.

Divide the zucchini 'noodles' among four plates or bowls, then top with one-quarter of the stir-fried beef and vegetables. Scatter the cashews evenly over the top and serve immediately. (Alternatively, add the stir-fried beef and vegetables to the zucchini 'noodles' and toss gently to combine, then divide among four plates or bowls.)

> **WEEKS 7–12 CARB EXTRAS**
>
> For an extra 10 g carbs per serve, add 160 g (40 g per person) baby corn, halved lengthways, to the wok when adding the asparagus.

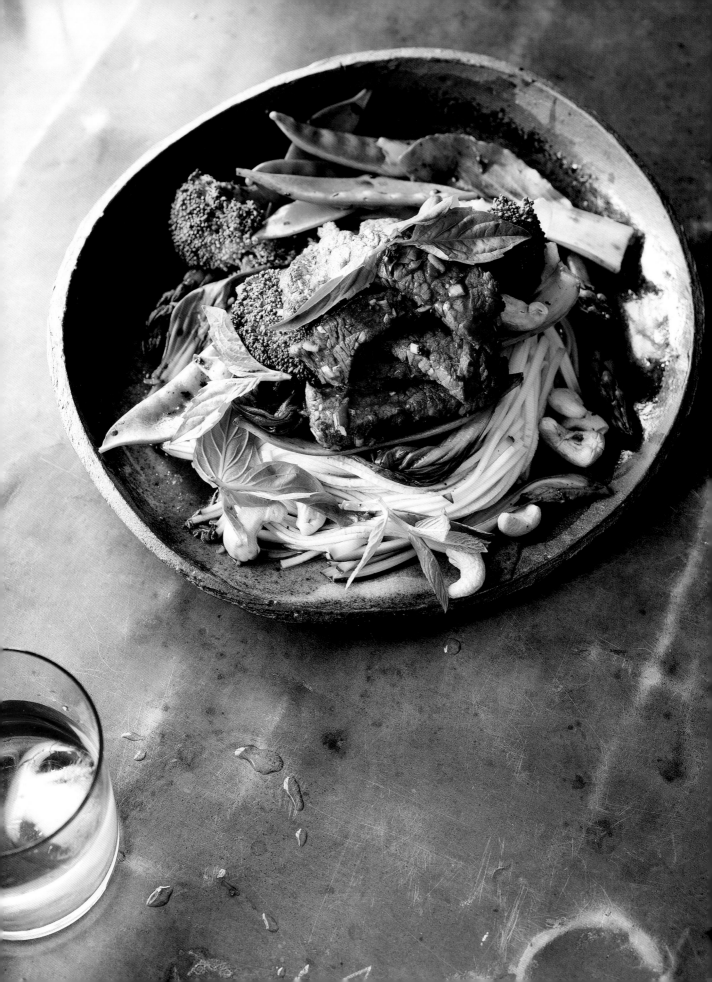

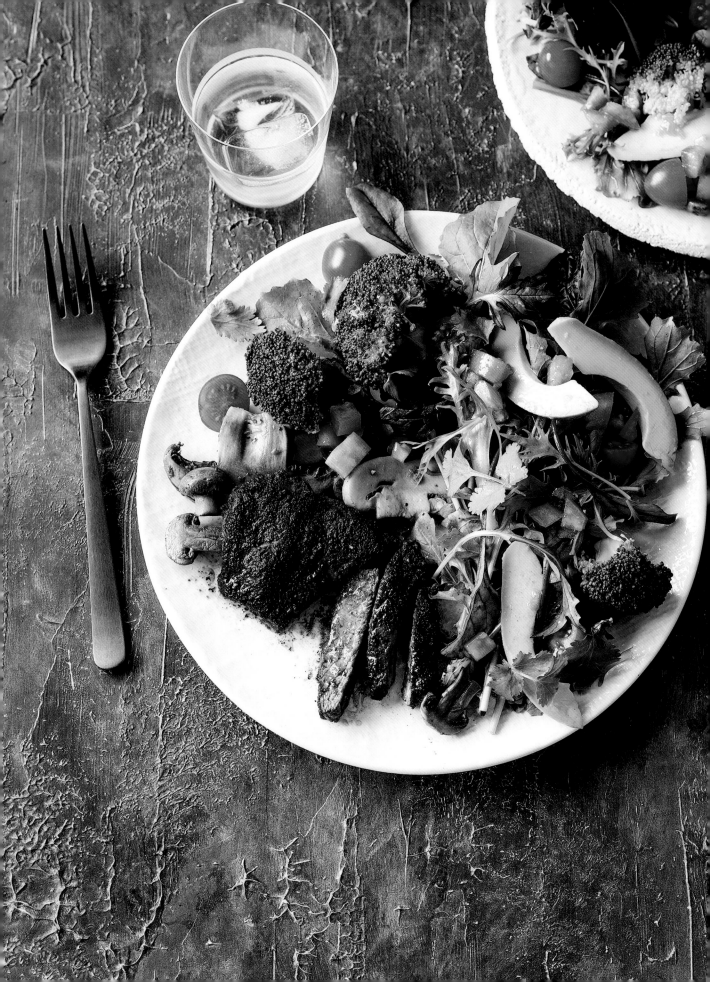

UNITS PER SERVE
Lean meat, fish, poultry, eggs, tofu **1.5**
Low-carb vegetables **3**
Healthy fats **2.5**

Spice-rubbed steaks with sauteed mushrooms

7 G CARB PER SERVE

🍴 Serves 4   🕐 Preparation: 20 minutes, plus resting time
〰 Cooking: 15 minutes

1 tablespoon sweet paprika
1 tablespoon garlic powder
1 tablespoon onion powder
½ teaspoon smoked paprika
½ teaspoon ground allspice
4 × 150 g scotch fillet steaks,
    all visible fat removed
2 teaspoons extra virgin olive oil,
    plus 1 tablespoon extra for brushing
500 g mixed mushrooms, thickly sliced
2 cloves garlic, crushed
3 teaspoons red wine vinegar
½ cup (125 ml) salt-reduced beef or
    vegetable stock
4 cups mixed salad leaves
3 cups rocket leaves
375 g cherry tomatoes, halved
80 g avocado, sliced

CORIANDER AND LIME DRESSING

1 tablespoon extra virgin olive oil
2 teaspoons lime juice, or to taste
¼ teaspoon ground cumin
2 tomatoes, finely chopped
¼ cup roughly chopped
    coriander leaves

To make the dressing, place all the ingredients in a small bowl and stir to combine, then season to taste with freshly ground black pepper. Set aside.

Place the sweet paprika, garlic powder, onion powder, smoked paprika and allspice in a shallow bowl and stir to combine.

Tie the outside of each steak with kitchen string to keep a uniform shape, if desired. Brush the steaks with olive oil, season well with pepper, then press the steaks into the spice mixture to coat.

Heat 1 teaspoon of the olive oil in a large heavy-based frying pan over medium heat. Add the mushrooms, garlic and vinegar and stir to mix well, then cover and cook, stirring occasionally, for 5 minutes or until slightly softened. Add the stock and bring to the boil, then simmer for 1–2 minutes to reduce slightly. Transfer to a bowl and keep warm

Wipe out the pan, if desired, then add the remaining olive oil and heat over medium–high heat. Add the steaks and cook, turning halfway through cooking, for 6–7 minutes for medium or continue until cooked to your liking. Transfer to a plate, cover loosely with foil and set aside to rest for 10 minutes.

Place the salad leaves, rocket and tomatoes in a large bowl, add half of the dressing and toss gently to mix.

Divide the mushrooms, steaks and salad among four plates and top with the avocado. Spoon the remaining dressing evenly over the steaks and serve immediately.

> **WEEKS 7–12 CARB EXTRAS**
>
> For an extra 10 g carbs per serve, add 160 g (40 g per person) drained tinned salt-reduced corn kernels, kidney beans or four-bean mix to the salad.

UNITS PER SERVE

Lean meat, fish, poultry, eggs, tofu **1.5**
Low-carb vegetables **3**
Mod-carb vegetables **0.5**
Healthy fats **3**

1½ tablespoons ground coriander
3 teaspoons ground cumin
½ teaspoon brown mustard seeds
½ teaspoon ground turmeric
½ teaspoon chilli powder
¼ teaspoon ground cardamom
¼ teaspoon freshly ground
    black pepper
2 tablespoons rice vinegar
1½ tablespoons extra virgin olive oil
600 g beef rump steaks, all visible
    fat removed, cut into 2 cm cubes
½ small onion, finely chopped
2 cloves garlic, crushed
1 × 2 cm piece ginger, peeled
    and finely grated
1 × 50 g sachet salt-reduced
    tomato paste
1 cup (250 ml) salt-reduced beef stock
150 g small button mushrooms,
    trimmed and halved
300 g spinach leaves

CAULIFLOWER AND BROCCOLI 'RICE'

½ small head (130 g) cauliflower,
    cut into small florets
300 g broccoli, cut into small florets
olive oil spray, for cooking
40 g flaked almonds

TOMATO AND CORIANDER SALAD

2 cups watercress sprigs
2 tomatoes, finely diced
2 teaspoons finely chopped red onion
⅓ cup coriander leaves, roughly
    chopped or torn
½ teaspoon cumin seeds, toasted
squeeze of lime juice

Madras beef curry with cauliflower and broccoli 'rice'

🍽 **Serves 4**   🕐 **Preparation: 25 minutes**   ♨ **Cooking: 1 hour**

Place the ground coriander, cumin, mustard seeds, turmeric, chilli powder, cardamom and pepper in a small bowl and stir to mix well. Stir in 1½ tablespoons of the vinegar to form a paste and set aside.

Heat half of the olive oil in an enamelled cast-iron casserole dish over medium heat, then add the beef and cook, stirring, for 3–4 minutes or until browned all over. Transfer to a heatproof bowl. Add the onion, garlic and ginger to the dish and cook, stirring, for 4 minutes or until softened and translucent. Add the spice paste and cook, stirring, for 2 minutes or until fragrant, then stir in the remaining vinegar. Return the beef to the dish, add the tomato paste and stir to coat the beef in the spice paste and tomato paste. Add the stock and ½ cup (125 ml) water and bring to the boil, then cover and simmer over low heat for 45–50 minutes or until the beef is tender.

Meanwhile, heat the remaining olive oil in a frying pan over medium heat, add the mushrooms and cook, stirring for 4–5 minutes or until browned all over. Transfer to the dish to cook with the beef; add a little water if a thinner sauce is preferred. When the beef is tender, stir in the spinach leaves until wilted.

Meanwhile, to make the cauliflower and broccoli 'rice', working in batches if necessary, place the cauliflower and broccoli in a food processor and process until finely chopped to resemble rice grains. About 10 minutes before serving the curry, heat a heavy-based non-stick frying pan over medium heat and spray with olive oil. Add the cauliflower and broccoli 'rice' and cook, stirring for 5 minutes or until warmed through. Cover and keep warm. Stir in the flaked almonds just before serving.

To make the relish, place the watercress, tomato, onion and coriander leaves in a bowl and mix to combine. Add the cumin seeds and lime juice to taste and mix to coat.

Divide the curry among four bowls and serve with the cauliflower and broccoli 'rice' and the relish alongside.

WEEKS 7–12 CARB EXTRAS

For an extra 10 g carbs per serve, add 480 g (120 g per person) frozen peas to the curry with the spinach and cook for 3 minutes or until tender.

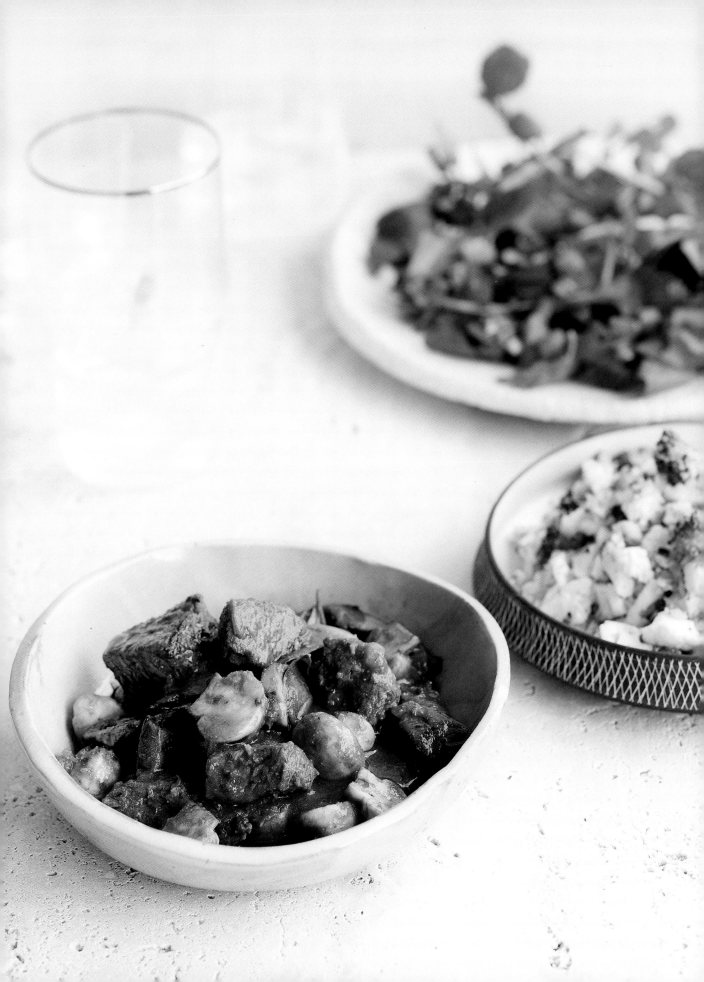

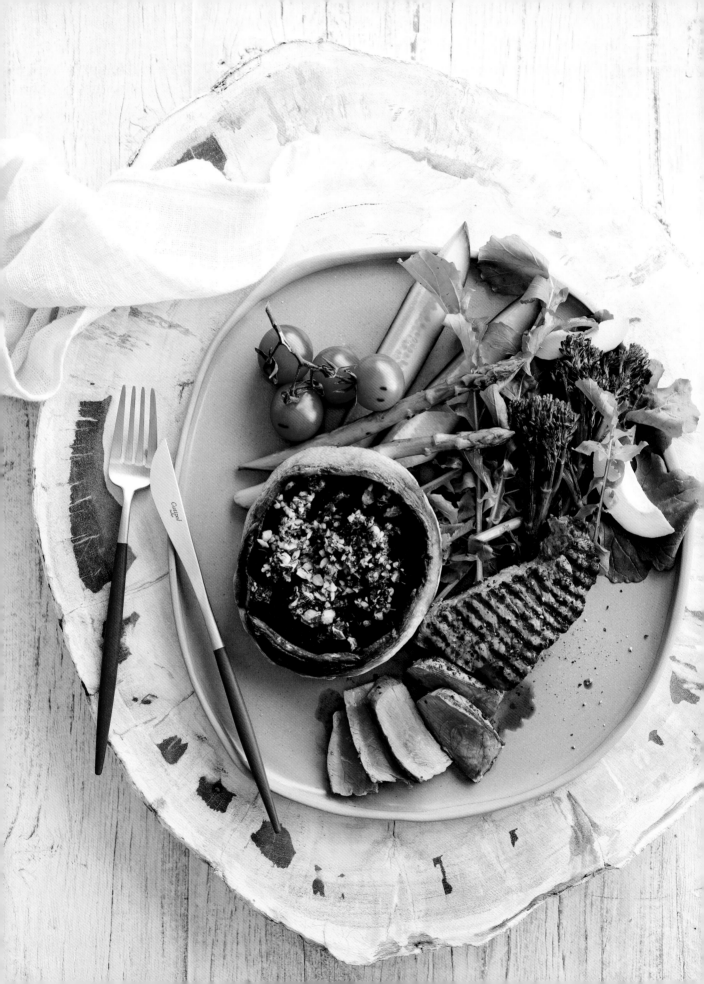

UNITS PER SERVE
Lean meat, fish, poultry, eggs, tofu **1.5**
Low-carb vegetables **3**
Healthy fats **4**

Barbecued fillet steaks with stuffed mushrooms

🍴 **Serves 4**   🕐 **Preparation: 15 minutes, plus resting time**
🍲 **Cooking: 20 minutes**

1 tablespoon extra virgin olive oil,
   plus extra for brushing
1 bunch broccolini, trimmed
1 bunch asparagus, trimmed
250 g cherry tomatoes
4 × 150 g sirloin/New York steaks,
   all visible fat removed
2 cups rocket leaves
1 Lebanese cucumber, sliced lengthways
80 g avocado, sliced or diced
1 teaspoon white wine vinegar

STUFFED MUSHROOMS
¼ cup flat-leaf parsley leaves,
   finely chopped
1 tablespoon chopped thyme
2 cloves garlic, finely chopped
40 g raw almonds, toasted and crushed
finely grated zest of 1 lemon
1 tablespoon extra virgin olive oil
4 large field mushrooms,
   stems trimmed

Preheat the oven grill to high.

Heat 1 teaspoon of the olive oil in a chargrill pan over high heat. Chargrill the broccolini for 3 minutes or until tender and golden, then transfer to a plate and set aside. Add another teaspoon of the olive oil to the pan and chargrill the asparagus, sprinkling with water and turning occasionally, for 2–3 minutes or until tender but still crisp. Transfer to the plate and set aside. Add the tomatoes to the pan and chargrill for 2–3 minutes or until they are blistered. Add to the plate and set aside.

Brush the steaks with olive oil and season well with freshly ground black pepper. Chargrill the steaks, turning every 30–40 seconds, for 6–7 minutes for medium or continue until cooked to your liking. Transfer to a plate, cover loosely with foil and set aside to rest for 10 minutes.

Meanwhile, to make the stuffed mushrooms, place the parsley, thyme, garlic, almonds, lemon zest and olive oil in a small bowl and mix to combine. Spoon one-quarter of the herb stuffing into each mushroom cup, then place, filled-side up, on a baking tray and grill for 8–10 minutes or until the stuffing is golden and the mushrooms are tender.

Place the rocket, cucumber and avocado in a bowl, drizzle with the vinegar and remaining olive oil and gently toss to mix.

Place a steak and stuffed mushroom on each of four plates, then divide the chargrilled vegetables and salad evenly among the plates and serve.

WEEKS 7–12 CARB EXTRAS

For an extra 10 g carbs per serve, add 480 g (120 g per person) cooked frozen peas alongside the steak, vegetables and salad.

Veal and mushroom involtini with crunchy Italian salad

🍴 **Serves 4**   🕐 **Preparation: 25 minutes, plus cooling time**
🍲 **Cooking: 45 minutes**

1 tablespoon extra virgin olive oil
250 g button mushrooms,
    finely chopped
1 cup kale leaves, thinly sliced
2 teaspoons thyme leaves
2 cloves garlic, finely chopped
40 g macadamias, coarsely crushed
600 g veal steaks (about 12), flattened
    with a meat mallet or rolling pin
400 g salt-reduced tomato passata
½ teaspoon dried oregano
2 bay leaves

CRUNCHY ITALIAN SALAD

2 heads radicchio, leaves torn or cut
    into bite-sized pieces
2 heads witlof, trimmed and
    leaves separated
3 cups rocket leaves
2 cups watercress sprigs
1 bulb baby fennel, trimmed and shaved
2 zucchini, shaved lengthways
1 tablespoon extra virgin olive oil
2 teaspoons balsamic vinegar

Heat 2 teaspoons of the olive oil in a heavy-based non-stick frying pan over medium heat, add the mushroom and cook, stirring, for 3–4 minutes or until softened. Stir in the kale, thyme and 1 clove of the garlic and cook, stirring for another 1–2 minutes or until the kale has wilted. Transfer to a bowl, then set aside for 5 minutes to cool. Stir in the macadamias and season to taste with freshly ground black pepper.

Place the veal steaks on a chopping board, then place 2 tablespoons or so of the mushroom mixture in a line down the centre of each steak; the exact amount will depend on the size of the veal steak. Roll up to enclose the filling, using toothpicks to keep their shape.

Heat the remaining oil in a heavy-based frying pan over medium–high heat, then add the involtini and cook, turning occasionally, for 8–10 minutes or until well browned all over. Transfer to a plate and set aside.

Add the remaining garlic to the pan and cook for 30 seconds or until fragrant. Pour in the passata, add the oregano and bay leaves and season to taste with freshly ground black pepper. Bring to a simmer, then cover and cook for 15–20 minutes or until slightly reduced and thickened. Discard the bay leaves. Return the involtini to the pan, then cover and cook for 5 minutes or until warmed though. Stir in any remaining mushroom mixture and cook for 1 minute or until warmed through.

Meanwhile, to make the salad, place the radicchio, witlof, rocket, watercress, fennel and zucchini in a large bowl, drizzle with the olive oil and vinegar and toss to combine.

Place three involtini on each of four plates, along with some of the sauce, then serve with one-quarter of the salad alongside each serving.

> **WEEKS 7–12 CARB EXTRAS**
>
> For an extra 10 g carbs per serve, add 400 g (100 g per person) orange segments to the salad.

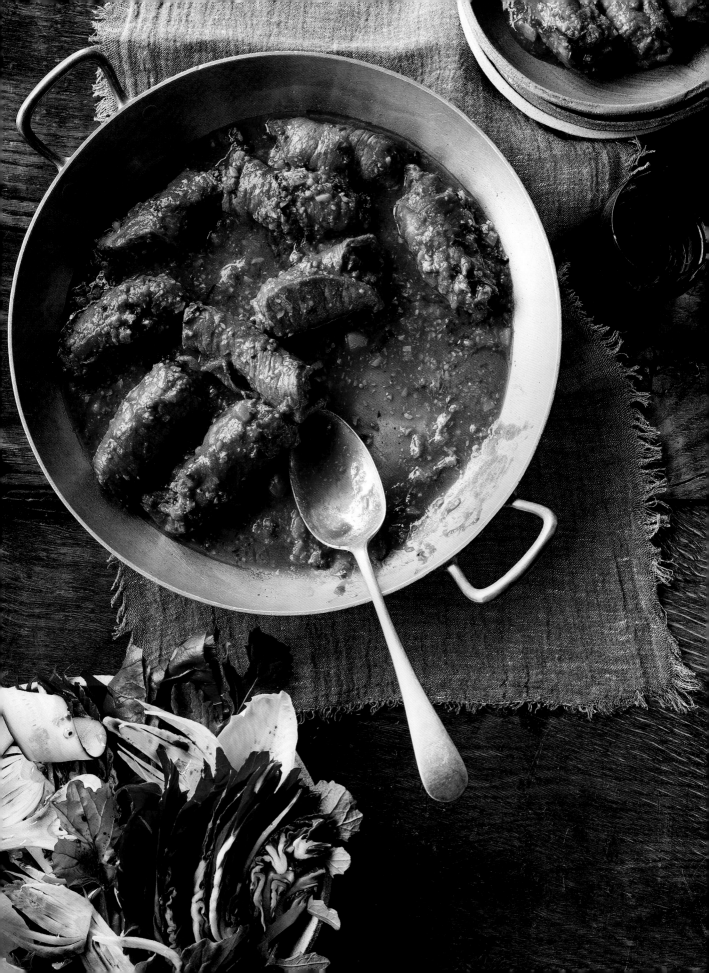

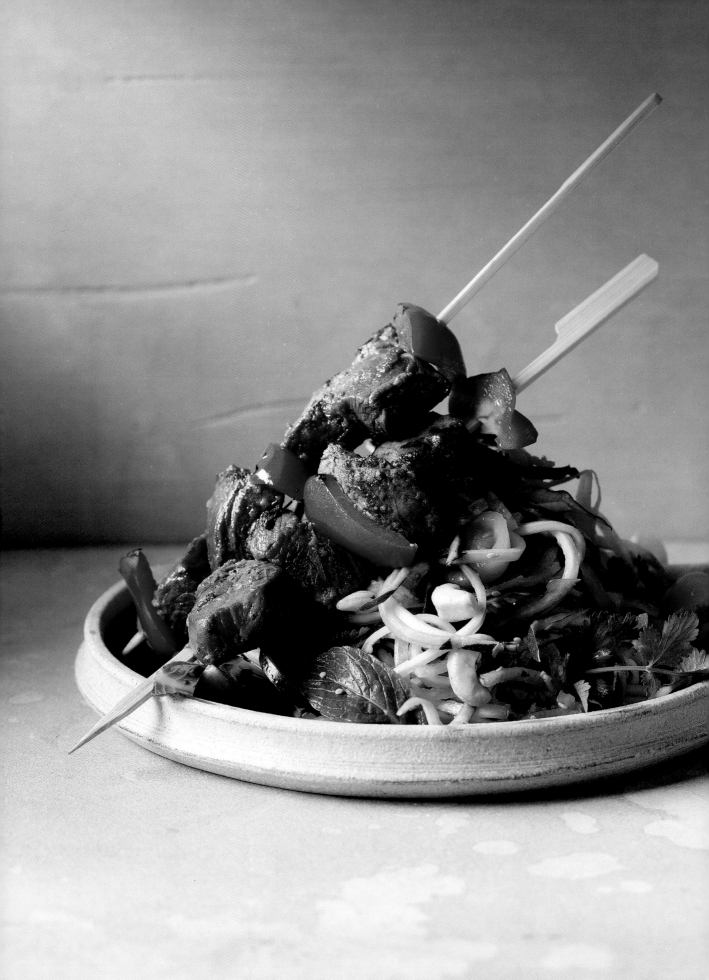

UNITS PER SERVE

Lean meat, fish, poultry, eggs, tofu **1.5**
Low-carb vegetables **2**
Mod-carb vegetables **1**
Healthy fats **2.5**

Ginger-soy beef skewers with zucchini 'noodle' salad

🍴 **Serves 4**   🕐 **Preparation: 20 minutes, plus marinating time**
〰 **Cooking: 10 minutes**

600 g beef rump steak, all visible
   fat removed, cut into 2 cm cubes
3 large zucchini, spiralised
2 carrots, spiralised
300 g mixed cherry tomatoes, halved
40 g raw unsalted cashews
   or raw almonds, toasted
large handful coriander leaves
handful mint leaves
1 tablespoon sesame seeds, toasted
1 tablespoon olive oil
1 tablespoon lemon juice
1 teaspoon sesame oil
1 large (300 g) red capsicum,
   seeded and chopped
olive oil spray, for cooking

GINGER-SOY MARINADE

2 teaspoons lemon juice
2 teaspoons salt-reduced soy sauce
1 clove garlic, crushed
1 teaspoon finely grated ginger
½ teaspoon five-spice powder

To make the marinade, combine all the ingredients in a bowl. Add the cubed steak, toss to coat, then cover and refrigerate for 1–2 hours to marinate.

Meanwhile, place the zucchini and carrot in a large bowl. Add the tomatoes, nuts, herbs, sesame seeds, olive oil, lemon juice and sesame oil and toss to combine. Cover and set aside for 20 minutes to allow the flavours to develop.

Thread the marinated beef and capsicum onto the skewers (see note). Spray lightly with olive oil.

Preheat a chargrill pan or barbecue grill to high heat, then reduce the heat to medium. Add the skewers, in batches if necessary, and cook for 5–6 minutes, turning occasionally, until just cooked through.

Divide the skewers and salad evenly among four plates and serve.

> **WEEKS 7–12 CARB EXTRAS**
>
> For an extra 10 g carbs per serve, chargrill 2 cobs sweetcorn with the skewers, then cut the kernels from the cob. Add 160 g (40 g per person) corn to the salad.

Note: You will need to soak eight long bamboo skewers in cold water for 30 minutes for this recipe.

Lean meat, fish, poultry, eggs, tofu **1.5**
Low-carb vegetables **2**
Mod-carb vegetables **1**
Healthy fats **1**

Thai beef and fried 'rice' lettuce wraps

10 G CARB PER SERVE

🍴 **Serves 4** 🕐 **Preparation: 20 minutes** 〰 **Cooking: 20 minutes**

150 g cauliflower florets
75 g broccoli florets
olive oil spray, for cooking
½ onion, chopped
1 clove garlic, crushed
1 teaspoon finely grated ginger
½ teaspoon dried chilli flakes
600 g lean minced beef
½ large (150 g) red capsicum,
    seeded and chopped
¼ cup (60 ml) lime or lemon juice
1 tablespoon fish sauce
2 teaspoons salt-reduced soy sauce
2 large handfuls coriander leaves
300 g cos lettuce leaves
2 Lebanese cucumbers, unpeeled,
    halved lengthways and cut
    into half-moons
2 tomatoes, chopped or 300 g
    cherry tomatoes, quartered
40 g raw almonds, toasted,
    roughly chopped
lime or lemon wedges, to serve

Working in batches if necessary, place the cauliflower and broccoli in a food processor and process until finely chopped to resemble coarse rice grains. Spray a large heavy-based deep frying pan with olive oil, add the cauliflower mixture and cook, stirring often, over medium–high heat for 3–4 minutes or until softened slightly. Transfer to a bowl and set aside.

Spray the frying pan with a little more oil, then add the onion, garlic, ginger and chilli and cook, stirring, for 1–2 minutes or until fragrant. Increase the heat to high, add the beef and cook, stirring occasionally, for 5–6 minutes or until browned. Add the capsicum and simmer for 3–5 minutes or until the capsicum is just tender.

Stir in the cauliflower mixture, lime or lemon juice, fish sauce and soy sauce and cook for 1–2 minutes or until heated through. Stir in the coriander.

Spoon the beef mixture into the lettuce leaves, top with the cucumber, tomato and nuts and serve with lime or lemon wedges on the side.

WEEKS 7–12 CARB EXTRAS

For an extra 10 g carbs per serve, add 200 g (50 g per person) steamed sweet potato or 480 g (120 g per person) steamed pumpkin or peas to the beef mixture.

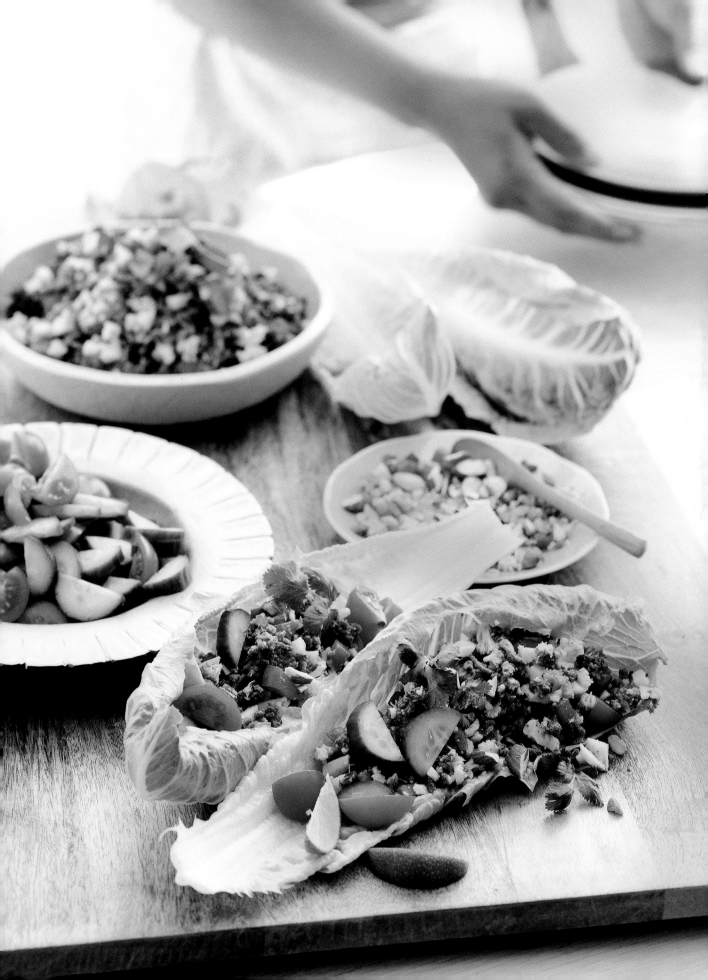

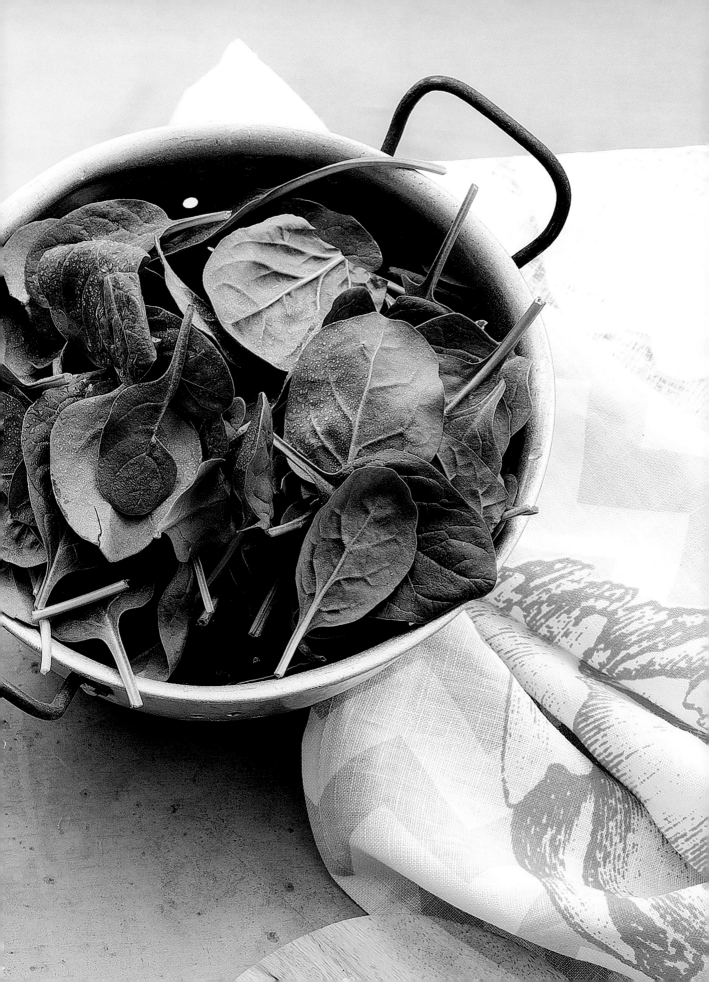

Lean meat, fish, poultry, eggs, tofu **1.5**
Low-carb vegetables **2**
Mod-carb vegetables **1**
Healthy fats **4**

Biryani-style lamb with spinach and mint salad

9 G CARB PER SERVE

🍽 **Serves 4**   🕐 **Preparation: 20 minutes, plus marinating time**
📖 **Cooking: 50 minutes**

2 teaspoons ground cumin
1 teaspoon garam masala
½ teaspoon ground fennel
¼ teaspoon ground cardamom
¼ teaspoon ground ginger
pinch of ground cinnamon
juice of 1 lime or ½ lemon
2 tablespoons extra virgin olive oil
600 g lamb leg steaks or backstraps,
    all visible fat removed, cut into
    2 cm dice
1 small onion, finely chopped
2 cloves garlic, crushed
1 × 1 cm piece ginger, peeled and
    finely grated
½ cup (125 ml) salt-reduced beef stock
1 quantity Cauliflower 'Rice'
    (see page 217)
¼ teaspoon ground turmeric
40 g flaked almonds

SPINACH AND MINT SALAD

4 cups mixed salad leaves
2 cups spinach leaves
250 g cherry tomatoes, halved
2 Lebanese cucumbers,
    halved lengthways and
    sliced on the diagonal
4 radishes, thinly sliced
½ cup small mint leaves
1 tablespoon extra virgin olive oil
2 teaspoons lemon juice

Place the cumin, garam masala, fennel, cardamom, ground ginger, cinnamon, lime or lemon juice and 1 teaspoon of the olive oil in a small bowl and stir to combine. Place the lamb in a bowl, add the spice mixture and stir to coat. Cover with plastic film and marinate in the refrigerator for at least 30 minutes or up to 2 hours.

Heat 2 teaspoons of the olive oil in a small enamelled cast-iron casserole dish over medium heat, then add the lamb and cook for 4–5 minutes, stirring until browned all over. Remove from the dish and set aside. Add 1 teaspoon oil to the dish, then add the onion, garlic and ginger and cook for 4–5 minutes or until softened. Return the lamb to the dish and stir to coat the lamb in the onion mixture. Pour in the stock and bring to the boil, then reduce the heat to low and simmer, partially covered, for 40 minutes or until the lamb is tender.

Just before serving, heat the remaining olive oil in a heavy-based non-stick frying pan over medium heat, then add the cauliflower 'rice' and turmeric and stir to mix. Cook for 5 minutes or until warmed through. Fold in the almonds.

Meanwhile, to make the salad, place the salad leaves, spinach leaves, tomatoes, cucumber, radish and mint in a large bowl and toss to combine. Drizzle with the olive oil and lemon juice and season to taste with freshly ground black pepper.

Divide the cauliflower 'rice' and lamb biryani evenly among four plates or bowls and serve with one-quarter of the salad alongside each serving. Alternatively, add the lamb to the cauliflower 'rice' and stir to combine, then serve with the salad alongside.

WEEKS 7–12 CARB EXTRAS

For an extra 10 g carbs per serve, add 320 g (80 g per person) drained and rinsed tinned salt-reduced lentils or 160 g (40 g per person) drained and rinsed tinned salt-reduced chickpeas to the biryani during the last 5 minutes of cooking to warm through with the cauliflower 'rice'.

Lean meat, fish, poultry, eggs, tofu **1.5**
Low-carb vegetables **3**
Mod-carb vegetables **0.5**
Healthy fats **4**

Mini herb and chilli lamb roasts with roasted vegetables

10 G CARB PER SERVE

🍴 **Serves 4**
🕐 **Preparation: 20 minutes, plus marinating and resting time**
🌀 **Cooking: 30 minutes**

1½ tablespoons finely chopped rosemary
2 sprigs thyme, leaves picked
2 teaspoons dried oregano
1 clove garlic, crushed
½ teaspoon dried chilli flakes (optional)
finely grated zest and juice of 1 lemon
2 tablespoons extra virgin olive oil
2 × 300 g lamb rumps, all visible fat removed
300 g broccoli, trimmed and cut into small florets
2 zucchini, quartered lengthways
100 g small brussels sprouts, trimmed
40 g blanched almonds
4 cups mixed salad leaves
1 cup lamb's lettuce or frisee
4 tomatoes, sliced or cut into wedges
2 teaspoons red wine vinegar
2 teaspoons Dijon mustard
80 g avocado, sliced

Place the rosemary, thyme, oregano, garlic, chilli flakes (if using), lemon zest and 2 teaspoons of the olive oil in a small bowl, season to taste with freshly ground black pepper and stir to combine. Place the lamb rumps in a glass bowl, then drizzle over the lemon juice, spoon the herb marinade over and rub in to coat well. Cover with plastic film and marinate in the refrigerator for at least 30 minutes or up to 24 hours.

Preheat the oven to 200°C (180°C fan-forced).

Heat a large ovenproof frying pan over medium–high heat. Add the lamb and cook, turning, for 8–10 minutes or until browned all over. Transfer the pan to the oven and roast the lamb for 15–20 minutes for medium-rare or continue until cooked to your liking. Loosely cover with foil and set aside to rest for 10 minutes.

Meanwhile, place the broccoli, zucchini and brussels sprouts in a roasting tin, drizzle with 1 teaspoon of the olive oil and roast in the oven for 20–25 minutes or until tender and golden around the edges; add the almonds to the tin in the last 8 minutes of roasting.

Place the salad leaves, lamb's lettuce or frisee and tomato in a large bowl and toss to combine. Place the vinegar and mustard in a small bowl, season with pepper and stir to combine, then stir in the remaining olive oil until emulsified. Add the dressing to the salad and toss to coat, then add the avocado.

Carve the lamb into slices, then serve 150 g per person with one-quarter of the roasted vegetables and salad to the side of each serving.

WEEKS 7–12 CARB EXTRAS

For an extra 10 g carbs per serve, add 480 g (120 g per person) pumpkin or 200 g (50 g per person) sweet potato cut into 1.5 cm cubes to the roasting tin of vegetables.

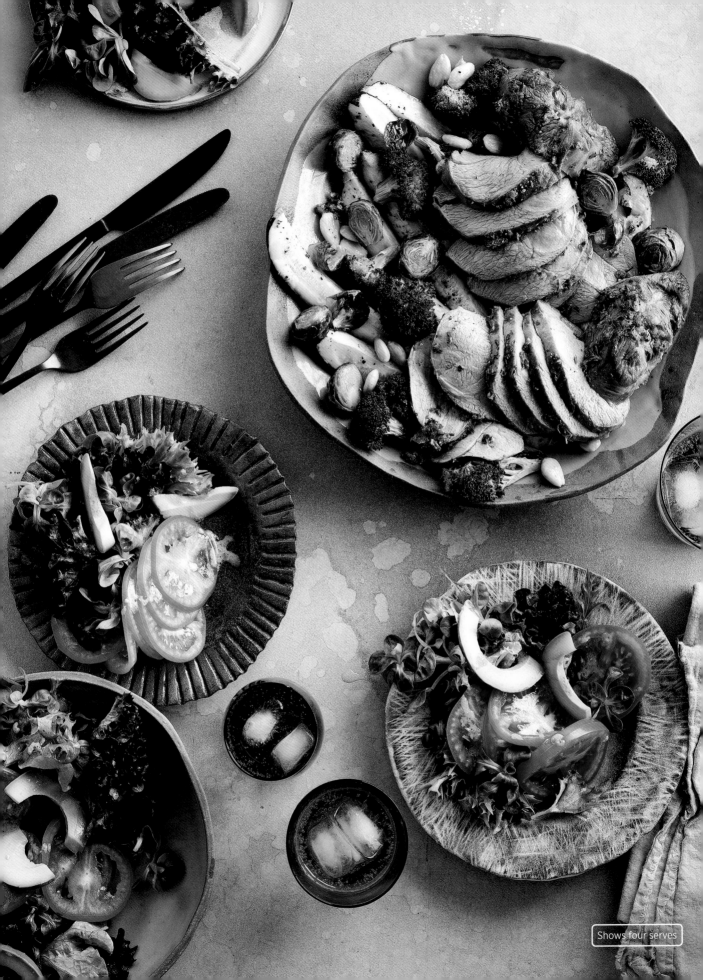

Shows four serves

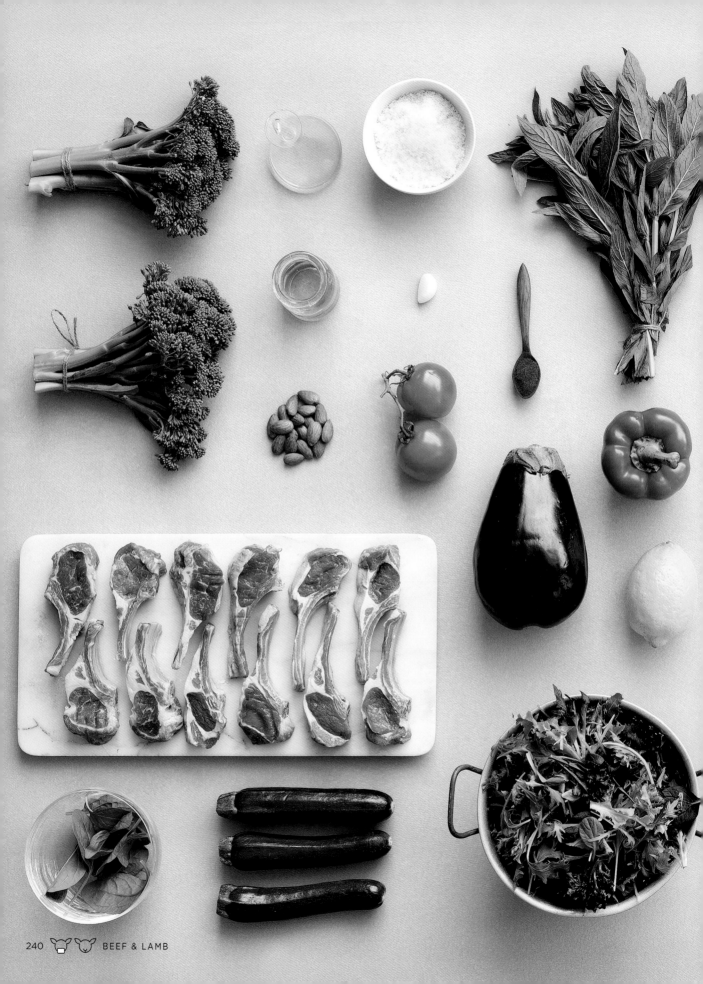

Lamb cutlets with chargrilled vegetables and mint pesto

🍴 **Serves 4**   🕐 **Preparation: 20 minutes, plus marinating time**
🍲 **Cooking: 25 minutes**

UNITS PER SERVE
Lean meat, fish, poultry, eggs, tofu **1.5**
Dairy **0.5**
Low-carb vegetables **2.5**
Mod-carb vegetables **1**
Healthy fats **3**

12 × 60 g French-trimmed lamb cutlets, all visible fat removed
1 teaspoon finely grated lemon zest
1 tablespoon lemon juice
1 teaspoon sweet paprika
olive oil spray, for cooking
3 zucchini, thinly sliced lengthways
1 eggplant (300 g), thinly sliced into rings
2 bunches broccolini, trimmed and halved lengthways if large
1 small (150 g) red capsicum, seeded and cut into strips
2 tomatoes, thickly sliced
100 g mesclun, rocket or baby spinach leaves

MINT PESTO
20 g raw almonds
1¼ cups (75 g) mint leaves
¼ cup baby spinach leaves
1 small clove garlic, crushed
2 tablespoons extra virgin olive oil
1 tablespoon lemon juice
½ cup (40 g) finely grated parmesan

To make the mint pesto, place the almonds, mint, spinach and garlic in a food processor and process until finely chopped. With the motor running, drizzle in the olive oil and lemon juice. Add the parmesan and pulse until just combined. Season to taste with freshly ground black pepper, then cover and set aside.

Place the lamb, lemon zest, lemon juice and paprika in a zip-lock bag and massage the flavourings into the lamb. Set aside to marinate for 5 minutes.

Heat a chargrill pan, barbecue or heavy-based frying pan over medium–high heat. Spray the lamb lightly with olive oil, then cook for 2–3 minutes on each side for medium-rare or continue until cooked to your liking. Transfer to a plate and cover lightly with foil to keep warm.

Spray the zucchini, eggplant, broccolini and capsicum lightly with olive oil and cook, in batches if necessary, for 3–4 minutes each until chargrilled and tender. Remove, spread with a little mint pesto if you like and set aside. Cook everything at the same time if you have enough room.

Divide the chargrilled vegetables, sliced tomato and mesclun, rocket or spinach evenly among four plates, top with 3 lamb cutlets each and serve with the remaining mint pesto.

> **WEEKS 7–12 CARB EXTRAS**
>
> For an extra 10 g carbs per serve, chargrill 160 g (40 g per person) baby corn or 200 g (50 g per person) thinly sliced sweet potato with the other vegetables.

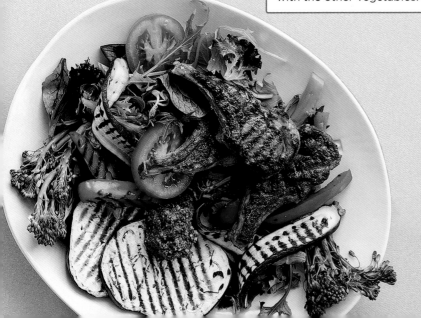

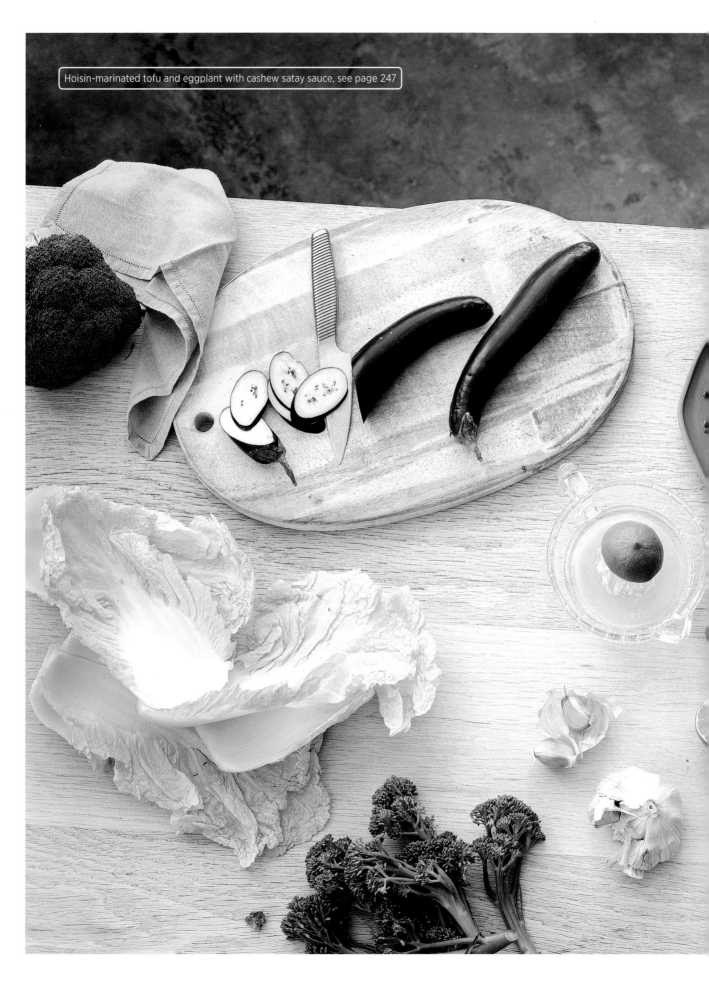

Hoisin-marinated tofu and eggplant with cashew satay sauce, see page 247

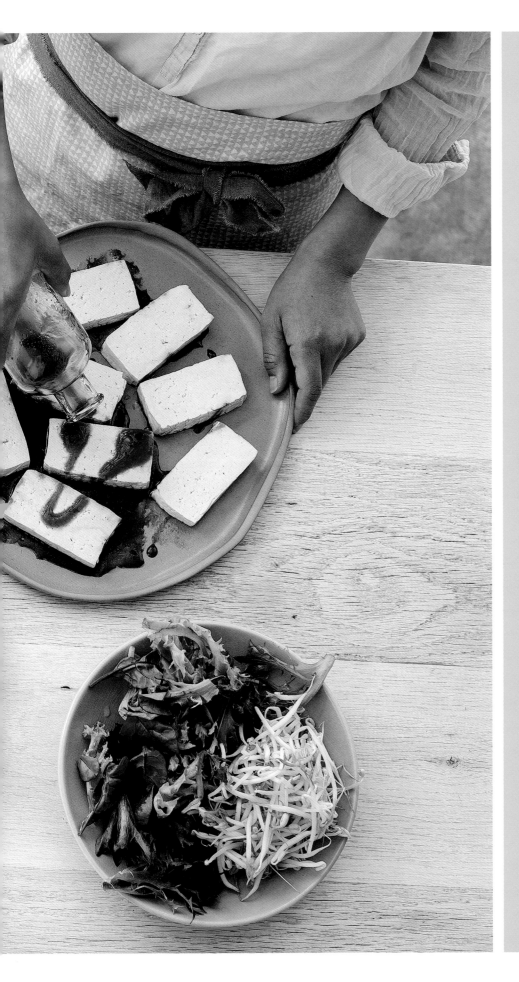

Sesame-crusted tofu with stir-fried Asian greens

5 G CARB PER SERVE

🍴 Serves 4   🕐 Preparation: 15 minutes   🌀 Cooking: 20 minutes

600 g firm tofu, drained

1 tablespoon sesame seeds

1 tablespoon extra virgin olive oil

3 baby bok choy, halved or quartered lengthways, depending on size

2 bunches broccolini, trimmed and halved widthways

2 bunches asparagus, trimmed and halved widthways

1 × 2 cm piece ginger, peeled and cut into julienne

1 clove garlic, finely chopped

1 small fresh red chilli, seeded (optional) and finely chopped

300 g fresh shiitake mushrooms

300 g enoki mushrooms

1 teaspoon mushroom/vegetarian oyster sauce

2 drops sesame oil

40 g raw unsalted cashews, toasted

TAHINI-SOY DRESSING

1 tablespoon tahini

1 tablespoon salt-reduced soy sauce

3 teaspoons seasoned rice vinegar

To make the dressing, place all the ingredients in a small bowl and stir until well combined. Set aside.

Pat the tofu dry with paper towel, then cut into 8 slices. Place the sesame seeds on a plate, then press on the tofu to coat evenly on one side.

Heat 2 teaspoons of the olive oil in a heavy-based non-stick frying pan over medium heat. Add the tofu, sesame seed-side down, and cook for 2 minutes or until light golden. Carefully turn and cook for another 2 minutes or until light golden. Transfer to a plate lined with paper towel to drain.

Heat 1 teaspoon of the oil in a wok over high heat, then stir-fry the bok choy for 2–3 minutes or until the stems are tender but still crisp. Transfer to a large bowl and set aside. Add the remaining oil to the wok, repeat with the broccolini and asparagus, then transfer to the bowl of bok choy. Add the ginger, garlic and chilli to the wok and cook for 30 seconds or until fragrant, then add all the mushrooms and stir-fry for 4–5 minutes or until softened. Add the mushroom/ vegetarian oyster sauce and sesame oil and return the vegetables to the wok, then turn off the heat and toss to combine.

Divide the stir-fried vegetables evenly among four plates or bowls, then scatter with the cashews. Top each serve with two slices of tofu and evenly drizzle over the dressing (or serve the dressing in a small bowl alongside). Serve immediately.

> **WEEKS 7-12 CARB EXTRAS**
>
> For an extra 10 g carbs per serve, serve with 200 g (50 g per person) cooked quinoa (this is 60 g raw quinoa; 15 g per person).

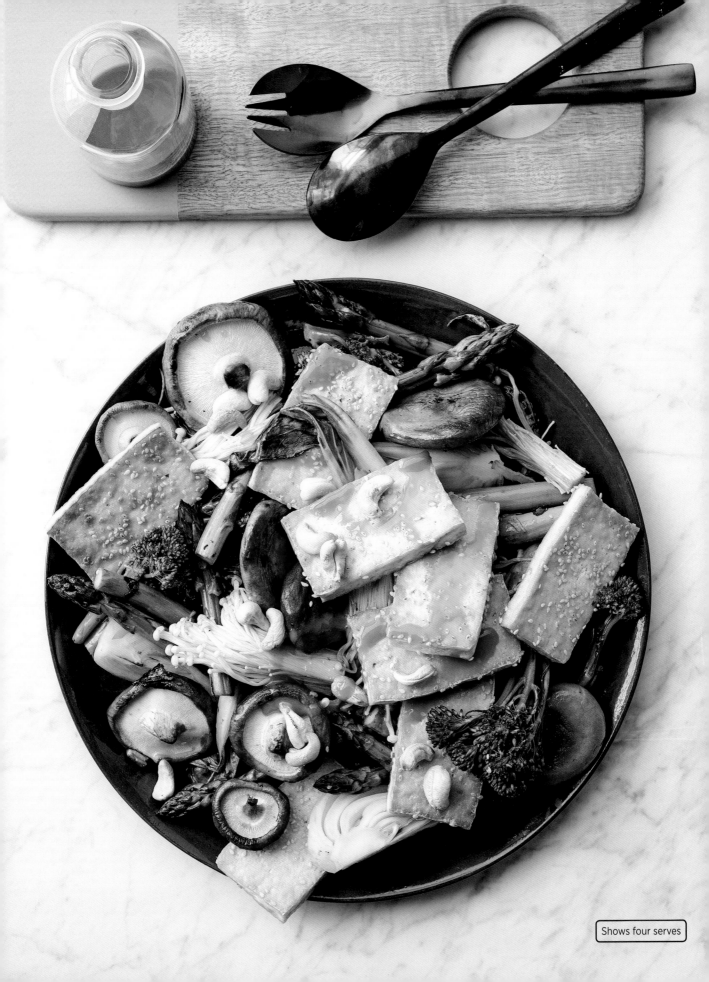

Shows four serves

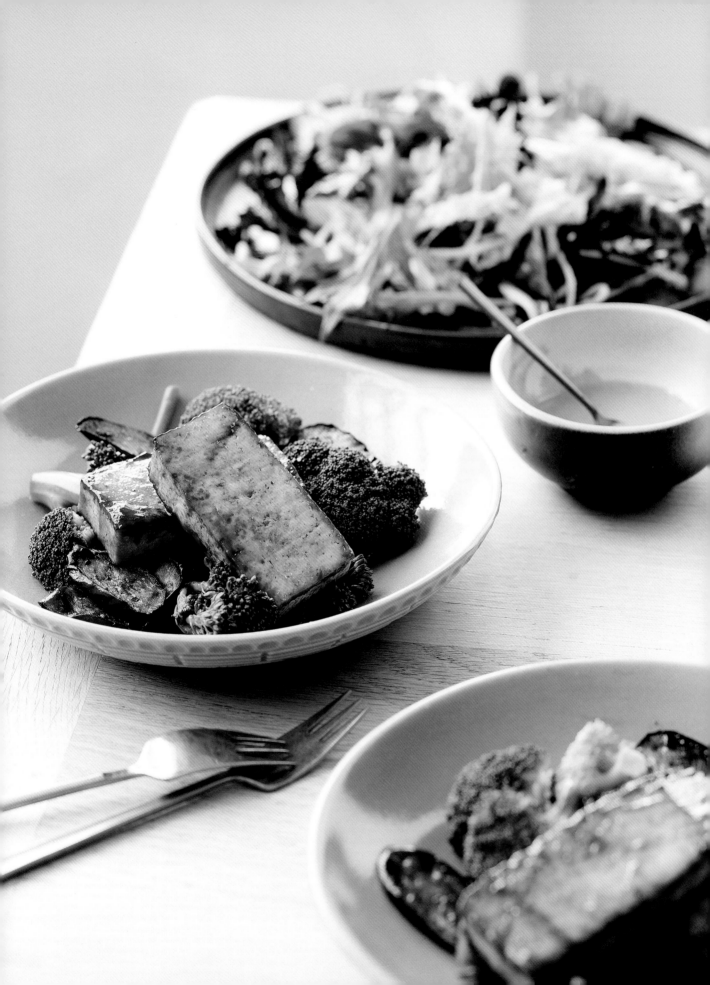

Lean meat, fish, poultry, eggs, tofu **1.5**
Low-carb vegetables **3**
Mod-carb vegetables **1**
Healthy fats **3.5**

Hoisin-marinated tofu and eggplant with cashew satay sauce

8 G CARB PER SERVE

🍽 **Serves 4**   🕐 **Preparation: 15 minutes**   ⓦ **Cooking: 20 minutes**

600 g firm tofu, drained
2 tablespoons hoisin sauce
2 teaspoons mirin
pinch of five-spice powder
2 tablespoons extra virgin olive oil
2 slender (Japanese) eggplants, thinly
   sliced lengthways
300 g broccoli, trimmed and cut into
   small florets
2 bunches broccolini, trimmed and
   halved lengthways
8 cups mixed Asian baby salad greens
   (including tatsoi, mizuna, watercress,
   red oakleaf lettuce and coral lettuce)
2 cups (160 g) bean sprouts, trimmed
1 cup shredded Chinese cabbage
   (wombok)
2 teaspoons salt-reduced soy sauce
2 teaspoons lime juice
2 drops sesame oil

CASHEW SATAY SAUCE

olive oil spray, for cooking
1 small clove garlic, finely chopped
1½ tablespoons raw unsalted
   cashew butter
2 teaspoons tahini
1–2 teaspoons lime juice, or to taste
1½–2 tablespoons boiling water
2 teaspoons salt-reduced soy sauce

To make the sauce, heat a small heavy-based non-stick frying pan over medium heat, then spray with olive oil. Add the garlic and cook for 30–60 seconds or until fragrant but not coloured. Transfer to a small bowl, then add the remaining ingredients and stir until smooth and well combined. Set aside until required.

Pat the tofu dry with paper towel, then cut into 8 slices. Place the hoisin sauce, mirin, five-spice powder and 1 teaspoon of the olive oil in a shallow bowl and stir to combine, then add the tofu and turn to coat evenly. Set aside.

Brush the eggplant lightly with olive oil and set aside.

Working in batches, steam the broccoli and broccolini in a steamer basket over a saucepan of simmering water for 3 minutes or until tender but still crisp. Leave to cool.

Place the salad leaves, bean sprouts and cabbage in a large bowl and toss gently to combine. Add the cooled broccoli and broccolini and set aside.

Heat another teaspoon of the oil in a heavy-based non-stick frying pan over medium heat and cook the tofu for 2–3 minutes on each side or until golden and warmed through. Transfer to a plate and set aside. Brush the eggplant with any remaining hoisin mixture in the bowl and pan-fry for 2–3 minutes on each side or until tender and light golden.

Place the soy sauce, lime juice, sesame oil and remaining olive oil in a small bowl and stir to combine, then pour over the salad and gently toss to coat.

Divide the salad evenly among four plates and add one-quarter of the tofu and eggplant to each plate. Serve with the satay sauce to the side.

> **WEEKS 7–12 CARB EXTRAS**
>
> For an extra 10 g carbs per serve, steam 160 g (40 g per person) baby corn with the broccoli and broccolini and add to the salad.

UNITS PER SERVE
Lean meat, fish, poultry, eggs, tofu **1.5**
Low-carb vegetables **3**
Mod-carb vegetables **1**
Healthy fats **1**

Vegetable fried 'rice' with tofu and egg

8 G CARB PER SERVE

🍴 **Serves 4**   🕐 **Preparation: 20 minutes**   ♨ **Cooking: 20 minutes**

2 teaspoons black mustard seeds

1 teaspoon ground coriander

½ teaspoon ground turmeric

4 eggs

olive oil spray, for cooking

400 g firm tofu, drained and cut into 2 cm cubes

1 bunch kale (400 g trimmed), stalks removed and leaves torn into bite-sized pieces

2 cloves garlic, crushed

2 teaspoons finely grated ginger

1 small fresh red chilli, thinly sliced (optional)

300 g cauliflower florets

150 g broccoli florets

2 baby bok choy, cut into 1 cm slices

2 cups (160 g) bean sprouts, trimmed

1 tablespoon salt-reduced soy sauce

40 g raw almonds, toasted and roughly chopped

Combine the mustard seeds, coriander and turmeric in a small bowl with 2 teaspoons water to make a paste.

Whisk the eggs with 1 tablespoon water. Spray a large heavy-based deep frying pan or wok with olive oil and place over medium heat. Add the egg mixture and cook, without stirring, for 2–3 minutes or until just firm on the top and the edge starts to loosen. Carefully flip over and cook the other side for 10 seconds. Transfer to a chopping board and allow to cool, then roll up and slice into 5 mm strips.

Reheat the same pan or wok and spray with a little more oil if necessary. Add the spice paste and tofu and gently stir-fry for 1–2 minutes or until well coated, lightly browned and fragrant. Remove the tofu from the pan and set aside.

Spray the pan with a little more oil, if necessary, and add the kale, garlic, ginger and chilli, if using. Stir-fry for 5 minutes or until fragrant and the kale is starting to soften.

Meanwhile, working in batches if necessary, place the cauliflower and broccoli in a food processor and process until finely chopped to resemble rice grains. Add to the pan with the kale mixture and stir-fry for 4–5 minutes or until almost tender.

Add the bok choy, bean sprouts and soy sauce and return the tofu to the pan. Toss gently until warmed through.

Divide the fried 'rice' evenly among four plates and top with the egg ribbons and almonds.

> **WEEKS 7–12 CARB EXTRAS**
>
> For an extra 10 g carbs per serve, add 160 g (40 g per person) drained and rinsed tinned salt-reduced chickpeas to the pan with the cauliflower and broccoli 'rice'.

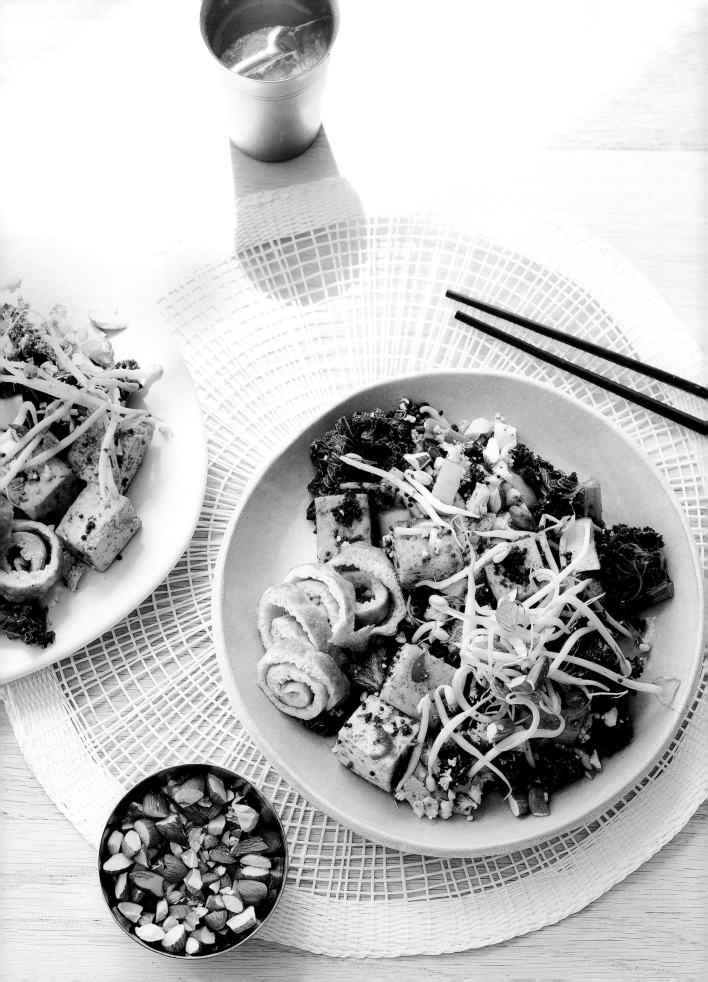

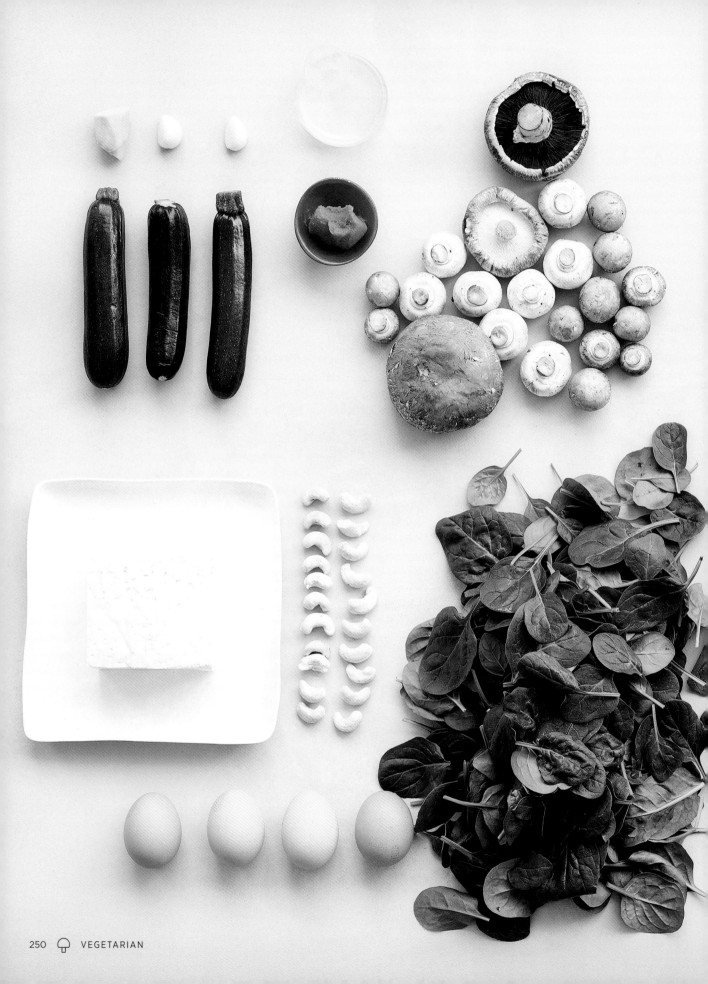

UNITS PER SERVE
Lean meat, fish, poultry, eggs, tofu **1.5**
Low-carb vegetables **3**
Healthy fats **1**

Mushroom, tofu and miso 'noodle' stir-fry

10 G CARB PER SERVE

🍽 **Serves 4** ⏱ **Preparation: 20 minutes** 🍲 **Cooking: 15 minutes**

4 eggs
olive oil spray, for cooking
400 g firm tofu, drained and cut into
   2 cm cubes
2 cloves garlic, thinly sliced
2 teaspoons finely grated ginger
300 g mixed mushrooms, sliced
300 g baby spinach leaves
3 zucchini, spiralised
40 g raw unsalted cashews
   or raw almonds, toasted

MISO SAUCE

1½ tablespoons white miso paste
2 tablespoons rice wine vinegar

To make the miso sauce, whisk the miso and rice wine vinegar together in a small bowl. Whisk in ¼ cup (60 ml) water and set aside.

Whisk the eggs in a bowl with 2 teaspoons of the miso sauce. Spray a large heavy-based deep frying pan or wok with olive oil and place over medium heat. Pour in the egg mixture and cook for 2–3 minutes. When the surface of the egg is just set, flip it over and cook for a further minute. Transfer the omelette to a chopping board and, when cool enough to handle, roll up and slice into ribbons. Set aside.

Spray the pan or wok with a little more oil if necessary, then add the tofu and half the garlic and ginger and stir-fry for 1–2 minutes or until lightly browned. Remove from the pan, cover with foil and set aside.

Spray the pan with a little more oil if necessary and add the mushrooms and the remaining garlic and ginger. Stir-fry for 5 minutes or until just tender. Add the miso sauce and then the spinach in two batches, allowing the spinach to wilt. Return the cooked egg to the pan and add the zucchini 'noodles'. Carefully fold in until all the ingredients are coated in the sauce and the 'noodles' are just heated through. Divide evenly among four bowls and top with the tofu. Scatter with the nuts and serve immediately.

WEEKS 7–12 CARB EXTRAS

For an extra 10 g carbs per serve, add 480 g (120 g per person) frozen peas or 160 g (40 g per person) corn kernels with the mushrooms.

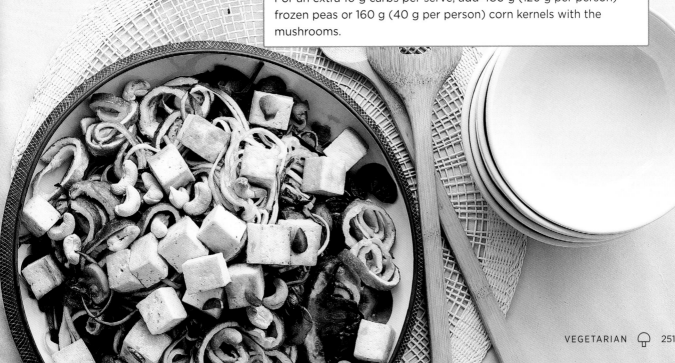

UNITS PER SERVE
Lean meat, fish, poultry, eggs, tofu **1.5**
Low-carb vegetables **3.5**
Healthy fats **4**

Moroccan tofu with grilled spiced-nut mushrooms

8 G CARB PER SERVE

🍴 Serves 4   🕐 Preparation: 20 minutes   ♨ Cooking: 20 minutes

2 tablespoons finely chopped
    flat-leaf parsley
2 tablespoons finely chopped
    coriander leaves
1 large clove garlic, crushed
2 teaspoons ground cumin
2 teaspoons sweet paprika
¼ teaspoon ground turmeric
1½ tablespoons extra virgin olive oil
600 g firm tofu, drained
2 bunches asparagus, trimmed and
    halved lengthways
8 cups mixed salad leaves
2 cups mixed baby spinach
    and rocket leaves
250 g cherry tomatoes, halved
2 Lebanese cucumbers, thinly sliced
2 teaspoons lemon juice
80 g hummus

GRILLED SPICED-NUT MUSHROOMS

4 large field mushrooms, trimmed
1 quantity (80 g) Spiced Nut Sprinkle
    (see page 120)
2 tablespoons roughly chopped
    flat-leaf parsley
olive oil spray, for cooking

Place the parsley, coriander, garlic, cumin, paprika, turmeric and 2 teaspoons of the olive oil in a shallow bowl and stir to combine.

Pat the tofu dry with paper towel, then cut into 8 slices. Add the tofu to the herb paste and turn to coat evenly. Set aside.

Steam the asparagus in a steamer basket over a saucepan of simmering water for 2–3 minutes or until tender but still crisp.

Preheat the oven grill to high. Line a baking tray with baking paper.

To make the grilled mushrooms, place the mushrooms on the prepared tray, cup-side down, and grill for 3–4 minutes or until starting to soften. Remove the tray from the grill, turn the mushrooms over, then spoon one-quarter of the nut crumble and parsley into each of the open mushroom cups and spray with olive oil. Grill for 5–6 minutes or until the mushrooms are tender and the crumble is golden. Set aside.

Place the salad leaves, spinach and rocket, tomatoes and cucumber in a large bowl and toss gently to mix. Set aside.

Heat another teaspoon of the oil in a heavy-based non-stick frying pan over medium heat and cook the tofu for 2–3 minutes on each side or until golden and warmed through. Transfer to a plate and set aside.

Drizzle the salad with the lemon juice and remaining olive oil and toss to coat, then divide evenly among four plates. Spoon the hummus evenly onto each plate in a little mound, then top with a grilled mushroom and place one-quarter each of the asparagus and tofu alongside each serving. Serve immediately.

> **WEEKS 7–12 CARB EXTRAS**
>
> For an extra 10 g carbs per serve, add 320 g (80 g per person) drained and rinsed tinned salt-reduced lentils or 160 g (40 g per person) drained and rinsed tinned salt-reduced chickpeas to the salad.

UNITS PER SERVE

Lean meat, fish, poultry, eggs, tofu **1.5**
Low-carb vegetables **3**
Mod-carb vegetables **0.5**
Healthy fats **2**

Tofu and turmeric 'scramble' with steamed greens

🍴 **Serves 4**   🕐 **Preparation: 15 minutes**   🍲 **Cooking: 15 minutes**

3 teaspoons olive oil
1 teaspoon sesame oil
1 small red onion, thinly sliced
3 tomatoes, chopped
2 cloves garlic, crushed
2 teaspoons finely grated ginger
1 teaspoon black mustard seeds
½ teaspoon ground turmeric
600 g silken tofu
3 spring onions, sliced on the diagonal
3 teaspoons salt-reduced soy sauce
1 cup (80 g) bean sprouts, trimmed
300 g choy sum, trimmed and cut
    into lengths
1 bunch broccolini, trimmed
100 g snow peas, halved on
    the diagonal
40 g raw almonds, toasted and
    roughly chopped

Heat the olive oil and sesame oil in a large heavy-based frying pan over medium heat. Add the onion and cook, stirring, for 2 minutes or until starting to soften. Add the tomato, garlic, ginger, mustard seeds and turmeric and cook, stirring occasionally, for 5 minutes or until the tomato has broken down to form a thick sauce.

Add the tofu, spring onion and 2 teaspoons of the soy sauce. Gently break up the tofu with the spoon as you combine the mixture. Do not over-mix as the idea is to keep some variation in the size of the tofu, not turn it to mush. Cook for 3–4 minutes or until well coated and heated through. Gently fold in the bean sprouts and season with freshly ground black pepper.

Meanwhile, steam the choy sum, broccolini and snow peas in a steamer basket over a large saucepan of simmering water for 3 minutes or until tender.

Divide the tofu scramble and steamed greens evenly among four plates. Scatter the almonds over the top and drizzle the remaining soy sauce over the greens.

> **WEEKS 7–12 CARB EXTRAS**
>
> For an extra 10 g carbs per serve, cut 200 g (50 g per person) sweet potato into wedges and steam for 8–10 minutes before you start cooking the scramble. Cover and keep warm, then serve on the side with the steamed greens.

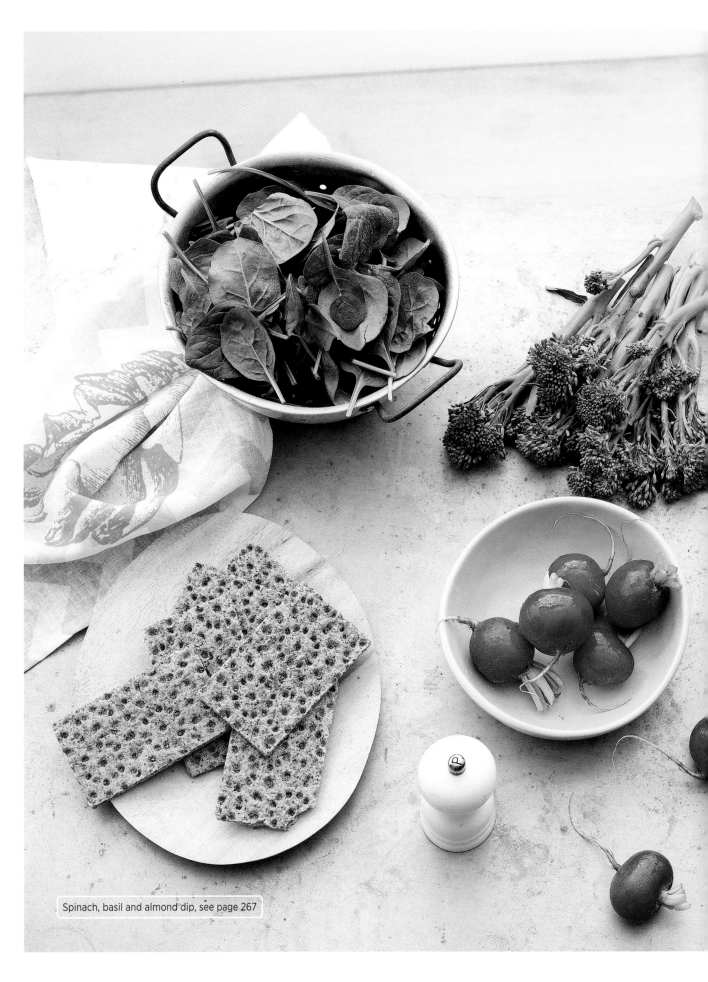

Spinach, basil and almond dip, see page 267

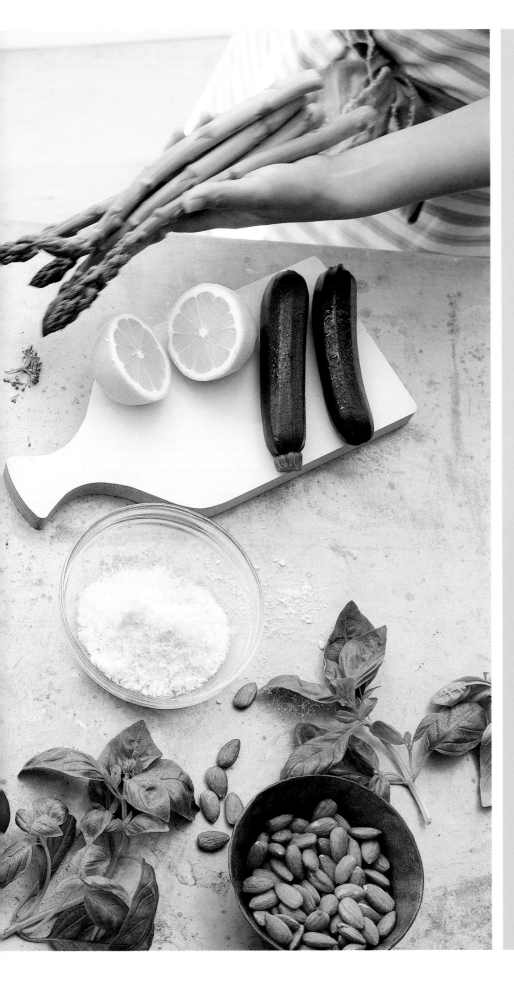

SNACKS & DESSERTS

Greek-style crispbread

7 G CARB PER SERVE

🍴 **Serves 4** 🕐 **Preparation: 10 minutes** 🍳 **Cooking: nil**

80 g salt-reduced low-fat feta
4 crispbreads (Ryvita)
2 tomatoes, sliced
1 Lebanese cucumber, sliced on the diagonal
8 olives, pitted and quartered lengthways

Crumble the feta into a bowl and mash with a fork to combine.

Divide the tomato and cucumber evenly among the crispbreads and season to taste with freshly ground black pepper. Spoon the feta evenly on top, add the olives and serve.

(Alternatively, if a smoother spread is preferred, place the feta and olives in a small food processor and process to form a paste. Divide among the crispbreads, then top with the tomato and cucumber, season with freshly ground black pepper and serve.)

UNITS PER SERVE

Breads, cereals, legumes, starchy vegetables **0.5**
Dairy **1**
Low-carb vegetables **1**
Healthy fats **0.5**

Caprese crispbread

7 G CARB PER SERVE

🍴 **Serves 4** 🕐 **Preparation: 10 minutes** 🍳 **Cooking: nil**

100 g baby spinach leaves, trimmed
¼ cup small basil leaves
4 tomatoes, sliced
100 g mozzarella, thickly sliced
2 tablespoons Pesto (see page 114)
4 crispbreads (Ryvita)

Divide the spinach, basil, tomato, mozzarella and pesto among the crispbreads. Season to taste with freshly ground black pepper and serve.

UNITS PER SERVE

Breads, cereals, legumes, starchy vegetables **0.5**
Dairy **1**
Low-carb vegetables **1**
Healthy fats **1**

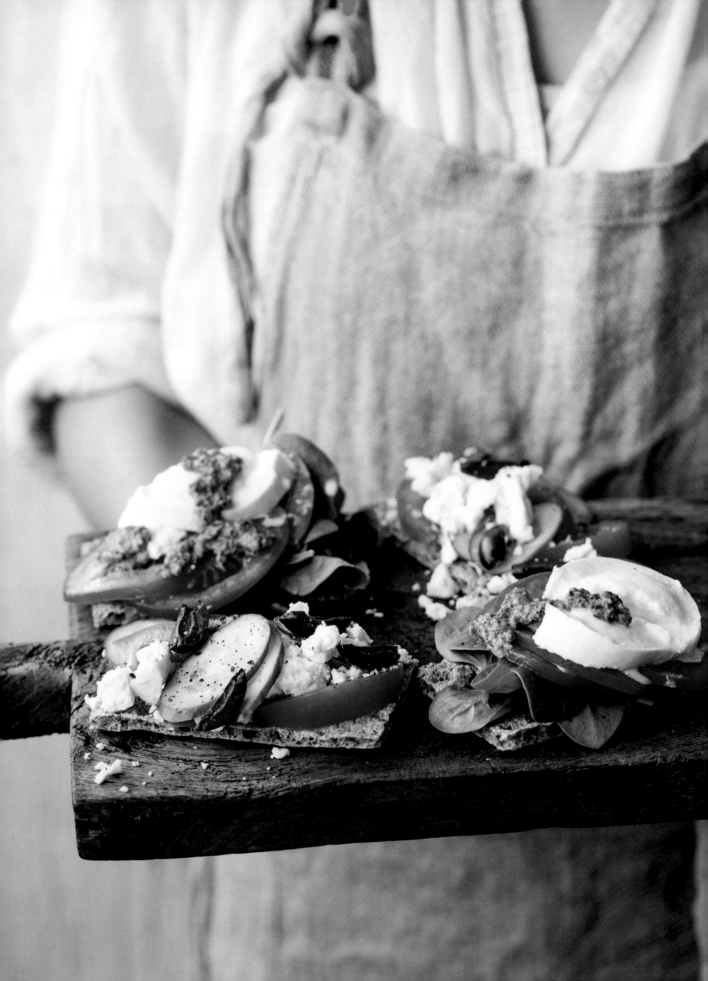

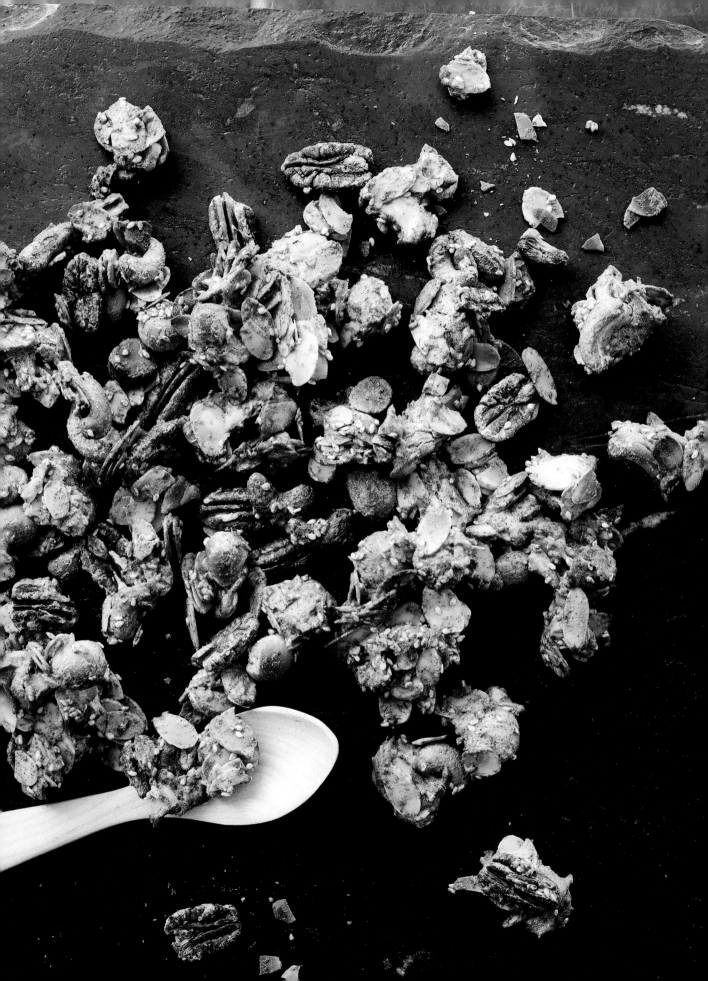

Sweet spiced nut clusters

1 G CARB PER SERVE

🍴 **Serves 25 (Makes about 255 g – 2¾ cups)**
🕐 **Preparation: 10 minutes, plus cooling time**
⊗ **Cooking: 15 minutes**

1 large egg white
pinch of cream of tartar
2 tablespoons tahini
1–2 teaspoons stevia granules
1 teaspoon ground cinnamon
½ teaspoon ground ginger
¼ teaspoon freshly grated nutmeg
60 g flaked almonds
40 g pecans or walnuts, roughly chopped
40 g raw unsalted cashews, roughly chopped
40 g macadamias, roughly chopped
2 tablespoons sesame seeds

Preheat the oven to 180°C (160°fan-forced) and line two baking trays with baking paper.

Beat the egg white in a bowl with a hand-held electric mixer until frothy. Add the cream of tartar and beat until soft peaks form, then beat in the tahini, stevia granules and spices until combined (the mixture will be thick but not airy). Fold in the nuts and sesame seeds until everything is coated.

Spread the mixture over the prepared trays in a single layer. Bake, stirring every 5 minutes, for 10–15 minutes or until golden.

Allow the nuts to cool completely on the trays. Break into smaller pieces, if necessary, and store in an airtight container for up to 2 weeks.

UNITS PER SERVE (5 TEASPOONS)

Healthy fats **1**

Grilled Swiss cheese and tomato toast fingers

9 G CARB PER SERVE

🍴 **Serves 4**   🕐 **Preparation: 5 minutes**
⊗ **Cooking: 5 minutes**

2 x 35 g slices mixed grain bread
Dijon mustard, for spreading
2 tomatoes, sliced
80 g Swiss cheese
100 g rocket leaves

Preheat the oven grill to high and line a baking tray with baking paper.

Lightly toast the bread in a toaster, spread with a little mustard, then top evenly with the tomato and Swiss cheese. Grill under the hot grill for 1–2 minutes or until the cheese has melted.

Cut into fingers, top with rocket and serve ½ slice toast per person.

UNITS PER SERVE

Breads, cereals, legumes, starchy vegetables **0.5**
Dairy **1**
Low-carb vegetables **0.5**

Zucchini and avocado 'fries'

Serves 4 **Preparation: 20 minutes** **Cooking: 15 minutes**

olive oil spray, for cooking

1 teaspoon ground coriander

1 teaspoon ground cumin

1 teaspoon sweet smoked paprika

2 zucchini (unpeeled), cut into
5 mm thick chips

80 g avocado, cut into 4 wedges

25 g flaked almonds, chopped

1 tablespoon finely chopped
pecans or walnuts

½ cup (40 g) finely grated parmesan

1 egg white

¾ cup (200 g) low-fat
Greek-style yoghurt

Preheat the oven to 220°C (200°C fan-forced). Line two large baking trays with baking paper and place an ovenproof wire rack on top of each. Lightly spray the wire racks with olive oil.

Put the spices in a large zip-lock bag and add the zucchini. Shake to coat the zucchini evenly in the spice mix. Remove the zucchini from the bag, shaking off the excess spice mix and tip any remaining spice onto a plate. Gently coat the avocado wedges in the remaining spice mix.

Combine the nuts and parmesan in a wide shallow bowl and season generously with freshly ground black pepper. Whisk the egg white with 1 tablespoon water in another bowl until frothy.

Working with one avocado wedge at a time, coat each wedge in the beaten egg white, shaking off the excess, and then roll in the nut and cheese mixture to coat lightly. Place on the wire rack, spaced well apart. Repeat this process with the zucchini, working with a few pieces at a time. Spray the 'fries' lightly with oil.

Bake for 13–15 minutes or until lightly browned. Remove from the oven and allow to cool for 5 minutes. Serve with the yoghurt.

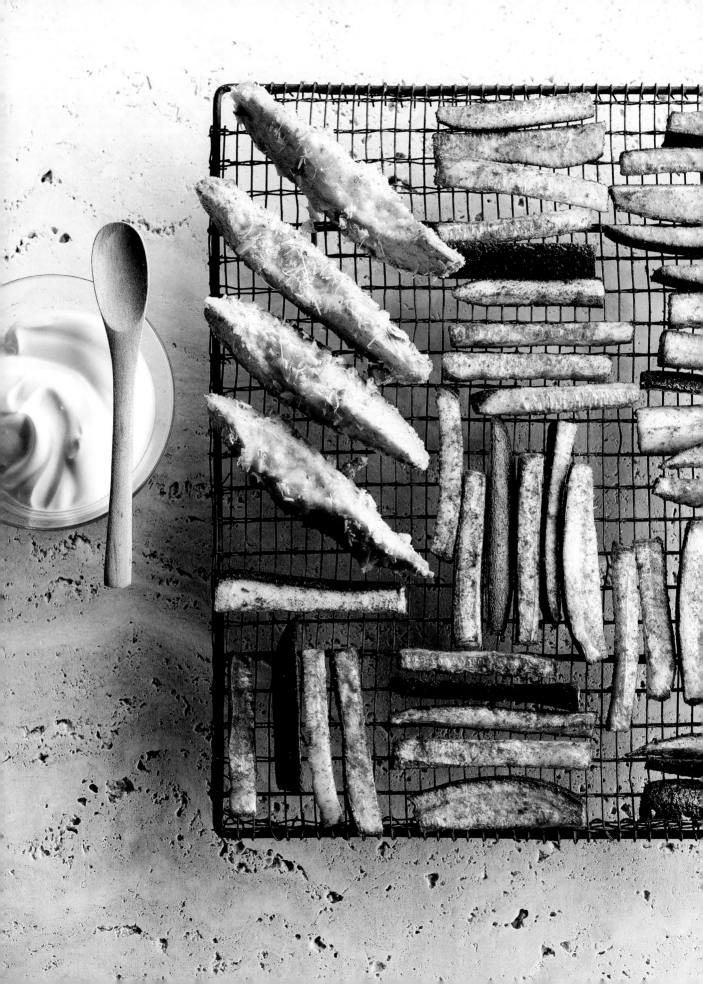

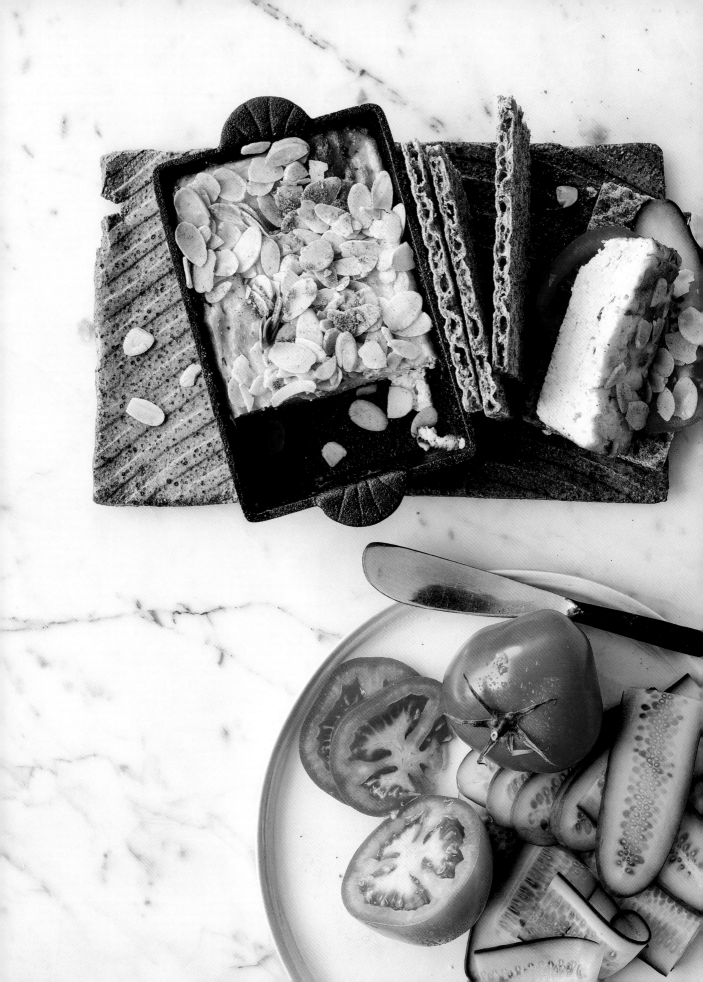

Spiced baked ricotta with almonds

UNITS PER SERVE
Breads, cereals, legumes,
starchy vegetables **0.5**
Dairy **1**
Low-carb vegetables **1**
Healthy fats **1**

---

olive oil spray, for cooking
40 g flaked almonds
¼ teaspoon ground coriander
¼ teaspoon ground cumin
200 g low-fat fresh ricotta
1½ tablespoons finely grated parmesan
1 egg
1 spring onion, chopped
4 wholegrain crispbreads (Ryvita)
2 tomatoes, sliced or
   300 g cherry tomatoes, halved
2 Lebanese cucumbers,
   halved widthways then
   thinly sliced lengthways

🍴 **Serves 4**   🕐 **Preparation: 10 minutes, plus resting time**
♨ **Cooking: 30 minutes**

Preheat the oven to 180°C (160°C fan-forced). Lightly spray 1 x 400 ml or 2 x 200 ml ramekins or ovenproof dishes with olive oil.

Toast the almonds in a small heavy-based frying pan over medium heat for 5 minutes or until lightly browned. Remove the pan from the heat and add the spices, shaking the pan to lightly toast the spices as well.

Sprinkle the nut and spice mixture evenly over the base of the ramekin.

Mash the ricotta in a bowl with a fork. Add the parmesan, egg and spring onion and mix well. Season lightly with freshly ground black pepper. Spoon the mixture into the prepared ramekin, smooth the surface and bake for 20–25 minutes or until puffed, golden and set in the centre. Set aside for 10 minutes to settle.

Loosen the edges of the baked ricotta and turn out onto a chopping board. Serve warm or store, covered, in the refrigerator for up to 3 days if you are not eating it straight away.

Cut the ricotta into even portions and serve with crispbreads, tomato and cucumber.

Indian-spiced kale chips with raita

🍴 Serves 4   🕐 Preparation: 15 minutes   🍳 Cooking: 15 minutes

1 bunch (about 350 g) curly kale
olive oil spray, for cooking
40 g salt-reduced low-fat
   feta, crumbled
2 cloves garlic, thinly sliced

MADRAS-STYLE SPICE MIX

1¼ tablespoons ground coriander
2 teaspoons ground cumin
1 teaspoon ground turmeric
1 teaspoon ground cinnamon
½ teaspoon ground ginger
½ teaspoon freshly ground
   black pepper
¼ teaspoon yellow mustard
   seeds, ground
pinch of ground cloves
pinch of ground cardamom
pinch of chilli powder

RAITA

200 g low-fat Greek-style yoghurt
1 Lebanese cucumber, grated (skin on)
   with the juice squeezed out
2 tablespoons shredded mint
½ small clove garlic, crushed (optional)

For the spice mix, combine all the spices together in a small bowl. Ideally, store in an airtight container out of direct sunlight for 24 hours before consuming to allow time for the flavours to develop.

Preheat the oven to 180°C (160°C) and line three large baking trays with baking paper.

Remove the leafy parts of the kale from the tough stalks and tear into bite-sized pieces. Wash and dry the kale very well. Use a salad spinner or a clean dry tea towel to dry the kale.

Spread the kale over the prepared trays in a single layer and spray with olive oil. Mix well with your hands, ensuring the leaves are lightly coated all over. Scatter over with the feta, garlic and 1½ teaspoons of the spice mix.

Bake for 12–15 minutes, swapping the trays around halfway through the cooking time, until the leaves are crisp.

Meanwhile, to make the raita, combine all the ingredients and ½ teaspoon of the spice mix in a small bowl. Cover and refrigerate until required.

Remove the kale chips from the oven and allow to cool. Serve immediately with the raita. Serve the raita with a spoon so that it can be dolloped onto the kale chips – they are not robust enough to 'dip'.

Note: The spice mix makes about ¼ cup; leftovers can be kept in an airtight container for several months. You can make the ground spices yourself from seeds where applicable. Grind in a spice grinder or use a mortar and pestle. If using a mortar and pestle, sieve the powder after grinding to remove any unground pieces.

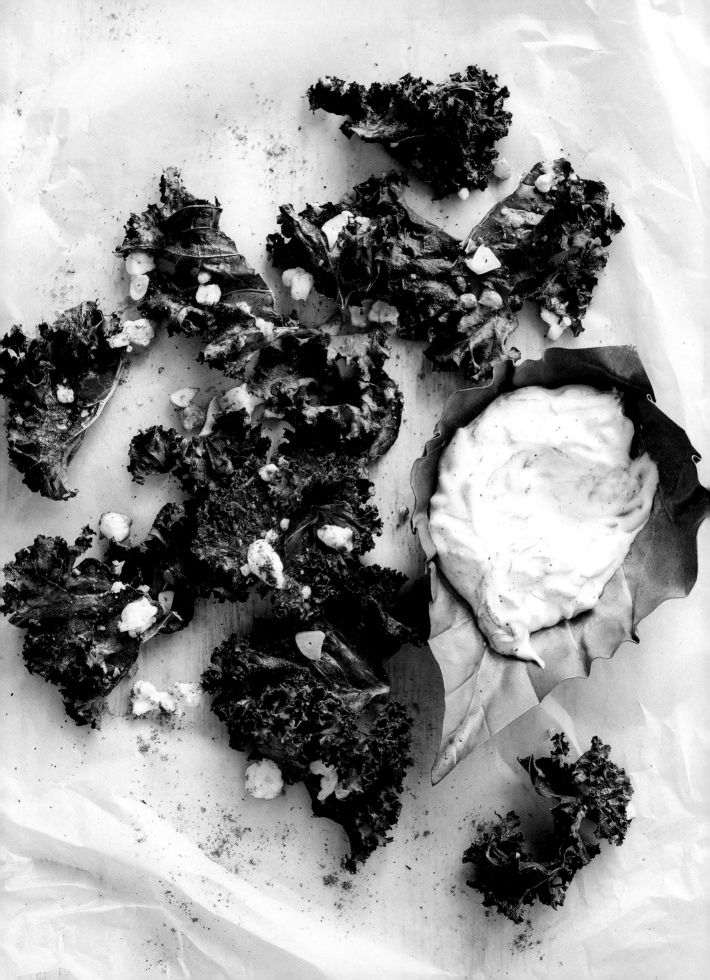

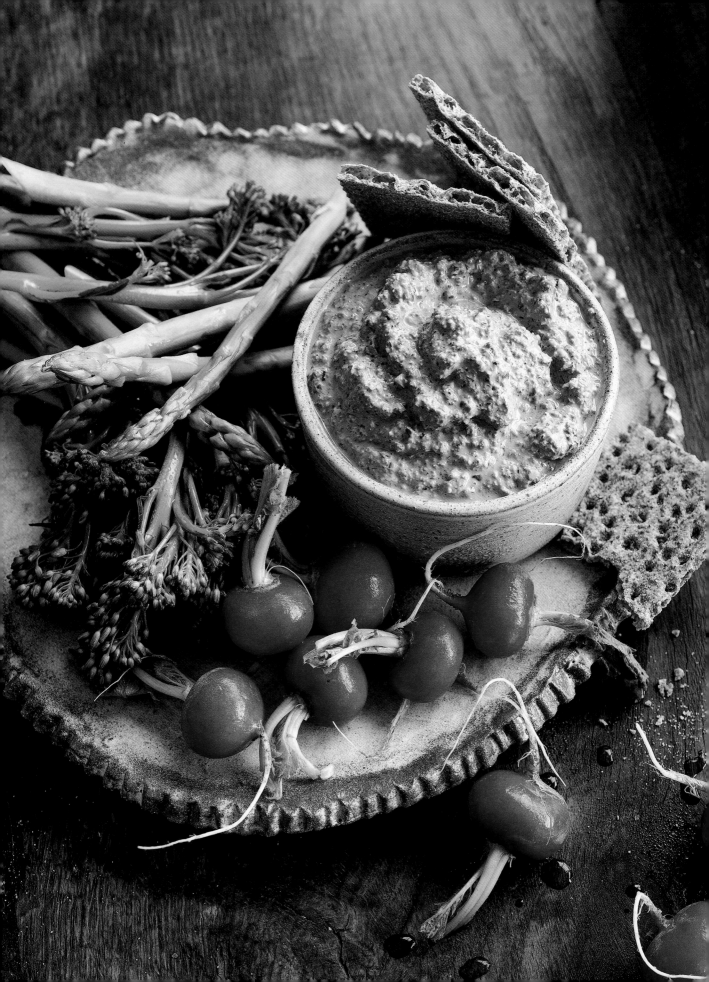

Spinach, basil and almond dip

UNITS PER SERVE
Breads, cereals, legumes,
starchy vegetables **0.5**
Dairy **1**
Low-carb vegetables **1.5**
Healthy fats **1**

---

100 g baby spinach leaves

1 zucchini, coarsely grated with
the juice squeezed out

½ cup (40 g) finely grated parmesan

large handful basil leaves

finely grated zest of ½ lemon

1 clove garlic, crushed

40 g raw almonds (optional)

110 g low-fat fresh ricotta or
200 g low-fat Greek-style yoghurt

1 bunch asparagus, trimmed

1 bunch broccolini, trimmed and
halved lengthways

4 wholegrain crispbreads (Ryvita)

1 bunch baby radishes,
tender tops intact

Serves 4   **Preparation: 10 minutes**   **Cooking: 3 minutes**

Put the spinach, zucchini, parmesan, basil, lemon zest, garlic and almonds, if using, in the bowl of a food processor and process until well combined and finely chopped. There will be some texture left in the almonds if you use them. Add the ricotta or yoghurt and blend until combined.

Steam the asparagus and broccolini in a steamer basket over a large saucepan of simmering water for 2–3 minutes or until just tender but still crisp.

Serve the dip with the crispbreads, steamed vegetables and radishes.

Coffee yoghurt with nut sprinkle

10 G
CARB
PER
SERVE

🍴 **Serves 4**   🕐 **Preparation: 15 minutes, plus setting time**
♨ **Cooking: 1 minute**

2 teaspoons powdered gelatine
400 g low-fat Greek-style yoghurt
1 teaspoon natural vanilla bean paste
¼ cup (40 g) Sweet Spiced Nut Clusters
    (see page 259)

COFFEE SAUCE
2 teaspoons stevia granules
1 teaspoon unsweetened cocoa powder
½ cup (125 ml) freshly brewed double-
    strength espresso or good-quality
    strong instant coffee

To make the coffee sauce, combine all the ingredients in a small heatproof bowl and stir until the stevia and cocoa powder have dissolved into the coffee. Remove ¼ cup (60 ml) of the coffee sauce and set aside for serving.

Sprinkle the gelatine over the remaining coffee sauce and whisk to combine. Set aside for 5 minutes for the water to absorb into the gelatine. Heat the gelatine mixture in the microwave in 10-second bursts on high until the mixture has dissolved and is translucent.

Combine the yoghurt and vanilla in a large bowl. Transfer ½ cup (140 g) of the yoghurt mixture to a separate bowl. Working quickly, whisk the coffee gelatine mixture into the smaller amount of yoghurt. Once combined, scrape this into the larger bowl of yoghurt and whisk until combined. Pour into four serving cups or glasses, then refrigerate for 2 hours or until set.

Sprinkle the nut clusters evenly over the yoghurts and serve with the reserved coffee sauce on the side.

WEEKS 7–12 CARB EXTRAS

For an extra 10 g carbs per serve, serve with 240 g (60 g per person) blueberries.

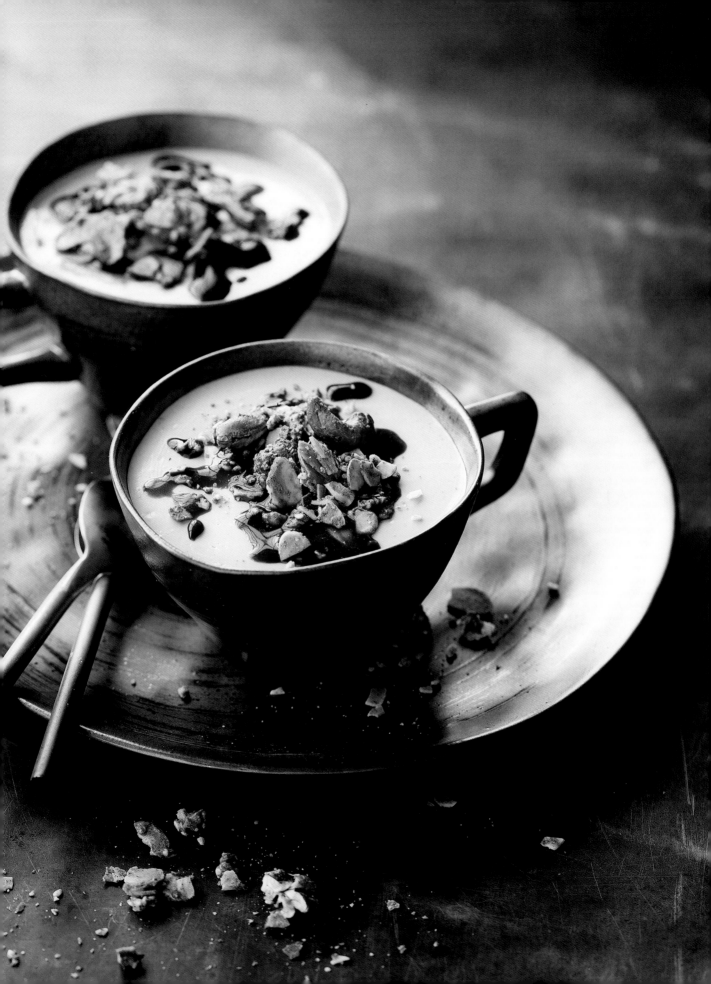

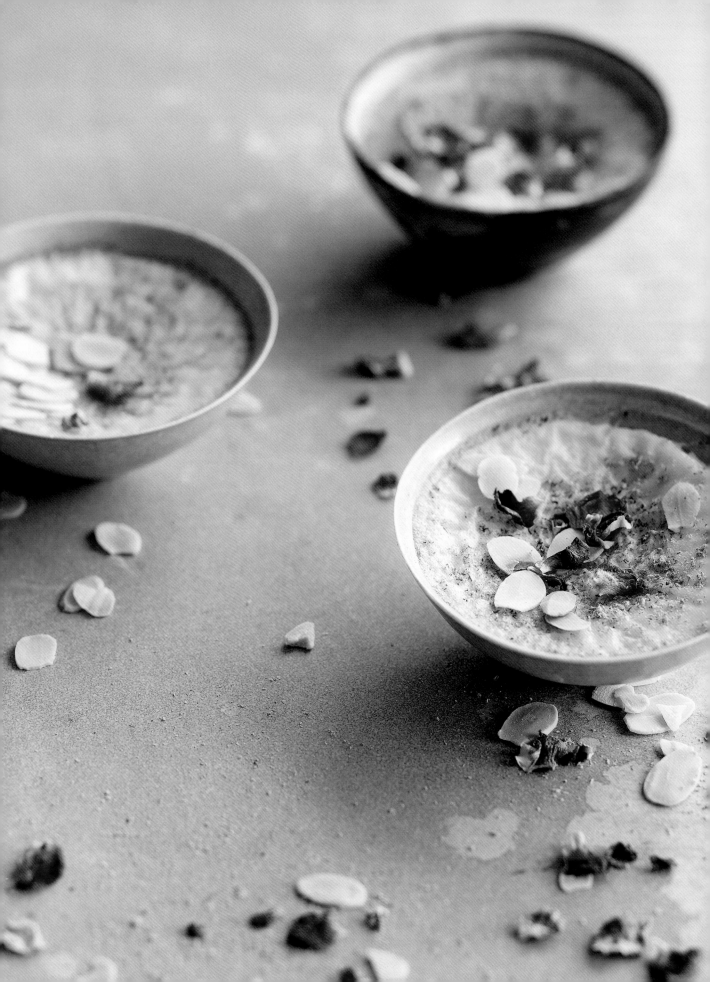

Lean meat, fish, poultry, eggs, tofu **0.5**
Dairy **1**
Healthy fats **0.5**

Baked orange blossom custards

10 G
CARB
PER
SERVE

4 extra-large eggs
3 cups (750 ml) skim milk
3 teaspoons orange blossom water
2 teaspoons stevia granules (optional)
freshly grated nutmeg, to taste
20 g flaked almonds, toasted
edible rose petals or flowers (optional),
    to serve

🍴 **Serves 4**   🕐 **Preparation: 5 minutes**   ♨ **Cooking: 35 minutes**

Preheat the oven to 160°C (140°C fan-forced). Place four 1 cup (250 ml) ramekins or ovenproof dishes on a baking tray.

Whisk together the eggs, milk, orange blossom water and stevia, if using, in a large bowl. Strain through a fine-mesh sieve into a large jug and pour evenly into the ramekins on the tray. Sprinkle with a little nutmeg.

Bake for 30–35 minutes or until lightly coloured on top and just set (the centre should wobble very slightly). Set aside to cool slightly. Serve warm or cold, scattered with the almonds and rose petals or flowers, if using.

WEEKS 7–12 CARB EXTRAS

For an extra 10 g carbs per serve, serve with 800 g (200 g per person) watermelon cubes or 400 g (100 g per person) orange segments, splashed with a tiny drizzle of extra orange blossom water.

Berry yoghurt jellies

6 G
CARB
PER
SERVE

🍴 **Serves 4**   🕐 **Preparation: 10 minutes, plus chilling time**
🍲 **Cooking: nil**

1 × 9 g packet lite strawberry or
  vanilla berry jelly crystals
  (Aeroplane jelly brand)
1 cup (250 ml) boiling water
1 cup (280 g) low-fat vanilla Greek-style
  yoghurt, plus 120 g extra, to serve

Place the jelly crystals in a heatproof bowl, add the boiling water and
stir until the crystals have dissolved. Stir in ¾ cup (180 ml) cold water.
Cover and refrigerate for 30 minutes or until lightly set.

Add the 1 cup (280 g) yoghurt, then whisk until the mixture is smooth
and well combined. Transfer to a measuring jug, if desired, as it makes
it easier to portion. Divide the yoghurt jelly among four 1 cup (250 ml)
capacity glasses, then cover with plastic film and refrigerate for
3–4 hours or until set.

Serve the jellies each topped with one-quarter of the extra yoghurt.

> **WEEKS 7–12 CARB EXTRAS**
>
> For an extra 10 g carbs per serve, accompany the jellies with
> 800 g strawberries (200 g per person) or 240 g blueberries
> (60 g per person).

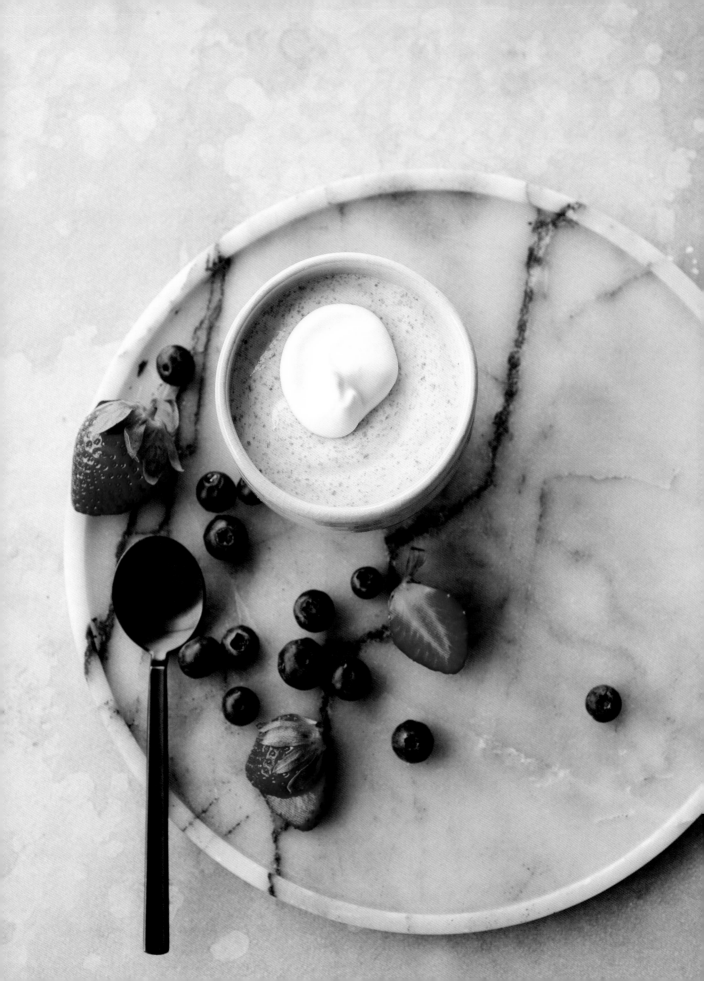

APPENDIX A:
HOW DOCTORS MANAGE TYPE 2 DIABETES

Doctors consider a range of short- and long-term factors to help manage diabetes to improve certain measurable health markers. The Low-carb Diet and exercise plan works because it results in a measurable improvement in these same health markers.

In the short term, medical management of diabetes means bringing its extreme highs of blood glucose safely under control, as interventions to control blood pressure and blood cholesterol. In the long term, medical treatments are aimed at preventing or slowing the complications of diabetes, which are grouped together into *macrovascular* (large blood vessel) diseases such as heart attack or stroke; and *microvascular* (small blood vessel) diseases, which involve poor circulation to other organs or the limbs, such as eye disease, kidney failure and nerve damage. These treatment strategies should be centred around long-term weight and dietary management, and physical activity, even if medications are required. Given that diabetes frequently goes undiagnosed, we urge you to ask your GP to check your blood glucose levels each year.

If you already have diabetes, your healthcare team will need to monitor your blood pressure, blood glucose and blood cholesterol levels regularly. Your healthcare team should always encourage you to learn how best to manage and control your diabetes yourself (under their supervision), as outlined below. If you find they don't support you in this way, perhaps seek a second opinion or a GP who can support you in making lifestyle changes.

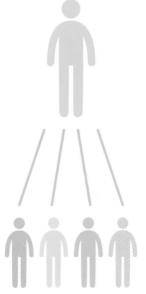

YOUR HEALTHCARE TEAM

If you have type 2 diabetes, you might want to expand your healthcare team, depending on your circumstances, to include a diabetes specialist (endocrinologist), a diabetes nurse and/or diabetes educator, an accredited practising dietitian, an exercise physiologist or physiotherapist with expertise in diabetes and weight management, your pharmacist, and perhaps even a counsellor. This team can monitor your health as you make changes to your lifestyle. If you need any medications, these could be prescribed by your endocrinologist, a diabetes nurse with prescribing rights or your GP.

Each year, many new studies are published exploring the best ways to manage diabetes and its complications. You should ensure that your healthcare team is keeping abreast of any new developments, and you may even enjoy keeping an eye on these yourself. You should feel confident enough to discuss your condition and any concerns with your endocrinologist or GP. If not, you have every right to build a new healthcare team.

The damage diabetes can do

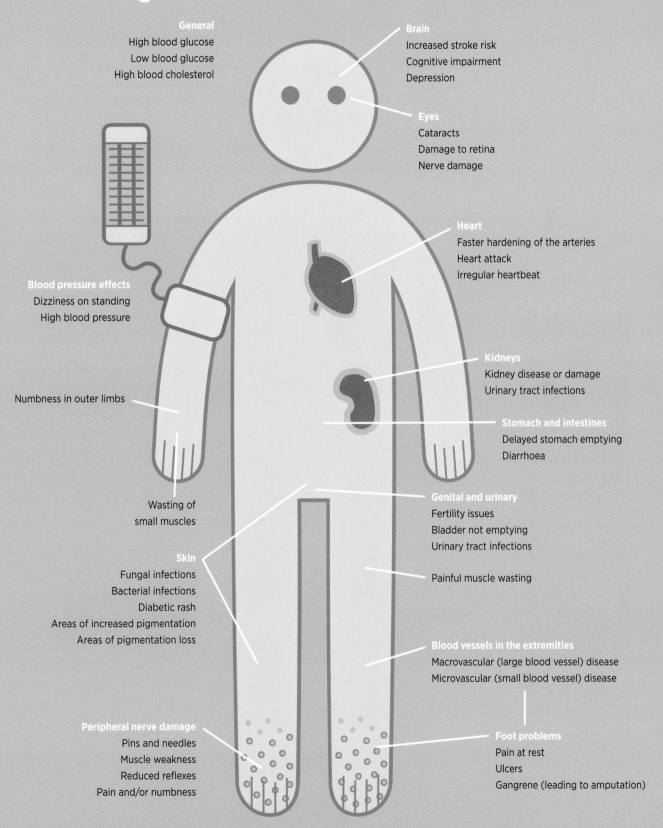

General
High blood glucose
Low blood glucose
High blood cholesterol

Brain
Increased stroke risk
Cognitive impairment
Depression

Eyes
Cataracts
Damage to retina
Nerve damage

Heart
Faster hardening of the arteries
Heart attack
Irregular heartbeat

Blood pressure effects
Dizziness on standing
High blood pressure

Numbness in outer limbs

Wasting of
small muscles

Kidneys
Kidney disease or damage
Urinary tract infections

Stomach and intestines
Delayed stomach emptying
Diarrhoea

Genital and urinary
Fertility issues
Bladder not emptying
Urinary tract infections

Painful muscle wasting

Skin
Fungal infections
Bacterial infections
Diabetic rash
Areas of increased pigmentation
Areas of pigmentation loss

Blood vessels in the extremities
Macrovascular (large blood vessel) disease
Microvascular (small blood vessel) disease

Peripheral nerve damage
Pins and needles
Muscle weakness
Reduced reflexes
Pain and/or numbness

Foot problems
Pain at rest
Ulcers
Gangrene (leading to amputation)

Your blood pressure

The higher your blood pressure, the greater your risk of developing one or more problems, such as heart attack, heart failure, stroke, kidney failure and poor circulation.

Good ways to control blood pressure include a diet low in salt, plenty of exercise, reducing your alcohol intake and, if you're overweight or obese, losing weight. The Low-carb Diet and exercise plan will help you achieve all of these. If you have type 2 diabetes as well, even if you make these lifestyle changes you might also need prescription medication to help keep your blood pressure down. If you don't make any changes to your lifestyle at all, you'll definitely need to take medication or you'll be putting your body at greater risk.

Measuring blood pressure

Blood pressure is usually given with an upper reading (which health practitioners call systolic blood pressure) and a lower reading (diastolic blood pressure), in millimetres of mercury (mmHg). Both readings are important, and adults should generally aim for a blood pressure of around 120/80 mmHg.

As you no doubt know, blood pressure is generally measured using an inflatable cuff around the upper arm. Assessing your blood pressure control relies on regular measurements. Portable blood pressure monitors are easy to purchase at a reasonable price, so that you can keep track of your blood pressure at home. This is especially useful if your blood pressure rises steeply when you visit your GP! Blood pressure can vary significantly during the day, so a 24-hour recording from an automated monitor or a diary of readings from a manual monitor, collected under the same conditions each time (e.g. after sitting quietly at a table for five minutes), can help your healthcare team understand your blood pressure control over time. This is especially important if you're losing weight, as blood pressure usually falls as weight is lost. An automated monitor can also identify people whose blood pressure doesn't fall while they sleep, a condition that requires particular treatment.

Blood pressure targets

You and your healthcare team should agree on a blood pressure target, but usually this will be around 120/80 mmHg (or a little higher in people over 70). If you have proteinuria (protein in the urine, an indicator of kidney damage), you'll probably be given a lower blood pressure target than this. A treatment is working if your blood pressure drops – as simple as that. This indicates good health outcomes, such as lower levels of protein in the urine and a reduction in the thickness of the heart muscle (which if necessary can be checked using an ultrasound of the heart). For older people, however, a lower blood pressure target may not be appropriate. This is because low blood pressure can increase the risk of a fall.

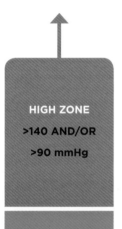

HIGH ZONE
>140 AND/OR
>90 mmHg

NORMAL TO NORMAL-HIGH ZONE
120–139 AND/OR
80–89 mmHg

OPTIMAL ZONE
<120 AND/OR
<80 mmHg

Monitoring blood pressure

If you're taking blood pressure medication and losing weight thanks to lifestyle modifications, your healthcare team will need to monitor your blood pressure levels particularly closely. This is necessary to prevent it falling too low, which can cause faintness or dizziness. If your blood pressure falls and you're still losing weight or maintaining a lower weight, your medication dose may need to be adjusted or stopped altogether. Since blood pressure medications can have side effects, reducing or stopping medication not only saves you money but may further improve your health and wellbeing.

If despite making lifestyle changes your blood pressure is still not fully under control, you may need antihypertensive (blood-pressure-lowering) medication.

Your blood glucose

If you have type 2 diabetes, controlling your blood glucose traditionally relies upon measurements taken using finger-prick blood tests at various times throughout the day, especially in the morning before breakfast – *fasting glucose* – and two hours after a meal – *post-prandial glucose*.

Monitoring blood glucose

You and your healthcare team will set specific targets for your blood glucose levels during the day, measured using a portable blood glucose monitoring kit. This uses a finger-prick blood test, which has the added advantage of telling you immediately whether any symptoms you might be experiencing are caused by hyper- (high) or hypoglycaemia (low blood glucose).

Hypoglycaemia – low blood glucose (less than 3.9 mmol/L) – can cause feelings of hunger, sweating, a racing heart, dizziness, poor memory or slurred or slow speech. Untreated, severe hypoglycaemia can cause blackouts. You can only have hypoglycaemia if you are on medications that lower blood glucose, such as insulin or sulfonylureas. Other types of diabetes medications do not cause hypoglycaemia.

Hyperglycaemia – high blood glucose (greater than 10 mmol/L) – causes no symptoms in many people until it's extremely high. When there are symptoms, they can include extreme thirst, frequent urination, tiredness and blurred vision. Hyperglycaemia indicates that the body is having difficulty processing the carbohydrates consumed during the preceding meal, and is associated with increased risk of diabetes complications.

If you have well-controlled diabetes, you should have your HbA1c checked every six months. If your diabetes is not well-controlled or is unstable, it should be checked every three months until good control is established. An HbA1c of less than 6.5–7 per cent (48–53 mmol/mol) is considered to indicate good control, but if you're older, an HbA1c level this low may not be appropriate. Aiming for too low an HbA1c target may result in too many low blood glucose levels, which can increase the risk of brain damage or heart attack.

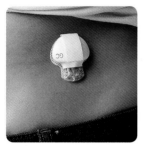

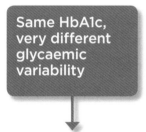

Figure reprinted with permission from Medtronic Australasia Pty. Ltd., NSW, Australia.

Same HbA1c, very different glycaemic variability

Continuous blood glucose monitoring devices

Non-invasive, wearable devices are now available that have a small, discreet glucose-measuring unit about the size of a 50-cent coin, and a sensor filament that sits just beneath the skin. These measure blood glucose levels every five minutes around the clock, allowing the wearer to track their blood glucose profile 24 hours a day. These devices are far less intrusive, painful and inconvenient than doing multiple finger-prick tests.

At the moment, these monitors are not cheap, but as they become more common, their price will fall. The less expensive devices capture information into a recording unit that can be subsequently downloaded and viewed, costing typically between $50 and $100 per trace. The latest continuous blood glucose monitoring systems are now Bluetooth-enabled, meaning the data is sent wirelessly to a device such as a smartphone so the results can be viewed instantaneously. These cost between $500 and $2000.

The measurements these devices take can be compiled into a daily graph such as the one below, indicating fluctuations in blood glucose throughout the day. Seeing your continuous blood glucose profile can help you manage your blood glucose by identifying when your highs and lows (your glycaemic variability) occurs, and the size of these peaks and troughs. This variability is largely determined by the amount of carbs eaten and the mismatch with the amount of insulin available in the body, which is why reducing the amount of carbs in your diet will reduce your glycaemic variability .

This is important because glycaemic variability gives different long-term information from Hb1Ac, and because widely oscillating blood glucose levels are associated with a greater risk of cardiovascular disease. As the graph below shows, two people with the same average blood glucose level could have very different glycaemic variability. The person represented by the green line has relatively stable blood glucose, while the person represented by the yellow line has blood glucose that fluctuates widely throughout the day, putting their health at much greater risk.

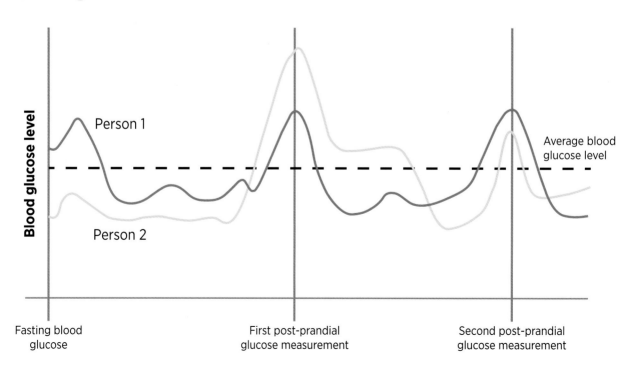

As the second graph below indicates, the continuous blood glucose monitor can help detect downward and upward swings in glucose levels into the hypoglycaemia and hyperglycaemia ranges respectively. This information is extremely useful when adjusting medications, diet and exercise habits to prevent these swings. **The dots on the graph indicate finger-prick tests, which would have provided no warning of these extremes or even indicated that they had occurred.** Research suggests that self-monitoring your blood glucose using one of these dynamic devices is a really effective means of achieving good blood glucose control, and can motivate you to stick with your diet and exercise plans.

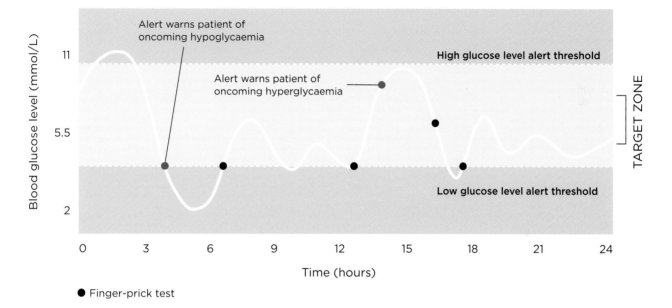

● Finger-prick test

Glucose-lowering medications

If you have type 2 diabetes, depending on its severity and stage, your healthcare team may have prescribed glucose-lowering medications such as insulin, insulin sensitisers and oral hypoglycaemic agents (e.g. metformin, diabex, diaformin, diamicron or melizide). Make sure you maintain a close relationship with your healthcare team. If you lose weight, reduce your carbohydrate intake and/or increase your exercise or activity levels – such as by following the Low-carb Diet and exercise plan – but your medication levels remain the same, your blood glucose levels could fall to dangerously low levels and become unpredictable. Conversely, if you reduce your exercise levels, perhaps due to a physical injury or a change in seasons, then your blood glucose levels may rise and you may need more medication. This is why, in addition to regular monitoring at home, you need to consult your healthcare team regularly.

Since hypoglycaemia is a distinct possibility if you're on some of these medications, you need to have a plan in place for dealing with it. This usually involves immediately ingesting easily absorbable glucose, for example by drinking orange juice or eating a few jelly beans. It might also include having handy a HypoKit pen, which injects glucagon, a hormone that opposes insulin and releases glucose from the liver to restore blood glucose levels. The pen is easy to use, so that if you collapse, a family member or any bystander can administer it. The effect of the glucagon lasts only 20 minutes, so you'll need to eat or drink as soon as possible and seek urgent medical assistance.

Your blood fats

High levels of blood fats – cholesterol and triglycerides – can increase the risk of cardiovascular disease, especially in people who have type 2 diabetes. Unhealthy blood fat levels can be influenced by genetics and a poor diet, but smoking and lack of exercise can also play a role.

What are blood fats?

Cholesterol and triglycerides are two forms of blood fats that are necessary for life itself. Both can either be produced within the body or come from dietary sources. The scientific word for fats is lipids, so you may hear your healthcare team talking about your blood lipid levels.

Cholesterol is a white, insoluble, waxy substance produced by the liver and most cells in the body. It's essential for many processes of daily life, including building cell membranes and brain and nerve cells, and producing the bile acids that absorb fats and the fat-soluble vitamins (A, D, E and K). The body also uses cholesterol to make vitamin D and key hormones that help our metabolism work efficiently.

Triglycerides are fats made up of groups of three chains of high-energy fatty acids produced in the intestine and liver from single fatty acids (small fat molecules). They provide body cells with fuel to function. If unused, triglycerides are stored in body fat deposits until required.

Cholesterol and triglycerides cannot circulate freely in the blood because blood is mostly water. Instead, they're packaged with proteins and other substances to form soluble particles called *lipoproteins*. There are several different types of lipoprotein, each with a different purpose. The two main types of lipoprotein we measure are:

- **low-density lipoprotein (LDL) cholesterol.** This delivers cholesterol to cells and is often called 'bad' cholesterol because when levels in the blood are too high, it builds up and sticks to the lining of the blood vessels. This stimulates the formation of plaques within the arteries and leads to atherosclerosis (hardening of the arteries).

- **high-density lipoprotein (HDL) cholesterol.** This helps remove excess cholesterol from the cells, including arterial cells, and is therefore called 'good' cholesterol.

Monitoring blood fats

A test of blood fat content, often a fasting blood test, can indicate the risk of a heart attack or stroke in the next five years. Treatment that lowers the levels of triglycerides and LDL cholesterol (bad cholesterol) reduces the risk of heart attack, while anything that elevates levels of HDL cholesterol (good cholesterol) also reduces the risk of cardiovascular disease. The great news is that the Low-carb Diet does exactly that. It will markedly improve your blood fat profile by reducing your triglyceride and LDL cholesterol levels and increasing your HDL cholesterol levels. This will significantly improve your diabetes control and reduce your risk of cardiovascular disease.

❝ Unhealthy blood fat levels can be influenced by genetics and a poor diet, but smoking and lack of exercise can also play a role. ❞

Blood fats target

Australian Government guidelines recommend that we have our health, and particularly our cardiovascular health, assessed every two years after the age of 45. This include having our blood glucose and blood fat levels checked. If your levels indicate a borderline–high risk of developing cardiovascular disease (see below), it is best to make changes to your diet and exercise habits (aiming for a modest weight reduction of around 5 kg) to help bring your blood fat levels down. If they remain elevated, and you are at high risk of heart disease, you may be prescribed lipid-lowering medication, most often statins. While these reduce the levels of LDL cholesterol in the blood, they can have side effects such as muscle aches, or can affect blood tests of liver function.

Blood fat (mmol/L)	Low risk	Borderline	High risk
LDL cholesterol	Less than 1.8	More than 2	More than 4.5
HDL cholesterol	At least 1	Less than 1	Less than 0.9
Triglyceride	Less than 2	2 or more	More than 6

A NOTE ABOUT MEDICATIONS

As we've already seen, there are many useful lifestyle strategies you can use if you need to control your blood pressure, blood glucose and/or blood fats, without having to resort to medication. In many cases, however, such medication is prescribed primarily to reduce the risk of diabetes complications. If you start the Low-carb Diet and exercise plan, we urge you to familiarise your healthcare team with its principles. In order to tailor your medications safely, your prescriber will need to monitor your blood pressure, blood glucose and blood fat carefully whenever you lose weight, alter your diet or change your exercise routine.

Note that most medications prescribed for diabetes should be taken at specific times of the day, often related to mealtimes. Extended-release medications, which deliver the active drugs over a prolonged period, can be very different from the quicker-acting formulations of the same drug. Their doses are often different, and they usually need to be taken fewer times during the day. Sometimes blood-pressure-lowering or blood-glucose-lowering drugs come in combined doses with other medications that have the same purpose and boost the lowering effect.

APPENDIX B:
CALCULATING
HEALTH MEASURES

What is your BMI?

If you prefer to use an online tool to calculate your BMI, visit:
healthyweight.health.gov.au/wps/portal/Home/helping-hand/bmi

Are you at risk of cardiovascular disease?

To complete the online Australian Absolute Cardiovascular disease risk
questionnaire, visit: cvdcheck.org.au. You'll need your latest blood pressure
and blood cholesterol readings.

Do you have type 2 diabetes?

The Australian type 2 diabetes risk assessment tool (AusDRISK) was created
by the Baker IDI Heart and Diabetes Institute to help health practitioners and
the general public determine their risk of developing the condition. Check
your risk now by answering the questions opposite, or complete the online
assessment at: diabetesaustralia.com.au/are-you-at-risk-type-2

Calculating your basal metabolic rate

To determine your BMR online, go to the Australian Government's
calculator at eatforhealth.gov.au/node/add/calculator–energy

Diabetes risk assessment

1. What is your age group?

Under 35	0 points
35–44	2 points
45–54	4 points
55–64	6 points
65 or over	8 points

2. What is your gender?

Female	0 points
Male	3 points

3. What are your ethnicity and your country of birth?

Are you of Aboriginal, Torres Strait Islander, Pacific Islander or Maori descent?

No	0 points
Yes	2 points

Where were you born?

Australia	0 points
Asia	2 points
Indian subcontinent	2 points
Middle East	2 points
North Africa	2 points
Southern Europe	2 points
Other	0 points

4. Have either of your parents, or any of your brothers or sisters, been diagnosed with diabetes (type 1 or type 2)?

No	0 points
Yes	3 points

5. Have you ever been found to have high blood glucose (sugar) in a health examination, during an illness or during pregnancy?

No	0 points
Yes	6 points

6. Are you currently taking medication for high blood pressure?

No	0 points
Yes	2 points

7. Do you currently smoke cigarettes or any other tobacco products on a daily basis?

No	0 points
Yes	2 points

8. How often do you eat vegetables or fruit?

Every day	0 points
Not every day	1 point

9. On average, would you say you do at least 2.5 hours of physical activity per week (for example, 30 minutes a day on five or more days a week)?

Yes	0 points
No	2 points

10. What is your waist measurement taken below the ribs (usually at the level of the navel, and while standing)?

For those of Asian or Aboriginal or Torres Strait Islander descent

Men	Women	
Less than 90 cm	Less than 80 cm	0 points
90–100 cm	80–90 cm	4 points
More than 100 cm	More than 90 cm	7 points

For all others

Men	Women	
Less than 102 cm	Less than 88 cm	0 points
102–110 cm	88–100 cm	4 points
More than 110 cm	More than 100 cm	7 points

Your risk of developing type 2 diabetes within 5 years

Check your total score against the three point ranges below. Note that if you're less than 25 years old, the overall score may overestimate your risk of diabetes.

5 or less: Low risk

Approximately one person in every 100 with a score in this range will develop diabetes.

6–11: Intermediate risk

Approximately one person in every 50 with a score in the range of 6–8 will develop diabetes. Approximately one person in every 30 with a score in the range of 9–11 will develop diabetes. Discuss your score with your GP and consider lifestyle changes to reduce your risk.

12 or more: High risk

Approximately one person in every 14 with a score in the range of 12–15 will develop diabetes. Approximately one person in every seven with a score in the range of 16–19 will develop diabetes. Approximately one person in every three with a score in the range of 20 and above will develop diabetes. You may have undiagnosed diabetes. See your GP as soon as possible for a fasting glucose test.

APPENDIX C:
TRAINING DIARY TEMPLATES

Resistance exercises

Week:			Date: ___ /___ /___		
Day: Monday Tuesday Wednesday Thursday Friday Saturday Sunday					
Session rating of perceived exertion (see page 91):					
General comments:					
Region	Exercise name	Body weight or dumbbell (kg)	Repetitions		
			Set 1	Set 2	Set 3
Upper body	**e.g. push-up**	**body weight**	**12**	**9**	**8**
Core					
Lower body					

Aerobic exercises

Week	Day (circle)	Date	Activity	Duration (mins)	Session rating of perceived exertion (see page 91)	General comments
1	M Tu W Th F Sa Su	__ /__ /__	e.g. walking	35	3	
	M Tu W Th F Sa Su	__ /__ /__				
	M Tu W Th F Sa Su	__ /__ /__				
	M Tu W Th F Sa Su	__ /__ /__				
	M Tu W Th F Sa Su	__ /__ /__				
2	M Tu W Th F Sa Su	__ /__ /__				
	M Tu W Th F Sa Su	__ /__ /__				
	M Tu W Th F Sa Su	__ /__ /__				
	M Tu W Th F Sa Su	__ /__ /__				
	M Tu W Th F Sa Su	__ /__ /__				
	M Tu W Th F Sa Su	__ /__ /__				
3	M Tu W Th F Sa Su	__ /__ /__				
	M Tu W Th F Sa Su	__ /__ /__				
	M Tu W Th F Sa Su	__ /__ /__				
	M Tu W Th F Sa Su	__ /__ /__				
	M Tu W Th F Sa Su	__ /__ /__				
	M Tu W Th F Sa Su	__ /__ /__				

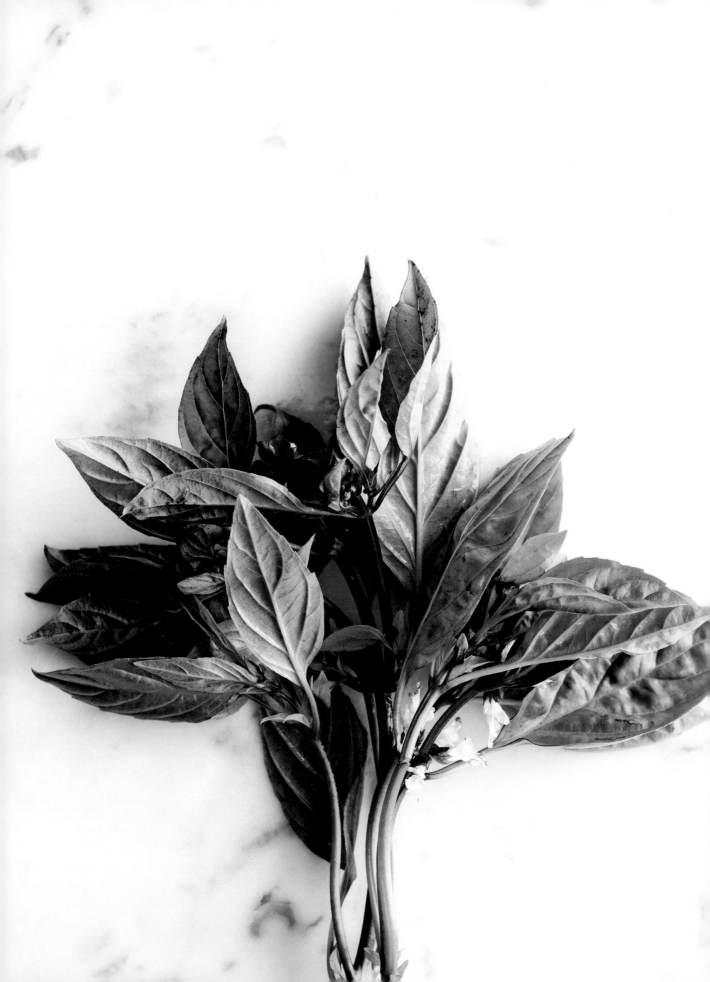

Acknowledgements

First, we'd like to thank our scientific chief and co-investigators for their contributions to our scientific ideas, their guidance and their commitment to this important research topic: Dr Jeannie Tay, CSIRO and Agency for Science Technology and Research (A*Star), Singapore; Professor Jon Buckley, University of South Australia; Professor Gary Wittert, University of Adelaide; Associate Professor William Yancy Jr, Duke University, United States; Professor Carlene Wilson, Flinders University, South Australia; Dr Vanessa Danthiir, CSIRO; Dr Ian Zajac, CSIRO; and Professor Peter Clifton, University of South Australia.

We thank the following individuals of the Clinical Research Team at CSIRO Health and Biosecurity, Adelaide, South Australia, for their tireless work in conducting the clinical research activities that underpin the contents of this book: Anne McGuffin, Julia Weaver, and Vanessa Courage for coordinating the research trials; Janna Lutze, Dr Paul Foster, Xenia Cleantheous, Gemma Williams, Hannah Gilbert and Fiona Barr for assisting in designing and implementing the dietary interventions; Lindy Lawson, Theresa McKinnon, Rosemary McArthur and Heather Webb for nursing expertise and clinical patient management; Vanessa Russell, Cathryn Pape, Candita Dang, Andre Nikolic and Sylvia Usher for performing biochemical assays and for other laboratory expertise; Julie Syrette and Kathryn Bastiaans for data management; Kylie Lange and Mary Barnes for assisting with statistical analyses; Andreas Kahl for communications; and our external fitness partners and health coaches for implementing the exercise interventions, including Luke Johnston and Annie Hastwell of Fit for Success, South Australia; Kelly French, Jason Delfos, Kristi Lacey-Powell, Marilyn Woods, John Perrin, Simon Pane and Annette Beckette of South Australian Aquatic Centre and Leisure Centre; and Angie Mondello and Josh Gniadek of Boot Camp Plus, South Australia.

We'd also like to thank Associate Professor Tim Crowe, Professor Katherine Samaras and Doctor Eugénie Lim for providing their professional expertise in reviewing and advising on the book content.

Thanks to the editorial and publishing team at Pan Macmillan Australia – Ingrid Ohlsson, who supported the writing of this book with great enthusiasm and encouragement; Virginia Birch, Nicola Young, Naomi Van Groll and Sally Devenish for their tireless work and support through the editorial and publication process. Thanks also to designer Daniel New, recipe developers Kathleen Gandy and Caroline Griffiths, recipe editor Rachel Carter, photographer Jeremy Simons, stylist Berni Smithies, home economist Tracy Pattison and exercise models Annie Smith and Evan Stillwell.

Finally, and most importantly, we'd like to thank the research volunteers for their participation in our research trials. It's only through their contributions that our research and these significant advancements in clinical practices for weight and diabetes management have been made possible.

References

Aucott L, Poobalan A, Smith WC, Avenell A, Jung R, Broom J & Grant AM, 'Weight loss in obese diabetic and non-diabetic individuals and long-term diabetes outcomes – a systematic review', *Diabetes, Obesity and Metabolism*, 2004, vol. 6, no. 2, pp. 85–94.

Brennan IM, Luscombe-Marsh ND, Seimon RV, Otto B, Horowitz M, Wishart JM & Feinle-Bisset C, 'Effects of fat, protein, and carbohydrate and protein load on appetite, plasma cholecystokinin, peptide YY, and ghrelin, and energy intake in lean and obese men', *American Journal of Physiology – Gastrointestinal and Liver Physiology*, 2012, vol. 303, no. 1, pp. G129–40.

Brinkworth GD, Buckley JD, Noakes M & Clifton PM, 'Renal function following long-term weight loss in individuals with abdominal obesity on a very-low-carbohydrate diet vs high-carbohydrate diet', *Journal of the American Dietetic Association*, 2010, vol. 110, no. 4, pp. 633–38.

Brinkworth GD, Luscombe-Marsh ND, Thompson CH, Noakes M, Buckley JD, Wittert G & Wilson CJ, 'Long-term effects of very low-carbohydrate and high-carbohydrate weight-loss diets on psychological health in obese adults with type 2 diabetes: randomized controlled trial', *Journal of Internal Medicine*, 2016, vol. 280, no. 4, pp. 388–97.

Brinkworth GD, Noakes M, Buckley JD, Keogh JB & Clifton PM, 'Long-term effects of a very-low-carbohydrate weight loss diet compared with an isocaloric low-fat diet after 12 mo.', *American Journal of Clinical Nutrition*, 2009, vol. 90. no. 1, pp. 23–32.

Brinkworth GD, Wycherley TP, Noakes M, Buckley JD & Clifton PM, 'Long-term effects of a very-low-carbohydrate weight-loss diet and an isocaloric low-fat diet on bone health in obese adults', *Nutrition*, 2016, vol. 32. no. 9, pp. 1033–36.

Cavalot F, Petrelli A, Traversa M, Bonomo K, Fiora E, Conti M, Anfossi G, Costa G & Trovati M, 'Postprandial blood glucose is a stronger predictor of cardiovascular events than fasting blood glucose in type 2 diabetes mellitus, particularly in women: lessons from the San Luigi Gonzaga Diabetes Study', *Journal of Clinical Endocrinology and Metabolism*, 2006, vol. 91, no. 3, pp. 813–19.

Farnsworth E, Luscombe ND, Noakes M, Wittert G, Argyiou E & Clifton PM, 'Effect of a high-protein, energy-restricted diet on body composition, glycemic control, and lipid concentrations in overweight and obese hyperinsulinemic men and women', *American Journal of Clinical Nutrition*, 2003, vol. 78, no. 1, pp. 31–39.

Faulconbridge LF, Wadden TA, Rubin RR, Wing RR, Walkup MP, Fabricatore AN, Coday M, Van Dorsten B, Mount DL & Ewing LJ, 'One-year changes in symptoms of depression and weight in overweight/obese individuals with type 2 diabetes in the Look AHEAD study', *Obesity* (Silver Spring), 2012, vol. 20, no. 4, pp. 783–93.

Foster GD, Wyatt HR, Hill JO, McGuckin BG, Brill C, Mohammed BS, Szapary PO, Rader DJ, Edman JS & Klein S, 'A randomized trial of a low-carbohydrate diet for obesity', *New England Journal of Medicine*, 2003, vol. 348. no. 21, pp. 2082–90.

Fuentes F, Lopez-Miranda J, Sanchez E, Sanchez F, Paez J, Paz-Rojas E, Marin C, Gomez P, Jimenez-Pereperez J, Ordovas JM & Perez-Jimenez F, 'Mediterranean and low-fat diets improve endothelial function in hypercholesterolemic men', *Annals of Internal Medicine*, 2001, vol. 134, no. 12, pp. 1115–19.

Gannon MC, Nuttall FQ, Saeed A, Jordan K & Hoover H, 'An increase in dietary protein improves the blood glucose response in persons with type 2 diabetes', *American Journal of Clinical Nutrition*, 2003, vol. 78, no. 4, pp. 734–41.

Gardner CD, Kiazand A, Alhassan S, Kim S, Stafford RS, Balise RR, Kraemer HC & King AC, 'Comparison of the Atkins, Zone, Ornish, and LEARN diets for change in weight and related risk factors among overweight premenopausal women: the A TO Z Weight Loss Study: a randomized trial', *JAMA*, 2007, vol. 297, no. 9, pp. 969–77.

Gentilcore D, Chaikomin R, Jones KL, Russo A, Feinle-Bisset C, Wishart JM, Rayner CK & Horowitz M, 'Effects of fat on gastric emptying of and the glycemic, insulin, and incretin responses to a carbohydrate meal in type 2 diabetes', *Journal of Clinical Endocrinology and Metabolism*, 2006, vol. 91, no. 6, pp. 2062–67.

Gibson AA, Seimon RV, Lee CM, Ayre J, Franklin J, Markovic TP, Caterson ID & Sainsbury A, 'Do ketogenic diets really suppress appetite? A systematic review and meta-analysis', *Obesity Reviews*, 2015, vol. 16, no. 1, pp. 64–76.

Jesudason DR, Pedersen E & Clifton PM, 'Weight-loss diets in people with type 2 diabetes and renal disease: a randomized controlled trial of the effect of different dietary protein amounts', *American Journal of Clinical Nutrition*, 2013, vol. 98, no. 2, pp. 494–501.

Keogh JB, Grieger JA, Noakes M & Clifton PM, 'Flow-mediated dilatation is impaired by a high-saturated fat diet but not by a high-carbohydrate diet', *Arteriosclerosis, Thrombosis, and Vascular Biology*, 2005, vol. 25, no. 6, pp. 1274–79.

Krauss RM, Blanche PJ, Rawlings RS, Fernstrom HS & Williams PT, 'Separate effects of reduced carbohydrate intake and weight loss on atherogenic dyslipidemia', *American Journal of Clinical Nutrition*, 2006, vol. 83, no. 5, pp. 1025–31.

Leidy HJ, Clifton PM, Astrup A, Wycherley TP, Westerterp-Plantenga MS, Luscombe-Marsh ND, Woods SC & Mattes RD, 'The role of protein in weight loss and maintenance', *American Journal of Clinical Nutrition*, 2015, doi: 10.3945/ajcn.114.084038.

Lim SS, Noakes M, Keogh JB, Clifton PM, 'Long-term effects of a low carbohydrate, low fat or high unsaturated fat diet compared to a no-intervention control', *Nutrition, Metabolism and Cardiovascular Diseases*, 2010, vol. 20, no. 8, pp. 599–607.

Look ARG, Pi-Sunyer X, Blackburn G, Brancati FL, Bray GA, Bright R, Clark JM, Curtis JM, Espeland MA, Foreyt JP, Graves K, et al., 'Reduction in weight and cardiovascular disease risk factors in individuals with type 2 diabetes: one-year results of the look AHEAD trial', *Diabetes Care*, 2007, vol. 30, no. 6, pp. 1374–83.

Ma J, Stevens JE, Cukier K, Maddox AF, Wishart JM, Jones KL, Clifton PM, Horowitz M & Rayner CK, 'Effects of a protein preload on gastric emptying, glycemia, and gut hormones after a carbohydrate meal in diet-controlled type 2 diabetes', *Diabetes Care*, 2009, vol. 32, no. 9, pp. 1600–1602.

Mayer SB, Jeffreys AS, Olsen MK, McDuffie JR, Feinglos MN & Yancy WS, Jr, 'Two diets with different haemoglobin A1c and antiglycaemic medication effects despite similar weight loss in type 2 diabetes', *Diabetes, Obesity and Metabolism*, 2014, vol. 16, no. 1, pp. 90–93.

Mensink RP, Zock PL, Kester AD & Katan MB, 'Effects of dietary fatty acids and carbohydrates on the ratio of serum total to HDL cholesterol and on serum lipids and apolipoproteins: a meta-analysis of 60 controlled trials', *American Journal of Clinical Nutrition*, 2003, vol. 77, no. 5, pp. 1146–55.

Nordmann AJ, Nordmann A, Briel M, Keller U, Yancy WS, Jr, Brehm BJ & Bucher HC, 'Effects of low-carbohydrate vs low-fat diets on weight loss and cardiovascular risk factors: a meta-analysis of randomized controlled trials', *Archives of Internal Medicine*, 2006, vol. 166, no. 3, pp. 285–93.

Parker B, Noakes M, Luscombe N & Clifton P, 'Effect of a high-protein, high-monounsaturated fat weight loss diet on glycemic control and lipid levels in type 2 diabetes', *Diabetes Care*, 2002, vol. 25, no. 3, pp. 425–30.

Rallidis LS, Lekakis J, Kolomvotsou A, Zampelas A, Vamvakou G, Efstathiou S, Dimitriadis G, Raptis SA & Kremastinos DT, 'Close adherence to a Mediterranean diet improves endothelial function in subjects with abdominal obesity', *American Journal of Clinical Nutrition*, 2009, vol. 90, no. 2, pp. 263–68.

Riccardi G, Giacco R & Rivellese AA, 'Dietary fat, insulin sensitivity and the metabolic syndrome', *Clinical Nutrition*, 2004, vo. 23, no. 4, pp. 447–56.

Rock CL, Flatt SW, Pakiz B, Taylor KS, Leone AF, Brelje K, Heath DD, Quintana

EL & Sherwood NE, 'Weight loss, glycemic control, and cardiovascular disease risk factors in response to differential diet composition in a weight loss program in type 2 diabetes: a randomized controlled trial', *Diabetes Care*, 2014, vol. 37, no. 6, pp. 1573–80.

Shai I, Schwarzfuchs D, Henkin Y, Shahar DR, Witkow S, Greenberg I, Golan R, Fraser D, Bolotin A, Vardi H, Tangi-Rozental O, et al., 'Weight loss with a low-carbohydrate, Mediterranean, or low-fat diet', *New England Journal of Medicine*, 2008, vol. 359, no. 3, pp. 229–41.

Sheard NF, Clark NG, Brand-Miller JC, Franz MJ, Pi-Sunyer FX, Mayer-Davis E, Kulkarni K & Geil P, 'Dietary carbohydrate (amount and type) in the prevention and management of diabetes: a statement by the American Diabetes Association', *Diabetes Care*, 2004, vol. 27, no. 9, pp. 2266–71.

Stern L, Iqbal N, Seshadri P, Chicano KL, Daily DA, McGrory J, Williams M, Gracely EJ & Samaha FF, 'The effects of low-carbohydrate versus conventional weight loss diets in severely obese adults: one-year follow-up of a randomized trial', *Annals of Internal Medicine*, 2004, vol. 140, no. 10, pp. 778–85.

Tay J, Luscombe-Marsh ND, Thompson CH, Noakes M, Buckley JD, Wittert GA, Yancy WS, Jr & Brinkworth GD, 'A very low-carbohydrate, low-saturated fat diet for type 2 diabetes management: a randomized trial', *Diabetes Care*, 2014, vol. 37, no. 11, pp. 2909–18.

Tay J, Luscombe-Marsh ND, Thompson CH, Noakes M, Buckley JD, Wittert GA, Yancy WS, Jr & Brinkworth GD, 'Comparison of low- and high-carbohydrate diets for type 2 diabetes management: a randomized trial', *American Journal of Clinical Nutrition*, 2015, vol. 102, no. 4, pp. 780–90.

Tay J, Thompson CH & Brinkworth GD, 'Glycemic variability: assessing glycemia differently and the implications for dietary management of diabetes', *Annual Review of Nutrition*, 2015, vol. 35, pp. 389–424.

Tay J, Thompson CH, Luscombe-Marsh ND, Noakes M, Buckley JD, Wittert GA & Brinkworth GD, 'Long-term effects of a very low carbohydrate compared with a

high carbohydrate diet on renal function in individuals with type 2 diabetes: a randomized trial', *Medicine* (Baltimore), 2015, vol. 94, no. 47, article e2181.

Tay J, Zajac IT, Thompson CH, Luscombe-Marsh ND, Danthiir V, Noakes M, Buckley JD, Wittert GA & Brinkworth GD, 'A randomised-controlled trial of the effects of very low-carbohydrate and high-carbohydrate diets on cognitive performance in patients with type 2 diabetes', *British Journal of Nutrition*, 23 November 2016: 1–9.

Westman EC, Yancy WS, Jr, Mavropoulos JC, Marquart M & McDuffie JR, 'The effect of a low-carbohydrate, ketogenic diet versus a low-glycemic index diet on glycemic control in type 2 diabetes mellitus', *Nutrition and Metabolism* (London), 2008, vol. 5, article 36.

Witte AV, Fobker M, Gellner R, Knecht S & Floel A, 'Caloric restriction improves memory in elderly humans', *Proceedings of the National Academy of Sciences*, 2009, vol. 106, no. 4, pp. 1255–60.

Wolfe BM & Piche LA, 'Replacement of carbohydrate by protein in a conventional-fat diet reduces cholesterol and triglyceride concentrations in healthy normolipidemic subjects', *Clinical and Investigative Medicine*, 1999, vol. 22, no. 4, pp. 140–48.

Wycherley TP, Moran LJ, Clifton PM, Noakes M & Brinkworth GD, 'Effects of energy-restricted high-protein, low-fat compared with standard-protein, low-fat diets: a meta-analysis of randomized controlled trials', *American Journal of Clinicial Nutrition*, 2012, vol. 96, no. 6, pp. 1281–98.

Wycherley TP, Thompson CH, Buckley JD, Luscombe-Marsh ND, Noakes M, Wittert GA & Brinkworth GD, 'Long-term effects of weight loss with a very-low carbohydrate, low saturated fat diet on flow mediated dilatation in patients with type 2 diabetes: a randomised controlled trial', *Atherosclerosis*, 2016, vol. 252, pp. 28–31.

Index

First published 2017 in Macmillan
by Pan Macmillan Australia Pty Limited
1 Market Street, Sydney, New South Wales
Australia 2000

A CIP catalogue record for this book is available from the National Library of Australia:
http://catalogue.nla.gov.au

Design by Daniel New / OetomoNew
Photography by Jeremy Simons
Prop and food styling by Berni Smithies
Recipe development by Kathleen Gandy and Caroline Griffiths
Editing by Nicola Young and Rachel Carter
Exercise plan by Tom Wycherley
Colour + reproduction by Splitting Image Colour Studio
Printed in China by 1010 Printing International Limited

10 9 8 7 6 5 4 3